Fat That Doesn't Come Back

Robert Ferguson & Krista Clarke

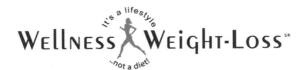

WELLNESS WEIGHT-LOSS℠

It's a lifestyle ..not a diet!

www.WellnessWeightloss.net

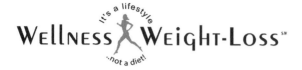

Robert Ferguson and Krista Clarke own and operate Wellness Weight-Loss℠ and they offer programs, materials and seminars to help people improve their health and fitness.

For more information on Robert and Krista's services, coaching, audio and visual programs, and their Wellness Weight-Loss℠ Support Network:

Phone: (805) 642-8440
e-mail: info@wellnessweightloss.net
Web site: www.WellnessWeightloss.net

ISBN 0-9742057-2

Printed in the United States of America

Book cover and design by Granite Mountain Graphics

Contents

Foreword

As a Holistic Healthcare practitioner (who was 75 pounds "over fat"), I had become very uncomfortable with my own ability to provide a model for my patients. I could clearly outline a weight-loss program for someone else to follow, but I somehow needed an outside 'accountability factor' to compel me toward a healthier body-fat percentage and lifestyle.

In line with that effort, I attended an evening lecture given by Krista Clarke, thinking, "If I just add one thing to my existing repertoire of knowledge, it will be worth my time." I was *so impressed* by Krista's handle on the subject of nutrition and her calm, self-assured manner that I found myself asking for her card. I soon enrolled into the Wellness Weight-Loss process and began my journey.

I quickly learned that the Wellness Weight-Loss process is nutritionally sound, and both Krista and Robert bring a personal joy and zeal to their work! After moving down from a size 18 to a healthier, more energetic size 10 in less than one year, I say to all of you—particularly all of you healthcare practitioners out there who could use some of your own advice—I highly recommend the services of the Wellness Weight-Loss team and this wonderful book, *Fat That Doesn't Come Back!*

— **Christine S. Hall, Ph.D.**

Preface

I have lost weight and repeatedly gained it back for most of my life. Although I can't tell you how much fat and muscle I have lost and gained over the years, I do know what it feels like to lose weight, relapse and battle with the emotional roller coaster that comes with dieting. I'm sure many of you can relate to my struggles; it is my goal to inspire you to read this book and learn how to avoid the pitfalls associated with dieting.

Early years

Fortunately, as a teenager I never thought about dieting because weight was never an issue for me. At the age of 18, I was 5'5" and weighed 125 pounds. I was no Ms. Fitness, but I wasn't considered fat either. However, shortly after high school and giving birth to my first child I became obsessed with the word "diet."

During my pregnancy I gained 75 pounds, and found myself an unhappy member of the "over 200 pound club." I became desperate and launched my diet career. After asking a few people how I could lose weight, I was introduced to diet pills, which were commonly referred to as "black beauties" or speed. At that time in my life, I fell in love with this amphetamine because of the way it made me feel and look.

Before long I was back to my pre-pregnancy weight of 125 pounds. Feeling energized and good about myself, I returned to what I felt was a normal weight. I soon discontinued the diet pills (which had suppressed my appetite) and revisited my old eating habits. Like most things we lose, I found my weight again. Before you could say, "all-you-can-eat buffet," I was once again over 200 pounds. Frustrated with myself, I returned to what I knew worked—diet pills. But then the health experts announced that such diet pills were causing health problems and were no longer legal. Still, I had enough diet pills to help me lose 70 pounds.

Down to about 140 pounds and beginning to feel good about my weight, I learned that I was once again pregnant. In no time I was back in the over 200 pound club. After Robert was born, I got back on my feet and decided it was time to lose this unwanted weight. It was during this time that the fitness and health craze was beginning to boom in the late 1960s, and I decided to jump on board and join a health club that offered a weight-loss program.

Exercise was something I hadn't done since high school and I found myself enjoying how good it made me feel. I still laugh when I think about that fat shaking contraption that you stood on, wrapped a belt around your waist and allowed it to jiggle the fat off your body. There was even a machine that you sat on to knock the cellulite off your butt. At any rate, I avoided these gimmicks and became addicted to dancing the fat off in the jazzercise class.

It was also during this time that I enrolled in the health club's weight-loss program where I was directed to purchase certain foods. This approach of combining exercise with their structured eating plan helped me lose nearly 70 pounds. However, my progress came to a screeching halt and I grew frustrated with the scale. After two months of stagnating at the same weight, I decided to deviate from the health club's weight-loss program and jump on the diet bandwagon.

Diet trap

Diets were very popular during this time, like they are today, and like everyone else who wanted to lose weight, I began my search for the ultimate diet. In little time I went from the high-protein diet to the banana diet—the water diet—the fruit diet—to *Weight Watchers,* and the list goes on and on. After working my way through more than 15 diets, I came to the realization that the greatest weight-loss success I'd achieved to date came by way of the diet pills. But then again, diet pills were no longer available.

Lost and running out of options, I stopped exercising and found myself going from one diet to the next until I fell in love with sweets. I became addicted to sugar. I couldn't eat a little. I had to eat a lot. So, in no time I was back up and over 200 pounds.

I am not the type of person who gives up easily, so I decided to avoid diets recommended by my friends and co-workers, and seek the advice of the medical industry instead. I then discovered a diet called "Opti-fast." Owned and operated by doctors and nurses, this diet helped me lose 100 pounds very quickly by drinking shakes, exercising and depriving myself of certain foods. However, during this particular transformation I took note of the effectiveness of exercise and how it helped to speed up the weight loss. Fed up with diet shakes, I decided to continue with the exercise, but went back to eating the food of my past.

Once more, I began gaining the weight back. I increased my exercise and still gained 50 of the 100 pounds I'd lost. Imagine the panic I was in when I stepped on the scale each week only to have it tell me I was going back to the "over 200 pound club." Exercising more than ever and still gaining weight caused me to doubt the effectiveness of working out.

The never ending saga

Although I had lost 100 pounds with the liquid drinks, I didn't want to go back to Opti-fast. I needed something different, something more satisfying. Then, I heard about this weight-loss clinic in town that guaranteed results.

Driving a total of two hours each week to spend an outrageous amount of money to lose weight proved to me that I was ready for permanent change.

Driving a total of two hours each week to spend an outrageous amount of money to lose weight proved to me that I was ready for permanent change. Upon arrival to this weight-loss clinic they would weigh me in and give me a shot that was supposed to curb my appetite. After leaving the clinic it became routine for me to reward myself with fast food after a week of deprivation.

To make a long story short, this weight-loss clinic was a joke and I felt like the biggest clown in town. So, after wasting a large amount of money, I went on my own and experienced another half-dozen or so diets. But, then came the "Eating Disorder Clinic." I liked what they had to offer. It was different and the idea of having more support in my life was inviting.

You see, the counselors felt I had an eating disorder that was a result of trauma that took place in my life. In short, I had lost my daughter in a tragic accident and I just couldn't seem to get myself together. Around this time I tipped the scales at a whopping 238 pounds. So, for 27 days I enlisted in their program. I allowed different therapists to get into my head. I was even eating three healthy meals per day. During my stay at this clinic I managed to lose 25 pounds. But once again it was time to return to reality and unfortunately I regained the weight plus a little more. I actually went up to 258 pounds.

Hitting rock bottom

At this point in my life I felt I had hit rock bottom. I felt desperate and considered stomach stapling. I didn't know what to do, but somehow I ended up enrolling into a program called "Physicians Weight Loss Center" and I lost over 100 pounds by replacing food with powdered drinks and exercising daily. Getting my weight down once again proved to me that I could succeed. I felt like I was a guru at losing weight. At the same time, I was equally skilled at gaining it all back. Full of confidence and believing that this was the last time, I found myself asking, "What happened?" as I gained all 100 pounds back.

Tired and fed up with programs and feeling beat up, I came to realize I was a compulsive overeater, and joined Overweight Anonymous where I lost 40 pounds. Not sure where to go, I took a major step in my journey and began a program called CEA-How.

The program was tightly structured and very restrictive. Like a soldier I adhered to what CEA-How advised and lost a total of 108 pounds. I felt confident with CEA-How and was able to keep the weight off for four years. I never wavered from the program. The discipline and structure of the program really worked and I had become a disciple of its laws and regulations. The only drawback for me was that I was faced with the feeling of being deprived of certain foods. The words "forbidden" and "illegal" were at the forefront of my mind when it was time to eat. But, I felt I was eating healthy and that was important to me.

The final straw

As I aged into my fifties, health issues began popping up. I've survived breast cancer and had both knees and one shoulder replaced. As tough as I was, cancer was the final straw. Here I was eating healthy, depriving myself of all the foods I loved and grew up on, and I ended up with cancer. It was at this point that I fell off the wagon and reverted to nurturing myself with food and eating what and whenever I wanted. As a result, I gained back that 108 pounds.

Now, as I enter my sixties, I have finally—I mean finally—moved into a healthier relationship with myself. Through all the diets, co-dependency of weight-loss programs and having lost and gained well over 1,000 pounds during my life, I now understand that leading a lifestyle that evolves is how you release fat that doesn't come back.

I used to pray that I wouldn't get buried in my own fat; I no longer have such thoughts. The Wellness Weight-Loss process has helped me become healthy and whole. I am no longer concerned with losing or gaining weight, but more interested in enjoying the journey of creating health. I do not feel deprived and I maintain a sense of power and control over the choices I make.

There are foods from my past that I enjoy and may crave at times, but I choose not to eat them. Knowing that there aren't any forbidden or restricted foods is what keeps me accountable and responsible for the choices I make. Because I am aware that I can choose what I want, I feel empowered and in control of my life.

One step at a time

As you read this book, notice that it has 24 chapters. Each chapter is symbolic to one hour in a day. The lifestyle that is promoted in this book is one that is based on 24 hours a day, 365 days per year. So, as you conclude each chapter, I encourage you to reflect on what you learn. I also stress that you read the chapters in sequence as they feed into one another.

The Wellness Weight-Loss process is truly a last step for those of you who are done with dieting.

I am forever grateful to have learned and lived what you are about to experience in this book. The tears and frustration I have experienced over the years do not have to be your experience. Take this opportunity that my son and his wife, Krista, have presented in this book and begin the process of releasing fat that doesn't come back. The Wellness Weight-Loss process is truly a last step for those of you who are done with dieting.

—Brenda A. Watson
Former lifetime dieter and mother of co-author, Robert Ferguson

Introduction

Each year Americans spend more than $40 billion on weight-loss programs, surgeries, products and pills. Unfortunately, much of this money is wasted on ideas and products that result in short-term success. These "quick-fixes" may promise an immediate solution, but they often eliminate important food sources, cut calories so low it's difficult to comply, or rely on one food group for the magic cure-all.

Fat That Doesn't Come Back, on the other hand, is not a diet. Written over the past few years and introduced to you by way of our business, Wellness Weight-Loss, it is a process to a lifestyle; one that more and more North Americans are choosing to embrace. We hope *Fat That Doesn't Come Back* will help you realize the power of change and enjoy the benefits of establishing life-long healthy habits.

Wellness Weight-Loss is a process—
not a fad, gimmick or new age method.

You may have come to this crossroad in your life previously, perhaps many times before. You want to release body fat. You want to improve your self-esteem. You want to establish healthy habits. You want to decrease your risk of illness or injury. These desires are certainly honest and genuine.

Your previous attempts at weight loss or healthy lifestyle changes may have come with some level of success. But if you're still looking for a program to help you reach your goals, you're probably overwhelmed by all the options available—low-fat, no-fat, high-protein, low-protein, cabbage soup, grapefruit, this zone and that zone, blood types—which diet and program do you choose? How do you know which approach works? This book will answer your questions, address your fears and give you the knowledge necessary to bring about the results you have been hoping to experience.

The Wellness Weight-Loss process is not a fad, gimmick or new age method. It is a process that helps you keep your healthy habits while replacing your unhealthy ones. Wellness Weight-Loss is about adopting and evolving with a healthy lifestyle by choosing to create health daily.

Moving beyond the event

Let's face it: the diet industry is an event-driven business. We all know someone who has purchased a fad or gimmick that extended the promise of a quick fix. Think of the vast number of people who go on diets to lose 10 to 15 pounds before the holidays, a reunion, anniversary or some other special occasion. Event-driven diets like these do not work long-term—*unless motivated by a process that leads them to, and then beyond, that event.* If that motivation is not there, people are most likely concerned only with the daily weigh-ins, consumed by the number on a scale or focused solely on reaching a certain point or preparing for a particular event. While the event may be important for one's career, social life or increased sense of self, what is even more important is the work done ahead of time, the steps taken to place someone at that particular event.

Let's use two world-class events as examples—the Super Bowl and the Olympics. Both are enormous productions that millions of people look forward to watching. Most people simply flip on the television to enjoy the show; few actually understand the amount of planning, decision-making and work that it takes to produce the final event that we see on the screen. Only a small number of us stop to think about the effort put forth by the athletes on a daily, weekly and monthly basis; however, those actually participating understand that the opportunity to play in the Super Bowl or to represent their country in the Olympics comes as the reward—after the work has been done. In the same way, we enjoy the rewards of fitness and health only after we've "paid our dues" through planning and hard work.

The process to health

It takes time to change unhealthy habits, which is why Wellness Weight-Loss is a process-driven lifestyle program. Our clients don't prepare for the next scale reading or a fancy party coming up in a few months. Our clients change their lives by improving their bodies and establishing healthy habits one step at a time.

Just like competitors in the Super Bowl and Olympics, in order to enjoy the fruits of our endeavors we first perform the necessary labor. While it's comforting to believe the old adage that if you work hard you will be successful, that's not always realistic. At Wellness Weight-Loss, we believe that hard work in the precise direction is crucial for success. How you work is just as important as how hard you work.

Let's talk about corn

Once upon a time a farmer planted a corn seed in the earth and covered it with soil. He then began the process of growing corn. Each and every day the farmer watered and fertilized this seed with nutrients; it was a daily routine that he went through. After several days, there was no sign of growth—no young seedling popping its eager head through the darkened earth. The farmer, however, continued to water and provide nutrients to this elusive seed daily.

One day the farmer noticed the seedling had pierced through the soil and soon after, it began to grow a stalk. This stalk's purpose was to provide the plant with a foundation of strength, one capable of supporting the bountiful and heavy ears of corn that would eventually mature.

Just when everything was looking bright and the stalk was apparently strong, the plant's appearance changed dramatically—the leaves turned brown and the top started to wilt and collapse. Most of the people who drove past the field felt sorry for the farmer, assuming that somehow his crop had been destroyed.

Now, picture yourself as that farmer; the process of planting new exciting seeds lies before you as you hold this book in your hands. In the beginning, releasing fat and establishing healthy habits may seem unreachable; that's because change can be a slow, drawn-out procedure.

The merit rule simply states that sometimes when you are closest to your goal, or your harvest, it feels as though you are farthest away.

Most people want results fast and many make the decision to avoid a hard, necessary approach to change and instead settle for the expediency option, or instant gratification. However, in nearly every situation those short-term gains result in long-term pain and disappointment.

Here's where the "merit rule" comes in. The merit rule simply states that sometimes when you are closest to your goal, or your harvest, it feels as though you are farthest away. During this period of stagnation, you might experience doubt and temptation. Lacking faith, you may simply give up, as many do, while unbeknownst to you, the harvest is waiting for you in the next cornfield.

You see, no one needs to feel badly for the corn farmer whose crops have turned brown, for the harvest is nearing. Where an inexperienced farmer throws in the towel, a wiser, more experienced grower watches and learns that the browning is the final step of the process. It is during this period of gestation that all the nutrients in the stalk are being funneled into the ear of the plant allowing the corn to fully develop.

When you have faith in and patience and knowledge of a particular process, you are more likely to push beyond the point of stagnation that so often stops many on the road to total health. The weight-loss breakthrough and lifestyle change you seek are right around the corner. The Wellness Weight-Loss process as provided in this book will guide you through the stages of nurturing, growth and development until finally, you arrive at your objective and reap the harvest of all your dedication and effort.

Getting started

The seeds of your personal weight-loss plan are planted during the first three chapters. Remember: avoid the instant gratification tendency of wanting to release body fat right now. The quick fix is not the way to achieve lasting weight loss and the healthier lifestyle you deserve.

Like any new seed, the beginnings are tough, but by the time you have read half the book, the stalk or strength of your commitment will have developed. As you continue to progress with **Fat That Doesn't Come Back** you will gain strength in your conviction as you grow intellectually, physically, emotionally, socially and spiritually.

Near completion of the book, you will find yourself making progress in both mind and body. The foundation will be established for your long-term growth and success. As subtle changes continue to take place, this lifestyle transformation may not be so obvious on the outside. You may feel tempted to stop reading or begin giving less than 100% of your attention and focus.

Know that changing negative behaviors and establishing new healthy habits are journeys well worth embarking on.

Remember the analogy of the farmer who believed in the process, and who honored his faith with his daily work and routine. Throughout the process, remember the corn and the farmer. Know that to grow—to change—takes time, and that changing negative behaviors and establishing new healthy habits are journeys well worth embarking on.

During this time your excitement will build as you develop the desire to evolve with your lifestyle. At the conclusion of this book you will be equipped with the knowledge, tools and action steps to begin releasing fat for the last time.

Take your time, read, reflect, take notes and enjoy the journey, as the experience that awaits you is priceless. It's your life. It's your health. It's all about you!

How to Use This Book

By Debi Mullens, *Wellness Weight-Loss Client*

If you are anything like the way I used to be—weary and fed up with dieting, losing a little but gaining it all back and not really knowing where to begin—this book is going to change your life. With each chapter your excitement about this process will grow and you will become stronger and more energized as a person. When you have finished reading this book, you will probably want to share it with a long list of friends and relatives.

My recommendations

Fat That Doesn't Come Back is both a reference book as well as a very practical workbook. It is theory and practice in one!

To totally benefit from this masterpiece, I recommend you begin by reading this book in its entirety. You might want to purchase a notebook or journal to document your thoughts along the way. You may also find it useful to highlight the areas of the book that inspire you to take action and evolve with your lifestyle.

In the last chapter of the book you will find a 24-step action plan. This plan describes in sequential order—steps you can take to maximize your efforts to create health and release fat that doesn't come back.

When creating health at your own pace, make sure that you go back to the relevant parts of the book as often as necessary. Both the logical structure as well as the glossary of common words and terms in Appendix D make it very easy to use this book as a general reference guide on healthy lifestyles. Keep using this book for inspiration and information. Since reading this book I have reflected and reviewed my notes, read parts again and most importantly taken actions to improve my lifestyle. The book has truly helped me remain focused and inspired.

Be open-minded

Read this book in sequence as each chapter builds on the previous one. To give you an introduction as to what to expect, the following synopsis is provided per my reflection:

- In part one, *"Opportunity Is Knocking,"* you will be introduced to what I regard as the foundation chapters. You will establish the frame of mind necessary to truly benefit from the subsequent chapters. It mentally prepares you for the journey ahead.

- In part two, *"It's All About You,"* Robert and Krista walk you through the benefits of being proactive and practical with your health.

- Part three, *"Removing Roadblocks,"* shows you why many people don't succeed at releasing fat even though they appear to be willing. I really connected with this part of the book as I could relate to many of the stories and examples given.

- You have done the groundwork and you are ready to plan your journey. You are ready for *"Defining Your Destination,"* the topic of part four. You will be empowered. Your dream to never diet again comes into focus and your vision to create change and improve the quality of your life becomes attainable. At the halfway point of this book you are totally motivated to succeed, and you know your destination. The subsequent parts give you the specifics on how to get there.

- Part five, *"Nutrition 101,"* provides you with authentic information about food. This in-depth part of the book brings clarity to the fiber-carb connection, the value of protein and the many faces of dietary fat.

- Once empowered with the facts on what makes for unhealthy and healthy foods, part six, *"The Skinny on Fat Loss,"* provides you with valuable information about your metabolism. Having the previously acquired knowledge of food made this part of the book easy to understand. Then, as I found myself beginning to wonder about exercise—BOOM—Krista and Robert provide you with specifics on both cardiovascular exercise and resistance training (i.e., weight lifting, strength training).

- Finally, in part seven, *"Resolve To Evolve,"* the book readdresses the mental connection once again by sharing with you how to bridge the gap between knowing what to do, and doing what you know. Great timing. Last but not least, Robert and Krista provide an entire chapter on conquering procrastination followed up with the bottom line and 24 action steps.

I know this first-hand

This book is your foundation for the truth. Say goodbye to the emotional ups and downs, because the blueprint to long-term success is available in *Fat That Doesn't Come Back.* Going beyond the call of duty, Robert and Krista provide appendixes that cover everything else you'll need to live a diet-free life. I know this first hand as I have experienced the Wellness Weight-Loss process—releasing nearly 50 pounds of fat that I can say with total confidence and assurance—*will never come back.* Good luck to you!

PART ONE

Opportunity Is Knocking

1

Fat That Doesn't Come Back

"A pessimist sees the difficulty in every opportunity;
an optimist sees the opportunity in every difficulty."
—**Sir Winston Churchill**

WARNING: If you are looking for a diet, you're not going to find one in this book. However, you can expect *Fat That Doesn't Come Back* to be enjoyable, informative and a way for you to discover purpose in your life, evolve as a person and never diet again. After all, we wrote this book to help you sort through the confusion surrounding weight loss—bringing clarity to how you can release fat that doesn't come back.

Over the years we have helped many people establish a lifestyle that not only lowers body fat, but also improves health and reduces stress. Because of our success and sincere desire to help as many people as possible, we decided to share with you the tools to take control of your life, release body fat and begin creating health daily.

As you read on and learn more about the Wellness Weight-Loss process and how it can guide you into a lifestyle that helps you manage your weight, improve your health, elevate your self-esteem and increase your energy, don't be surprised if other areas of your life are positively affected (i.e., marriage, career). The diets and weight-loss programs you have participated in up to this point have been practice for what you are about to experience. Today is definitely the first day toward a new feeling of peace and freedom.

Diet mania

It doesn't surprise us to learn that many of our clients, and probably many of you reading this book, may have in-depth knowledge and experience with dieting. Let's face it—diets are not difficult to find. For many people, diets are practically an American pastime. Pick up just about any

1

magazine, turn on the television or search on the Internet, and in no time you will have thousands to choose from. Because of this diet mania, it's not uncommon for most people we meet to have experienced a half-dozen or more diets.

To have lost 20, 50 and 100 or more pounds and then gain it back is not unusual either. As a matter of fact, it's significantly more common for people to re-gain weight than to keep it off. One of our clients summarized this well, saying, "I don't doubt that I can lose weight. I've done it before and I can do it again. My problem is keeping it off!" Most people know how to lose weight. Losing weight is not the problem. The bigger issue is what you lose (i.e., fat, water, muscle), how your health may be affected and how to keep the fat from coming back.

Sustainable success

Do you deserve more than a low-calorie, highly restrictive approach to merely losing weight and being faced with the threat of gaining it all back? We believe so! As your guides—your master coaches—we intend to help you bridge the gap between knowing what is in your best interest, and doing what is in your best interest. This will ultimately result in you being the person that leads a lifestyle that is forever evolving.

By "evolving," we mean that the changes you make over time will guide you to a healthier lifestyle. Don't expect to get there all at once. In fact, most people who make many radical changes in their lifestyle find that they can't sustain them over time. Instead, begin making healthier choices today, and learn to continually re-evaluate your habits. Over time, you'll replace unhealthy habits with new, healthier ones. Lifestyles that evolve over time are easier to sustain.

Delete "diet" from your vocabulary

We will not forbid you to eat certain foods. We aren't in the business of magic potions or supplements that promise instant results. We are experts in recognizing where you are, and helping you establish a lifestyle that doesn't include dieting. We do this by providing you with the necessary knowledge, tools and inspiration to create health daily. One of our goals is to heighten your awareness of how you can enjoy the benefits of exercise and keep the taste, convenience and satisfaction in your food choices.

From this day forward, we encourage you to think of diets as schemes—misrepresentations of healthy and vibrant living. In our opinion, dieting is nothing short of being misled, deceived and eventually disappointed. As you will learn in this book, diets diminish the very element that is responsible for an efficient metabolism. But before you learn more about how diets negatively affect your long-term success, let's first take a closer look at our approach to weight loss, and the crucial difference between *releasing* fat and *losing* fat.

The "non-diet" philosophy

What makes this book different from those that claim to be the best of the best when it comes to weight loss? First of all, let us remind you that the Wellness Weight-Loss process is not a diet, but a way of evolving in your life. There are no lifetime memberships, no pre-packaged foods and we do not recommend one group of food over another. Wellness Weight-Loss is purely a process to releasing body fat and keeping it from coming back. Furthermore, the Wellness Weight-Loss process encourages you to evaluate—not judge—the thoughts you think and the actions you take. This philosophy alone increases the likelihood that you'll experience long-term success.

The Wellness Weight-Loss process encourages you to evaluate—not judge—the thoughts you think and the actions you take.

Now that you have a clearer understanding of our beliefs, it's time to jump start your "resolve to evolve" by making the great exchange—substituting words that best describe the approach you take toward weight loss. For instance, instead of saying, "I am *losing* fat" we encourage you to say, "I am *releasing* fat." Believe it or not, there is a critical distinction between *losing* and *releasing* fat.

Consider the universal principle that says, "What we lose, we eventually find again." A great example of this principle is losing your car keys and finding them again. Your body fat is no different. As many people can attest, 10 pounds lost is often another 10 or 15 pounds gained. Fortunately, managing your weight does not have to be this way.

Think of releasing fat from your body as holding on to a string that is attached to a helium balloon. The helium balloon in this analogy is your body fat. Once you let go of the string, the balloon (body fat), it is gone forever.

Webster's New World Dictionary defines release as: **to let go—to set free.** We sincerely hope that you no longer lose body fat, but learn to release it. That's what we mean by "fat that doesn't come back."

Fit or fat?

When people first visit our office and inquire about the Wellness Weight-Loss process—almost always we hear, "I need to lose weight." If this is the case for you, ask yourself, "What makes me believe that I am overweight?" Is it the scale? Did your doctor inform you to lose weight? Did someone say you are fat? And for those of you who feel you aren't overweight, but need to lose weight—think again. Wanting to lose weight means there is an ideal weight (point of reference) that you are over. If you are over what you consider your ideal weight then you are indeed overweight.

Then again, being overweight does not necessarily mean you are over fat. For this reason, we refer to the term "over fat," rather than "overweight."

In conversation, we often use weight and body fat interchangeably. But the truth is, there is a significant distinction between what you weigh and the amount of fat on your body. Learning more about this distinction is of great importance and will prove more valuable than the confirmation you get from a bathroom scale.

The almighty scale

How do you know whether or not you are fat? Do you base being fat on how you feel or the way your clothes fit? What role has the scale played in gauging whether or not you are fat? Almost every person we meet says the scale is the almighty when it comes to indicating whether or not they are fat. One of our clients told us that as a teenager, in her house the scale was the "be all, end all" for gauging if she was fat.

We are happy to inform you that the scale is not the "be all, end all" for confirming whether you are fit or fat. The scale is good for merely one thing—providing you with your total body weight. The scale doesn't explain the difference between fat weight and lean body mass—your muscle, bones, blood, connective tissue, organs and water. It doesn't tell you how fit you are. Stepping on the scale does nothing but add to the confusion surrounding weight loss. However, most of us continue to step on the scale regularly to confirm whether or not we are making progress.

"The first inkling I got that the scale reflected how fat I was didn't take place at home, but at the doctor's office," explained our client, Norma. Like many of us, Norma felt she needed to routinely weigh herself after her doctor recommended she lose a few pounds. This doctor's recommendation sparked Norma's obsession with the scale and weighing herself became a morning ritual. Soon the obsession became a fixation that was reinforced by both *Weight Watchers* and *Jenny Craig* since each of these commercial programs rely on the scale to gauge weight-loss progress.

The truth about the scale

Whether it's at home, your doctor's office or some commercial weight-loss center, the scale does not reflect how much fat is on your body. Take the doctor's office, for instance. During each appointment you are weighed and your height is measured. These numbers are then compared to the forever-popular "Desirable Height-Weight Table." Commonly used by physicians, the height-weight table was statistically developed by Metropolitan Life Insurance Company in 1959 to correlate lower incidence of mortality. The height-weight table is outdated and we do not recommend that you use it to determine whether you are over fat or obese. A lot has changed since 1959!

In addition to the height-weight table, there are other methods typically used to gauge whether you are fit or fat. For example, the Body Mass Index (BMI) is the most common method used around the world to determine if you are overweight or obese. Surprisingly, the BMI dates back to 1835 when French mathematician Adolphe Quetelet developed it. Though useful to some degree, the BMI is not our first choice and we do not recommend it for gauging your progress. Our preferred method is the body composition analysis—learning how much of your total body weight is fat and how much is lean body mass. By relying on a body composition analysis, you are better able to track your progress by measuring your percentage of body fat. As a result of reading this book you will also learn how to conduct one in the privacy of your home *(see Appendix A)*.

Although we can share various methods of gauging whether you are fit or fat, nothing compares to a body composition analysis—monitoring your percentage of body fat. Knowing how much of your body weight is fat is the truest determining factor for whether you are fit or fat—healthy or unhealthy—not some mathematical equation that dates back to the 19th century.

Presuppositions can hold you back

If you visited our office for a body composition analysis, and you stepped on our scale and weighed 10 pounds more than your bathroom scale, would you be shocked? You'd probably say something like, "Is this scale accurate?" or "My scale at home says that I am lighter." No matter what you say, the reality is that you have a presupposition with what makes you fat when it comes to the scale.

Presuppositions are assumptions or preconceptions—when we believe or suppose things to be a certain way in advance. For example, prior to learning that the scale is not an accurate indicator for whether you are fit or fat, you may believe that if the number on the scale is higher than the last time you stepped on, you're getting fat. So, the presupposition in this scenario is concluding before you even step on the scale that if the number is higher—you are fatter.

Consider our client Lesley who enrolled into Wellness Weight-Loss with hopes of going from 150 to 135 pounds. At 38 years of age, Lesley has been conditioned since her teenage years to compare her total body weight to the last time she stepped on the scale. As a result of this mindset, even if she gained lean muscle tissue rather than fat, if the numbers on the scale didn't go down she was discouraged and flabbergasted. You see, Lesley felt that if she ate healthy, exercised regularly and did everything we recommended—the numbers on the scale would go down. As we explained to her the importance of the ratio between total body weight to pounds of fat, she seemed to understand, but her reaction each time she stepped on the scale was to the contrary.

Four weeks after beginning the Wellness Weight-Loss process, Lesley stepped on the scale so that we could establish her total body weight and she was not happy. Even though she went from being sedentary to exercising three times per week and eating healthier than ever before—the scale read the same. When she enrolled, Lesley weighed 150 pounds and four weeks later she still weighed 150. She couldn't believe it. She was quick to say things like, "I might as well be doing the Atkins' diet." As we completed her body composition analysis we learned that Lesley had released five pounds of fat and gained five pounds of lean body mass. We were excited for Lesley, but she didn't share our enthusiasm because she was fixated with what the scale said.

Because of her presuppositions about weight, Lesley had a difficult time accepting that the scale is not a true indicator of her progress. She was frustrated, so she decided to cut back on her calories rather than sticking to the Wellness Weight-Loss process. Two weeks later she stepped onto the scale and her total body weight shifted from 150 to 147 pounds. Lesley was relieved that she was now making progress, but unbeknownst to her, she had digressed. She gained one pound of fat and lost four pounds of lean body mass (mostly in the form of water and lean muscle tissue). In short, she was beginning to lose her all-important muscle that she had gained as a result of her exercise efforts.

As we explained to Lesley that losing muscle meant a slowed metabolism and reduced fat-burning potential, she made the connection. She finally realized that if muscle is essential for burning fat—to lose muscle was out of the question. Lesley was fortunate enough to grasp the reality that the scale was only good for measuring her total body weight. She came to the realization that what makes up that total body weight is more important than the number on the scale.

Fortunately, Lesley is no longer living with a diet mentality. She is more interested in keeping the muscle and releasing the fat. We are happy to share with you that she is no longer fixated with the scale. As a matter of fact, she only steps on a scale for the purpose of conducting a body composition analysis.

What makes up total body weight is more important than the number on the scale.

Sharon's story

Meet Sharon. Prior to going through the Wellness Weight-Loss process she had a fixation with the scale, which was reinforced by the BMI and what her doctor believed to be a healthier weight for her height. Standing 5'4" and weighing a total of 160 pounds, Sharon felt she was overweight. When she came to us, there was nothing we could say or do to help her realize the importance of reducing her body fat and keeping her lean body mass—specifically her muscle. All Sharon wanted to do was to lose 40 pounds.

After hearing Sharon complain about the size of her legs, we jokingly suggested she take six weeks off from work and have her lower body put in a cast. Surprised that we would say such a thing, she asked why? Just as when someone breaks their arm, six weeks in a cast will cause the arm to reduce in size. Having her lower body in a cast for six weeks meant she would finally have smaller legs. As Sharon pondered the idea, she realized that muscle atrophies, not fat. In short, after six weeks of not using her legs she would reduce the size but her legs would still be fat...actually, even more fat.

As we captured her attention and caused her to be more interested in the importance of muscle, we took advantage of the opportunity and explained to Sharon that muscle is metabolically active. Muscle is primarily responsible for our body's ability to burn fat. And losing muscle meant reducing her fat-burning potential, which in the long-term meant she was more likely to gain the fat back. Our goal with Sharon and also with you is to help you realize the importance of a body composition analysis to determine the amount of body fat and lean body mass you have. If you want to release fat—fat that doesn't come back—it is to your benefit to keep your lean muscle tissue. And no, that does not mean you must build up large muscles or look like a bodybuilder. It simply means that you need muscle to burn fat. We will explain this in greater detail later.

Today, more than three years later, Sharon maintains a body-fat percentage of 22 percent. Her total body weight is 140 pounds which consists of 30.8 pounds of fat and 109.2 pounds of lean body mass. She wears a size four and looks very fit and healthy. Now when her doctor recommends she lose a few pounds, she laughs and educates him about the importance of body composition.

What is an ideal body-fat percentage?

Knowing that excess body fat is associated with an increased chance of cardiovascular heart disease . . . it is to your benefit to establish a healthy range of body fat.

Don't worry—we are not going to compare you to a predetermined chart. And we're not going to tell you to reduce your body fat to zero. Actually, fat plays an important role. It cushions your brain and allows your cell membranes to transport nutrients in and out of the cell. In fact, you wouldn't be able to survive without body fat.

However, because excess body fat is associated with an increased risk of cardiovascular disease, Type 2 diabetes and many other chronic illnesses, it is to your benefit to establish a healthy percentage of body fat. In addition, the process of lowering your body fat to a healthy level actually speeds up your metabolism.

So here it goes: for men who aspire to achieve optimum health, we recommend a body-fat percentage of no more than 15. If a man weighs 200 pounds that would mean he has 30 pounds of fat. With regard to women, we recommend no more than 22 percent. If a woman weighs 160 pounds that would mean she has 35.2 pounds of fat. Now, if you are breastfeeding, taking hormone replacements, beta-blockers, birth control pills or any other medication that may affect your hormonal balance, we recommend that you add up to five percent body fat to the baseline for optimum health.

How low do you go?

Once you get your body-fat percentage down to a optimum range and you decide to continue reducing your body fat, the lower you go, the higher the risk for reduced health. For this reason, we recommend men stay above six percent and women 12 percent. Just as with having excess body fat, there are also health risks associated with having too little body fat. Some of these include hypothermia, vitamin toxicity, cessation of menstrual cycle and osteoporosis.

Going forward

We believe that this can be your last time reducing your waistline. Take a closer look at your lifestyle and choose to evolve. It will be the choices you make that determine whether or not you experience long-term success. You won't find lasting success through fads and creative shortcuts that promise weight loss. It's about accepting what's real and what's not. It's about leading a lifestyle that progresses and evolves.

The first major difference so far is that you have decided to release body fat and not merely lose it. Secondly, since you are reading this book, we assume that you have decided to take control of your life, and that means being responsible for the actions you take and the thoughts you think.

Weed your garden, change your life

Have you ever heard the saying, "Where the mind goes, the body follows?" It's true—your life is merely an expression of your dominant thoughts. As you may have experienced already, the mind is a powerful tool. The people and circumstances that come into your life are without question the result of the thoughts you think about most of the time. So, in order to begin changing your life, begin changing your thoughts.

After you're done reading **Fat That Doesn't Come Back,** a great addition to your personal library would be James Allen's magnificent book, *"As A Man Thinketh."* In this book he helps the reader understand that the mind can only hold one thought at a time—either positive or negative. He explains that the mind is very much like a garden, and just like in a garden, either weeds or flowers will grow. He maintains that if you don't consciously, deliberately and purposely plant flowers, weeds will grow automatically. The point he makes is that weeds do not need any encouragement, nutrition, or fertilizer—weeds just grow automatically. And if your mind is not filled with flowers, you are likely to have your mind occupied with such negatives as worries, anxieties, doubts and fears. So, consciously and deliberately fill it with thoughts consistent with the direction you want your life to move.

To ensure your thoughts are positive, ask yourself, "Is my mind filled with weeds or flowers?" If your focus is on positive thoughts (i.e. circumstances, goals) you have flowers. If your thoughts are negative (i.e. self-doubt, concern with what others think about you) you have weeds. If you have weeds, then it's time to pull them out!

The most common reason people are so unhappy in life is not due to economic struggles or being over fat, but because their minds are filled with weeds. The thoughts or "battles" that take place in your mind can be reversed if you practice filling your mind with positive thoughts. Become skilled at weeding negative thoughts out of your head as you keep things in perspective and remain focused on where you are going, not where you are now or where you have been.

Think for yourself

Even when we're independent in most areas of our lives, look at how easy it is to become co-dependent on others for weight loss. Like many people, you may have enrolled in a commercial weight-loss program that restricted your calories through a point system, provided prepackaged foods or liquid drinks. If it wasn't a weight-loss program, maybe you at one time or another purchased a diet book at the recommendation of a friend. In short, your goal was to lose weight and you didn't know how to do it, so you went with an established, credible approach that promised success.

Sorry to say it, but when you began your quest to lose weight, you probably stopped thinking for yourself with hopes of having someone tell you what to do because you were fed up with feeling and looking out of shape. Sound about right so far? If the diet book said to stop eating carbohydrates (carbs), you followed the directions and stopped eating our body's primary source of fuel. If the diet book said to eat only protein and fat, like a soldier, you and many others took action—following the orders with hopes of getting rid of the unwanted body fat.

Now, we aren't suggesting you drift through life and never seek the advice or guidance of others (i.e. professionals, experts, authors). When releasing body fat, it is in your best interest to take an approach that is conducive to a lifestyle that evolves. For example, if a diet says to avoid carbs, ask yourself, "What kind of life is it to never eat carbs again?" or "How will no longer consuming carbs affect my health?" What we propose is a process that leads to a lifestyle developed and designed for you. If you're ready for that lifestyle, you're ready to take the next step forward.

We had a 71-year-old client once share with us that she lived more than 50 years as an adult not knowing she was in the dark. Not until she discovered Wellness Weight-Loss did she realize she could lead a lifestyle that consistently redefined her age. For instance, instead of not eating carbs (i.e. bread), she learned to choose bread that tastes great, but wasn't made with the ingredients that caused her to gain excess body fat. The same went for chocolate, pizza and hundreds of other food and snacks that get a bad rap for making us fat.

There are millions of people like our 71-year-old client who go through life not knowing that it could have been lived differently. Your lifestyle can empower you to eat healthy, exercise regularly and think positively. Your lifestyle can be framed around the freedom to choose. Being held to liquid drinks, point systems and prepackaged foods is not freedom, but restriction.

Believe it or not, you can enjoy the entire process of releasing body fat. It will be your lifestyle that will take you to your destination. Whether you want to release 25, 75 or 150 pounds, simply choose to begin creating health daily, and it's only a matter of time before you reach your personal goal. As with sports, business and many other activities, your secret weapon in this journey is taking charge of what thoughts occupy your mind. The truth is that what we believe in our mind and expect with confidence becomes our own self-fulfilling prophecy.

Points to remember:

- As your guides—your master coaches—we intend to help you bridge the gap between knowing what is in your best interest, and doing what is in your best interest. This will ultimately result in you being the person that leads a lifestyle that is forever evolving.
- Diets are schemes—misrepresentations of healthy and vibrant living.
- Wellness Weight-Loss is a lifestyle—not a diet.
- Instead of saying, "I am losing fat" we encourage you to say, "I am releasing fat."
- There is a significant distinction between your total body weight and body composition—your body's pounds of fat and pounds of lean body mass (which consists of muscle, bones, blood, connective tissue, organs and water.)
- The scale is good for merely one thing: providing you with your total body weight. It does not reflect how much fat you have.
- You cannot survive without some body fat.
- For optimum health, we recommend a body-fat percentage of no more than 15 for men, and 22 for women. However, if you are

breastfeeding, taking hormone replacements, beta-blockers, birth control pills or any other medication that may affect your hormonal balance, we recommend a body-fat percentage of no more than 22 for men, and 27 for women.

- Taking control of your life starts with being responsible for the actions you take and the thoughts you think.

2

Lifestyle

*"So many people spend their health gaining wealth,
and then have to spend their wealth to regain their health."*
—A. J. Reb Materi

Over the years we have shared with thousands of people in our seminars, in magazines and newspapers, on television and radio, and now in this book, that it is your lifestyle that enables you to create health and release the body fat that doesn't come back. Now, "lifestyle" is a word that takes on many meanings. A perfect example is the once-popular television show, "Lifestyles of the Rich and Famous." However, according to Webster's New World Dictionary, lifestyle is defined as, "An individual's whole way of living." We concur with this definition, however, we would like to share with you how others define its meaning. This will help you bring this chapter into perspective. But, first, we would like to take a closer look at Webster's definition and what we mean by lifestyle.

The word "individual" in Webster's definition of lifestyle confirms that it's personalized. Further, when you look at the definition of "whole" you quickly discover that its meaning points to words such as "entire," "all" and "total." The reason for this is simple: lifestyle branches out to include everything we as individuals think, do and believe. Lifestyle encompasses everything from our personal religion to our profession, hobbies, eating and exercise habits, family and the people we associate with.

Another empowering note: the word "whole" is often defined as health. Likewise, the root meaning of health gives us the word "wholeness." As a matter of fact, wholeness comes from the same root that gives us the word "holy." With this said, it is apparent that you cannot talk about lifestyle without referring to personal health.

Truth is: the essence of the word lifestyle is not how much money you have or what type of home you reside in—it is your health. That television show could have easily been titled, "Health of the Rich and Famous." So from this day forward, when you think of lifestyle, keep in mind that health is a major component of its meaning.

Defining lifestyle

To help you bring the meaning of lifestyle into perspective, we surveyed well over 100 people and asked them to define what lifestyle meant to them. We then randomly chose 15 responses to share with you. Although names are withheld, the responses are provided in their entirety.

- Male (insurance agent), age 38, says, "Lifestyle is the way you conduct yourself on a daily basis, including habits, attitudes and beliefs."
- Female (technical advisor), age 33, says, "Lifestyle is how you live your life day to day, how values that you hold important are demonstrated in your daily life."
- Male (medical doctor), age 48, says, "Lifestyle is a description of the choices one makes in their life. For example, I could choose to party and drink a lot, which would be one type of lifestyle with its consequences. Alternatively, I might choose a lifestyle of careful eating, exercise, yoga, etc., which requires a certain commitment and generates its own benefits, analogous to the 'consequences' above."
- Female (graphic designer), age 37, says, "Lifestyle is a combination of many things, and kind of a culmination of all your life's experiences to date. It's how you choose to live your life; your beliefs, your personality, your health, your spirituality, the good and the bad things about you. A lot of times when people talk about lifestyle, it seems like they focus on one or two small parts of a lifestyle (such as using 'lifestyle change' for changing one's church or diet plan). But to me, 'lifestyle' is bigger than that. In order to significantly change something about you, you first need to look at ALL the parts of your life that make up WHO you are, and why you are that way."
- Male (personal fitness trainer), age 46, says, "Lifestyle means life-habits to me. We'd like to think our life has style, but it doesn't. It just has habits, some good and some bad. Same question can be asked of class. What makes or gives a person class? Some think it's breeding and some think it's money, still others think it's the people you hang out with. I think its demeanor."
- Female (writer), age 47, says, "Lifestyle means the way in which people 'live their life' and all that entails. For example, I am now

leading a healthier lifestyle, exercising more, eating the right foods, and taking time for r & r *[rest and relaxation]*. Others that I associate with are leading stressful lifestyles, gulping food on the go and not taking time to care about their appearance. Lifestyles are also particularly relevant to the world of beauty. For instance, salons generally categorize clients by the lifestyles they lead; i.e., active, classic, avant-garde, etc., and then design hairstyles and beauty treatments accordingly."

- Male (realtor), age 41, says, "Lifestyle is doing what you want, when you want, and being able to afford it."
- Female (high school student), age 14, says, "Lifestyle is something that you follow to make yourself happy and make you feel good about the things you do."
- Male (retired lawyer who currently works as a personal trainer), age 58, says, "Lifestyle means absolutely nothing! Just another buzzword full of sound and fury, but signifying nothing! Anyway, whatever definition the dictionary gives for the word, I'll go with that. Sorry, but the word has zero meaning to me."
- Female (school teacher), age 43, says, "Lifestyle is how you choose to live, not just what you do or buy or how much money you make. People choose to be giving and caring, to take care of their health and their bodies without caring who is looking at them. People choose to help others, to make a difference in people's lives and to make the planet better for all of us. That is lifestyle for me. It is not how extravagant your home or wardrobe or car(s) are, how much jewelry you can wear or how much you can order others around. It is the whole picture, inside and outside, for me. Are you healthy? Do you love to live, to give, to share? Do you like to share ideas, your time, your knowledge? These are the things that are important in a lifestyle."
- Female (office manager), age 50, says, "Lifestyle is a choice for some but not for others. If you are financially secure, you can choose your lifestyle. If you're not financially secure and want a certain lifestyle, you have no other choice but to work really hard to have the lifestyle you want. Lifestyle is living the way you want to live given what you can afford."
- Female (engineer), age 54, says, "Lifestyle at its most basic level is the way one styles their life. My lifestyle is how I choose to format my daily existence, with all of the complex variables that I have available to me."
- Female (homemaker), age 42, says, "Lifestyle is the manner in which we choose to live our life. The way we dress, the food we eat

and the people we choose to associate with are indications of our lifestyle."

- Female (weight-loss coach), age 39, says, "Lifestyle is the way in which I choose to live my life. I believe life is all about choices. The choices I make now affect my quality of life today and in the future."
- Female (nurse), age 38, says, "Lifestyle is a way of living that reflects a person's attitudes and values."

Lifestyle, value and self-esteem

As you have read, lifestyle can be defined many ways. The reality is that it's largely determined by what we value most. We believe that lifestyle is intertwined with our self-esteem. Think about it. What you have, what you do and your physical appearance is often the motive for the lifestyle you uphold and seek. Unfortunately, when our lifestyle is based on what we do, what we have and our physical appearance, we often find ourselves depressed, unsure and empty.

To get a clear picture of what we are saying, take a look at the early 1900s—the depression. Many people who based their lifestyle on what they had (i.e., money, stocks), committed suicide when it was gone. Then you have those who put their stock in stardom—what they do. Proof positive, many celebrities find themselves lonely at the top. The reality is that when we find ourselves defining who we are by external accomplishments and gratification, the outcome is more often than not a lowered self-esteem and a pressured lifestyle that says, "If I lose what I have or what I do, my worth, importance and value is zilch." The same goes for weight loss. Many people who are obese or wanting to release body fat have this belief that once the weight is gone, then, they will be happier. Guess what? Not true, unless being healthier is the primary reason for the weight loss.

Meet Betty, who at 49 percent body fat weighed nearly 300 pounds when we first met her. With a vision to one day have a body-fat percentage under 25 and weigh 140 pounds, Betty's work ethic proved to be the foundation of her future success! Two years later, Betty was at her goal weight, but unfortunately, her happiness was temporary. You see, Betty felt that after losing the weight, what we refer to as "Hunting Trim," she would find a man and in her words, "Have a life."

Eventually Betty met someone and found love, but not until she grew past measuring her importance and self-worth by her physical appearance did she begin to discover the beauty within herself. Betty has always been beautiful, but since the fourth grade she was trapped into believing her physical appearance was the deciding factor in how she felt and what she was worth.

*What we encourage you to do is to come in contact
with who you are as a person and to live a life
that brings out the beauty that lies within.*

Please take note that we are not saying physical appearance isn't important. We are not saying living a life of financial wealth is not of value. What we encourage you to do is to come in contact with who you are as a person and to live a life that brings out the beauty that lies within. So, as you create health and build your self-esteem, you are guaranteed long-term success.

Lifestyle is largely affected by self-esteem

We once read a nationwide study that surveyed more than 10,000 single people. In this study, participants were asked, "What is the worst thing about being single?" Astonishing enough, 85 percent of those that responded said, "Loneliness is the worst part about being single." They took the same questionnaire and mailed it to married couples, asking, "What is the worst thing about being married?" You guessed correctly. Eight-five percent of those who responded said, "Loneliness is the worst thing about being married." Sadly, more than 50 percent of those who were single and didn't want to be lonely anymore got married, thinking they would no longer have to deal with loneliness.

Whether rich or poor, healthy or unhealthy, when we asked more than 100 people, "What area of your life do you dislike most?" again, "loneliness" topped the list. What we have learned through our research and working with people who want to lead a lifestyle that creates health daily, is that feeling lonely is a silent cry for self-discovery.

If you think self-esteem does not play a role in feeling lonely and not experiencing lasting weight loss, pay close attention to the rest of this chapter, because it does. The truth is, your self-esteem is affected by your lifestyle and vice versa. Living proof, it is your lifestyle that serves as the source for whether you release or gain body fat.

Lifestyles that exist

After hearing "lifestyle" defined hundreds of ways, it has become apparent to us that a person's lifestyle is easily placed into one of two categories: those that evolve and those that exist. We start by explaining the difference between the two.

In short, a lifestyle that exists is the opposite of a lifestyle that evolves. Having a lifestyle that evolves refers to people looking to improve their overall health. Whether it is creating health through exercise, nutrition or reducing body fat—progressing in these areas is a confirmation that you are evolving in your lifestyle. On the flip side, having a lifestyle that exists refers to people who live life based on the philosophy, "If it isn't broke, don't fix it." Sadly, it may already be broke. And if it isn't, it's just a matter of time before health begins to diminish and chronic diseases become a permanent fixture in these people's lives.

It is more common than not for people to live for today and worry about their health only if and when they become ill.

There are many people who see no need to adopt healthier habits, because they are comfortable and complacent with their current lifestyle. For instance, we have heard people say time and again, "We are all going to die of something, so why change or worry about it now?" Basically, it is more common than not for people to live for today and worry about their health only if and when they become ill.

You would think the possibility of being faced with a life-threatening disease like Type 2 diabetes or cancer would be enough to provoke a person to evolve with their lifestyle. Unfortunately, the thought of losing health and quality of life because of the way we live is not a real enough threat for many people to trigger a change in eating habits and begin exercising.

In our research we visited a cancer ward and learned that even when patients were shown lungs of a non-smoker compared to those of a long-time smoker, it wasn't enough to motivate smokers to stop. We even spoke with smokers who viewed a television commercial that displayed a smoker with a hole in her throat. Still, the visual of watching her take a puff through the hole in her neck wasn't enough to motivate smokers to end the habit of smoking.

We didn't give up however, and soon after we learned that practically every cancer patient we met wished they had lived life differently. One lung-cancer patient said, "If I could turn back time and live my life over, I would never smoke." Unfortunately, we can't turn back the hands of time. We can only live life going forward, and that means being proactive, not reactive.

George's surprise

At most parties, events and dinners we attend, once people learn of our profession, sooner or later we get bombarded with nutrition and exercise questions. When it's not questions, we are confronted with statements from people who are determined to inform us that their approach to weight loss and health is the best.

Even when people don't know of our profession, by the time we sit down to eat, it becomes obvious to those at the dinner table that what we choose to eat differs from most everyone else. Socializing in an environment that caters to the consumption of food is a guarantee that, at one point or another, we will stand out and bring attention to our lifestyle. As a result, we end up talking about Wellness Weight-Loss.

While at our friend's dinner party, we welcomed the opportunity to entertain questions about nutrition, exercise and various types of diets. During this time we met George. Standing 6'2" and weighing approximately 260 pounds, George quickly became the life of the party—making himself loud and clear as he expressed to everyone that he had a perfect bill of health. Waving his arms around and explaining how his doctors were amazed at how healthy his heart was and how his cholesterol levels were perfect—he went on to explain how health and longevity was all about genetics.

George must have read every diet book on the market. He had answers and solutions for every dilemma. According to George, it doesn't matter which diet you choose to follow—when it is all said and done, he believed it comes down to genetics. George explained how his parents were fat and that is why he is overweight. He also raved about all the people he knew that ate fried foods and drank hard liquor and lived to be 100 years of age.

After hearing George ramble for more than 20 minutes, it became apparent that he would be a great politician. Then, we learned that he was a lawyer. Fortunately, we didn't fall into his trap and debate with him. Instead, we remained neutral and respectful of his choice of lifestyle. Then, George ran out of topics and ended his outrageous claims about nutrition and exercise and everyone grew bored and became more interested in dancing and chatting with others.

About a month after the dinner party we ran into our friend who hosted the event. After some small talk, we asked, "How is George doing?" To our dismay, George fell into a diabetic coma about a week after the dinner party. Saddened, but not surprised, it was apparent to us that George had three major risk factors: over fat, over 40 and out of shape. You see, until his coma incident, George had no idea that he had Type 2 diabetes.

Before you begin to judge George for not being aware of his Type 2 diabetes, consider this: The National Institute of Health and the American Diabetes Association (ADA) report that 33 million adults have blood glucose that is higher than normal, 16 million in the pre-diabetic stage and 17 million already diagnosed with diabetes. Up to 25 percent of Americans have pre-diabetes, previously referred to as insulin resistance. An expert panel of the ADA and U.S. Department of Health and Human Services estimates that without lifestyle changes, insulin resistance will result in Type 2 diabetes within 10 years.

At the youthful age of 56, George, like many Americans, felt he was in decent health and believed that genetics was responsible for diseases like Type 2 diabetes. Prior to his surprise attack with a diabetic coma, George would have been the first to argue that such diseases are hereditary. And if you had met George prior to his face-to-face confrontation with losing his health, unless you knew differently, George may have convinced you of his beliefs.

What makes George's situation even more profound is that he must have had Type 2 diabetes for more than a year. Once at the hospital and after waking out of the coma, George was informed that his blood glucose was much higher than what is considered normal. For example, a normal fasting blood glucose level is 70 to 110 mg/dL, or milligrams of glucose per deciliter of blood. After eating a meal, a reading of 150 mg/dL is considered high.

The shocker

George was in shock as he learned that his blood glucose levels were over 1,500 mg/dL. It was a miracle that George was still alive. The doctors and nurses never witnessed a patient living with such a high level of sugar floating around in their blood. To put this into a broader perspective, most people fall into a coma when there blood glucose levels are 500 mg/dL. Furthermore, it is not uncommon for someone with a blood glucose of 1000 to die. But George, who announced at the dinner party that diabetes was hereditary and it didn't run in his family, learned the hard way. As a nurse explained to George, "When you play (i.e., eat unhealthy), you pay." George didn't refute her statement, for he was happy to be alive and given an opportunity to change his lifestyle.

Shortly after he was released from the hospital, we spoke with George and he shared with us how frightened he was. He was then ready to make a lifestyle change. He was definitely a different man from the one we met at the dinner party. We invited him to come in for a free consultation with Wellness Weight-Loss and he accepted.

George is a prime example of someone who led a lifestyle that merely existed. Although he excelled in his profession and as a father, George neglected to evolve with his health. After coming face to face with losing his life, George was ready, willing and able to begin creating health daily. No more living on the edge and neglecting his health. George has decided to resolve and evolve in all areas of his life—specifically his health.

If you want to confirm whether or not you lead a lifestyle that evolve, ask yourself, "In one year will I be doing the same things?"

Lifestyles that evolve

If you want to confirm whether or not you lead a lifestyle that evolves, ask yourself, "In one year, will I be doing the same things (i.e., eating habits, exercise routine) and expecting a different result?" If so, you are most likely in denial or you have been deceived. Case in point, if you continue to do the same things like sticking to the same workout routine three to four times per week, year after year—wanting to reduce your body fat, but each year being no better or worse—you are not evolving in that area of your life. The reality is that you are simply drifting through life with the mindset that heart attacks, strokes and diseases like Type 2 diabetes happen to other people. But, like George, the day may arrive where you come face to face with the true value of health.

Consider George's situation. Prior to his diagnosis with Type 2 diabetes, he basically led a lifestyle that existed. He had no interest in eating foods labeled as healthy. Exercise was for people who had time. George was a prime example of how many Americans live.

Since George's episode, what do you think resulted from his lifestyle change? The first thing that happened is that George released over 60 pounds of fat. He now eats more vegetables and fruit, and exercises a few times per week. George now looks at fast food restaurants as though they are crack houses. No longer tired after a full day's work, George's energy has increased and his health has drastically improved. When we asked George if it cost more to eat healthy and live in a fit body, he said, "When I traded in my lifestyle of unhealthy choices, I did spend quite a bit of money buying a new wardrobe."

Next step

Being in a different place a year from now is the confirmation that you have evolved.

"How can I improve?" There isn't a week that goes by that George doesn't ask himself this question. We consider questions like this to be tools that ensure you are evolving. By honestly answering this question and then following up with an action step, you are sure to evolve with your lifestyle. For example, if you are currently drinking whole milk, ask yourself, "What's a healthier choice?" and then take action. The question keeps your awareness heightened and puts you in a place where you're constantly in search of making progress. So, in place of whole milk, the next step forward would be to drink two percent milk. A year or two later you may find yourself drinking one percent or non-fat milk. Ultimately, the day may come where your preference is organic soy milk. Being in a different place a year from now is the confirmation that you have evolved.

Gym goers

A couple of years before writing this book, we began touring fitness centers and lecturing on how to release fat that doesn't come back. To our surprise, most of the people we met in gyms and fitness centers were complacent. They talked a big talk, but very few people appeared to be making progress. We thought to ourselves, "At least at *Weight Watchers* and *Jenny Craig* people lost weight. You would think people working out in gyms would be the perfect picture of health." But, as we visited and lectured in fitness and health clubs, we discovered that gym goers aren't in tip-top shape, and many of the owners of these facilities count on their clientele being inconsistent.

We are sure fitness and health club owners would love it if everyone who enrolled at their facility made exercise a habitual part of their life. However, the reality is that nearly 80 percent of those who enroll never, if ever, use their membership and workout. With this being the case, it only makes sense that a club owner wants to enroll thousands of people—collect a monthly membership fee electronically from those who never use the facility. Makes sense, doesn't it? But don't get upset with the club owners. Keep in mind that it's not their responsibility to make sure you use your membership.

Going inside

Before we developed our seminars, we asked ourselves, "What do we know about our audience?" It was apparent that our audience would consist of people who use the gym often; therefore, we would be speaking to fitness-minded people. However, we felt inclined to focus more on nutrition since everyone attending would have general knowledge about exercise.

After facilitating a half-dozen seminars in fitness centers, it didn't take long before our prediction proved true. Time and time again we were asked questions like, "Why is it that I workout everyday but I'm not losing weight?" Each and every time we lectured to people in these fitness centers, the questions and results people were experiencing were the same. And each time, we felt nutrition was the key reason why most of these people remained stuck—not getting the results they hoped to acquire.

After working in and around the fitness industry for many years, we are not surprised to see the same people, doing the same thing and getting the same results year after year. As we expressed in many of the seminars we presented, "A year from now, many of the people you see in the gym will look the same." Most people didn't know how to take such a statement, and we would always follow up with asking those in attendance, "Are you going to be one of those people who continues doing the same thing day after day expecting a different outcome?" Though most of the group appeared shocked and not sure how to answer the question, it was quite obvious that no one wanted to remain stuck. They wanted to evolve.

Following a particular seminar we scheduled a couple of consultations and this is when we met Susan. At 5'1" and weighing in at 181 pounds at 38 percent body fat, Susan was fed up with not getting results. When we sat down with Susan we inquired about what motivated her to meet with us and she said, "I do **not** want to be one of the people you talked about." Basically, Susan was saying she wanted to evolve.

Susan went on to release more than 50 pounds of fat. No longer was Susan falling prey to exercising two and three hours a day. Susan quickly learned that exercising four or five times per week for a maximum of one hour and enjoying healthy, yet tasteful foods was the lifestyle she always wanted. Today, Susan leads a lifestyle that evolves. When a new cereal becomes available and she knows we would enjoy it, she contacts us. When she comes across a new recipe that keeps the fat from coming back, she contacts us.

Both Susan and George have taken control of their lifestyles and now enjoy never having to think about dieting again. And like Susan and George, you can begin asking yourself on a daily basis, "What can I do today to evolve in my health—my lifestyle?" With a strong belief and confidence that you are forever moving into a healthier relationship with yourself, the fat that you release will be gone forever.

Points to remember:

- Webster's New World Dictionary defines lifestyle as, "An individual's whole way of living."
- Lifestyle branches out to include everything we as individuals think, do and believe.
- Many people who are obese or want to release body fat believe that once the weight is gone, they will be happier. Guess what? Not true, unless being healthier is the primary reason for the weight loss.
- We have learned through our research that feeling lonely is a silent cry for self-discovery.
- After hearing "lifestyle" defined hundreds of ways, it has become apparent to us that one's lifestyle is easily placed into one of two categories: those that evolve and those that exist.
- People who live life based on the philosophy, "If it isn't broke, don't fix it" lead lifestyles that exist.
- People who are conscious of the choices they make and the opportunity to improve their health lead lifestyles that evolve.
- We can only live life forward, and that means being proactive, not reactive.
- Up to 25 percent of Americans have pre-diabetes, previously referred to as insulin resistance. An expert panel of the ADA and U.S. Department of Health and Human Services estimates that without lifestyle changes, insulin resistance will result in Type 2 diabetes within 10 years.

3

The Choice Is Yours

"Choice—not chance—determines human destiny."
—Anonymous

What if you knew you were going to suffer a heart attack—and you could prevent it? Sounds like an easy choice, right? You'd do everything in your power to stop it from happening. But what if you found out the number one cause of heart attacks was lifestyle? Would you alter your lifestyle to avoid a heart attack? As you learned with George in Chapter 2, most people avoid changing their lifestyle until someone like a medical doctor puts the fear of death in their hearts. Even then, many people go into denial–choosing not to accept or believe it will happen to them.

Continuing on a path of destruction is not an uncommon choice. You may find it difficult to believe, but most people will not alter their lifestyle to prevent disease. Consider this: many people smoke cigarettes knowing it's harmful to their health. People eat deep fried foods knowing they're linked to various types of cancer. But guess what? People will continue to choose cigarettes and eat fried foods. **The reality is that 25 percent of the American population smokes cigarettes and the fast food industry earns billions of dollars annually.**

Did you know that the McDonald restaurant franchise serves over 40 million people daily? In our opinion McDonald's doesn't love to see us smile. Apparently, they love to see us waddle.

Nonetheless, the business of weight loss has grown by leaps and bounds, just like the average American waistline. Since the early 1990s it has climbed from a $30 billion- to a $40 billion-a-year business. Whether it is publishing, entertainment or advertising, practically all have cashed in on our desire to shed body fat. In contrast, the food industry has added to the bulge by selling super-sized meals and foods comprised of more fat, sugar and salt (above and beyond what most health and fitness advocates believed possible for human consumption) while the marketing and advertising of these unhealthy foods are packaged in a way to make us think we are getting a bargain and eating healthy.

Fortunately, we live in a world where information is rampant and even though getting control of your health and weight may seem like an unsolvable riddle, you can succeed and you can do it at any age. Once you meet the prerequisite of being willing and able, you are only choices away from lasting success. That's right! You are always one choice from moving forward or backward when it comes to your lifestyle supporting the progress you make.

Whether you are over fat or under fat, sick or in great health, you have a choice to begin creating health or diminishing it.

Choices

Whether you are over fat or under fat, sick or in great health, you have a choice to begin creating health or diminishing it. If it's not apparent that you have a choice in every moment of your life—please take our word for it—you do! You are not locked into a pre-destined outcome. As you take control of your lifestyle through implementing change where necessary, it will be the choices you make today that move you closer to the outcome that best suits your desired results.

A great example of the role choice plays in our life is embodied in the movie Minority Report. Directed by Steven Spielberg and starring Tom Cruise, this film shows us that our fate is largely determined by the choices we make in life. The movie takes you to Washington D.C. int the future. Detective John Anderton (Cruise) leads an elite law enforcement agency known as the Pre-crime Unit, which uses the abilities of three psychic beings (dubbed "Pre-cogs") to see murders before they happen and bring the potential killers to justice before they can carry out their crime. With no murders having been committed in six years, the system seems perfect—until Anderton himself is tagged as a future killer and must go on the run to either clear himself or carry out his pre-destined fate. Fortunately, Anderton uncovers the fact that the Pre-crime Unit is not perfect and that we are not locked into a pre-destined decision. In the movie, when Anderton is faced with making a decision that was pre-destined by the "Pre-cogs," he chooses differently. The choice Anderton makes goes against what was predicted, and this proved that we always have a choice. We have a choice to change what was previously chosen.

In the end, regardless of what a situation looks like, we are in charge of the decisions we make.

Brainpower

Have you ever wondered about which area of our mind is responsible for how we make choices? Recognized as your brain's executive center, the frontal cortex is the area of the brain that allows us to consciously choose what to pay attention to. The frontal cortex is what separates us from other living creatures. For instance, even though there is a genetic similarity between humans and apes—apes do not have a frontal cortex. Only humans are gifted with the ability to choose with logic and reason.

There's no doubt that having a frontal cortex is a blessing, however, it can also be a misfortune for those who choose recklessly. Whether positive or negative, it is the choices we make on a daily basis that determine the direction our lives take. Choosing which direction your life moves in is not something you put on autopilot. Ultimately, each one of us is responsible for the choices we make and the actions we take. So gaining control over our thoughts and the words we use is a major step in being able to choose wisely.

Thought power

Have you ever noticed yourself thinking about something negative for long periods of time? Maybe it's time for your monthly body composition analysis, and in your mind you hear yourself asking, "What if my body-fat percentage went up?" If it isn't a question, maybe you will make a statement like, "I hate getting a body composition analysis conducted." When you ask yourself a question or make such a statement, your brain responds. For instance, your brain may respond by saying, "You aren't consistent and it won't be surprising if your body fat has gone up." Or, "Accept yourself for who you are. You're fat and that's just the way it is."

What can you do to avoid the pitfalls of negative questions, statements and labels you place on yourself? As we will discuss in Chapter 6, it begins with getting control of your internal dialogue. These voices in your head can make all the difference between long-term and short-term success. To get control of your thoughts, you want to begin filtering information that is presented to you. Furthermore, it helps to ensure that the questions you ask yourself are going to help you, not discourage your ability to progress.

If you want to change your life, change your thinking. The most powerful tool you have is your mind, and where the mind goes, the body follows. Remember, it's getting control of your thoughts that put you in charge of your life.

Word power

As you heighten the awareness of your thoughts it is also beneficial to become conscious of your vocabulary. The way we think and the words we use have a tremendous impact on our quality of life. Certain words are destructive; others are empowering.

Did you know that most people we meet describe their eating habits as good or bad? At first glance, the words good or bad may not seem like a big deal, but such words may have a negative effect on self-esteem. For instance, judgments are made when we use words like good and bad. When something is good or bad it can be translated into right and wrong. If someone says it is good, that's saying it's better than something else. If they say it's bad, that's saying it's worse in comparison. In short, using words like good or bad, right or wrong, clarifies that a judgment is being made. For example, you may be judging yourself if you say things like, "My eating habits are bad."

Instead of labeling a food or meal as good or bad, we encourage you to use words such as healthy and unhealthy. For instance, say to yourself, "I was bad this weekend," and then say, "I made unhealthy choices this weekend." Feel the difference? Being bad is one thing, but eating unhealthy is another.

At the same time, what one person defines as healthy, another may consider unhealthy. One of the most common statements we hear from new clients is, "I eat pretty healthy." After about six weeks into the Wellness Weight-Loss process and learning more about creating health, the same person who said, "I eat pretty healthy" gets dumbfounded when they think back to those early statements. The reason for this is simple: what they once identified as healthy and unhealthy often proves to be just the opposite.

Making healthy choices are largely based on heightening your awareness. For instance, if you are not knowledgeable about the damage trans fatty acids and highly refined and processed sugar may cause to your health, you might as well consider yourself in the dark. This doesn't mean you are stupid, just unaware. Once you make the decision that you want to create health daily—day after day, month after month, and year after year—you will learn more about which foods empower your body and which products diminish your health. Over time your options will expand and soon you will be empowered and forever progressing and evolving toward a healthier you.

To help you remain focused and on track, we would like to share empowering alternatives for some of the most common words and statements verbalized that take power away from those wanting long-term success:

Instead of saying ...	*Say ...*
I can't	I won't
I'll try	I will
I hope	I know
I should	I could
It's a problem	It's an opportunity
I have to	I prefer to
I should be	I choose to
It's not my fault	I'm totally responsible
Why can't I?	How can I?

As you have noticed, the goal is to replace poor quality questions and statements with words that help you remain empowered. As you begin putting into practice what we term "word replacement therapy," we would like to share with you the words that offer you a choice in every moment of your life. The moments when you feel threatened with sabotage refer to the following words and statements in your vocabulary:

Instead of saying ...	*Say ...*
I have to	I would rather
I need to	I want to
I should be	I prefer to be
I can't	I choose not to

Most people who are on a diet say things like, "I can't have that," "That's not legal," and "I have to eat one apple a day." It's statements like these that lower self-esteem and take their power away without them noticing it. So, instead of saying, "I have to eat one apple a day," we recommend you say, feel and think, "I prefer to have one apple a day." The same goes for when someone approaches you at a dinner party and insists you have a piece of cake. Instead of saying, "I can't have cake," we recommend you say, "Thank you. I would rather eat some fruit."

Also, when someone offers you a food you do not want or inquires why you are the only one not eating fried food, we recommend that you use these words of power. If not, it is almost a guarantee that you will be defending yourself. For instance, if you say to someone, "I can't eat fried foods," you better get ready because they are going to ask why. And before you know it, you will be debating with this person—defending why you are adhering to the process or lifestyle that you have chosen to follow.

Unfortunately, most people want to feel good and in order for that to take place, it's important that they are right. Being right means if you are doing something different from what they are doing, they must be wrong. In order to avoid such debates or conflicts, we encourage you to use words of power and present your preferences with grace and love.

Doing this will prove quite rewarding because you will feel empowered and better able to remain true to the promises you have made to yourself.

Winning words

If there was one thing that we hope everyone reading this book would grasp, it would be the importance of honoring the boundaries you set with words of power. As we have said, using words like "I can't" implies you have no control over your life, whereas "I won't" puts a situation in the realm of choice. Verbalizing words like "try" is a safe approach to putting off a decision. When you catch yourself saying things like, "I'll try," ask yourself the question, "What decision am I putting off?"

Using winning words is not just adding to your positive word bank, but learning to avoid negative words. For instance, instead of saying, "I can't," in its place you can choose words that are empowering. For example, after being asked to attend a dinner party, one of our clients said, "I can't come." This statement was untrue. They could go to dinner, however, they were choosing to do something else. If you don't want to hurt someone's feelings, you simply invest some time and effort in evoking your power with grace and love. After our client thought about it, she realized she could have simply responded by saying, "I appreciate the offer for dinner, but I have an important meeting tomorrow that I have to prepare for. I would love to get together another time."."

As you come to learn and apply winning words to your life, you will feel empowered and in control of how your life unfolds.

Another group of words to replace is, "I should" and "I think." When you say, "I should" you are implying a judgment—meaning there is no choice available. When you say things like "I think" you are choosing to be safe and giving the impression that you don't know. It is imperative that you understand that there is a choice in every moment of your life. As you come to learn and apply winning words to your life, you will feel empowered and in control of how your life unfolds.

Situations of choice

We could go on and on about which words are damaging and which words empower you. However, to help you better understand that there is a choice in every moment of your life, we would like you to become familiar with the three situations of choice that plague us all.

1. Positive versus positive—the first situation of choice involves being faced with a decision to choose between two positives. In this exercise we want you to choose between "a" and "b":
    a. Get your groceries paid in full for an entire year.
    b. Have your very own personal chef cook all your meals for an entire year.

Which do you prefer?   a   or   b   *(circle your answer)*

FOLLOW UP: Some people will choose "a" and others will choose "b." Regardless of which choice you make, it is a win-win situation. Both outcomes are positive. Unfortunately, situations like this seem to be rare.

2. Positive versus negative—the second situation of choice involves being faced with a decision to choose between a positive and a negative. Consider the following and choose between "a" and "b":
    a. Eat every two to three hours and release two pounds of fat each week.
    b. Eat one meal a day and gain two pounds of fat each week.

Which do you prefer?   a   or   b   *(circle your answer)*

FOLLOW UP: Unless you want to gain fat, choosing "a" is the option that would be considered positive. This situation is somewhat easy because of the extremes. When we ask people this question, it doesn't take much thought to decide which outcome to choose.

3. Negative versus negative—the third situation of choice is a tough one. Take your time and choose between "a" and "b":
    a. Your best friend is getting married and expects you to eat cake and drink champagne at the wedding reception. You made a promise to yourself to stick to the Wellness Weight-Loss process, so you decide not to go to the wedding reception. *(Before you choose, think of how your best friend is going to feel if you don't attend the wedding reception.)*
    b. You decide to go to the wedding reception, but stick to the Wellness Weight-Loss process. This means choosing not to eat cake or over indulging in food and alcohol. *(Before you choose, think of how your best friend is going to feel seeing you sober and somewhat of a party-pooper. How do you think others will feel if you don't eat cake and be merry, so that you can honor your self-promise?)*

FOLLOW UP: If you don't attend the wedding, your friend will be hurt. If you do attend the wedding, but choose not to drink alcohol and eat cake and other tasty treats, your best friend and many others may be offended and somewhat bewildered and concerned that you are not having a good time. Either way, your friend will most likely be upset. Even though you don't like, enjoy or want to go with "a" or "b," you still have a choice in the matter. It is consciously being aware that you have a choice that empowers you!

The choice is yours

Have you ever done something you didn't want to do? Maybe you didn't want to go to work, attend a dinner or visit your doctor for an annual checkup. We have all been in such situations. What is important is to remember it's our choice to do these things.

Consider the reality that you may find yourself working a job you don't like or enjoy. Ask yourself, "If I did not work, how would my life change?" By not working you may lose your car, have your home repossessed and not be able to eat. So, when you think about it, going to work is something you choose to do because you prefer to have a car, shelter and food to nourish your body. Say to yourself, "I have to go to work" and then say, "I choose to go to work." Feel the difference?

When most of new our clients walk into our office, they want us to tell them what to eat, when to exercise and basically, how to think. We are quick to share with them that this is not what Wellness Weight-loss is all about. The Wellness Weight-Loss process is designed to educate, empower and create independence—not make a person co-dependent.

Most weight-loss programs may not realize it, but they groom people to be co-dependent. They take the ability to choose away from those wanting to lose weight and be empowered. Think about it. You start a weight-loss program and successfully lose weight through prepackaged or liquid foods for instance, and the next thing you know you are back to shopping for yourself and unaware of the foods that cause excess body fat. Then, months later you are back where you started and gearing up to begin the process all over again.

Have you ever heard the saying, "Give a man a fish, you feed him for a day. Teach a man how to fish and you feed him for life?" This is our philosophy. By providing you with options—variety—making it easier to choose the food and exercise methods that make for a lifestyle you're happy to live with, you can succeed in long-term weight management and health. At first, when you are in the process, your range of options to choose from seems limited, but in a short amount of time as you gain more knowledge, your options expand and you feel confident and assured because you chose your way to a healthier lifestyle.

If you live your life not realizing you have a choice in every situation, you may find yourself dependent on others and feeling restricted and unsure of most things you do. When you choose water over soda, that in itself can be an empowering experience. When you "have to" drink water instead of soda, it's just a matter of time before you rebel against the rules and regulations that are typical of diets and most weight-loss programs.

Make a conscious effort to heighten your awareness that you are choosing every thing you do on a daily basis.

Make a conscious effort to heighten your awareness that you are choosing every thing you do on a daily basis. Make a commitment to use winning words that empower your choices and soon you will be living a healthier lifestyle—by choice!

Points to remember:

- You are always one choice away from moving forward or backward when it comes to your lifestyle.
- You are not locked into a pre-destined outcome.
- The frontal cortex is the area of the brain that allows us to consciously choose what to pay attention to. The frontal cortex is what separates us from other living creatures.
- If you want to change your life, change your thinking. The most powerful tool you have is your mind, and where the mind goes, the body follows. Remember, it's gaining control of your thoughts that puts you in charge of your life.
- The way we think and the words we use have a tremendous impact on our quality of life. Certain words are destructive; others are empowering.
- If you live your life not realizing you have a choice in every situation, you may find yourself dependent on others and feeling restricted and unsure of most things you do.
- When most of our new clients walk into our office, they want us to tell them what to eat, when to exercise and basically, how to think. We are quick to share with them that this is not what Wellness Weight-loss is all about. The Wellness Weight-Loss process is designed to educate, empower and create independence —not make a person co-dependent.

Wellness Weight-Loss

It's a lifestyle ..not a diet!

PART TWO

It's All About You!

4

Creating Health Daily

"The doctor of the future will give no medicine, but will interest
his patient in the care of the human frame,
in diet and in the cause and prevention of disease."
—Thomas A. Edison

What if you could eat whatever you wanted and never gain an ounce of
body fat? What if there was a pill you could swallow that would cause
you to release body fat without effort? What if you could eat chocolate,
fast food and everything in between and never get sick; never get fat;
never feel fatigued; never be concerned or diagnosed with disease?

What a wonderful world it would be if we didn't have to be responsible for our well being. Eat, drink and be merry 24 hours a day, 365 days
a year. Wouldn't this guilt-free life of ice cream, fried foods and soda be
great? Maybe—maybe not.

We can choose to live a sedentary life and eat whatever and whenever we want. That's right. We don't have to do anything. No one is going
to put a gun to your head and force you to eat tomatoes for the sake of
reducing the risk of cancer. No one is going to disown you for eating
highly processed and sugar-loaded foods that have proven to increase
your risk of Type 2 diabetes.

If you're sedentary, that's your choice. If you exercise, that's your
choice. Not liking, enjoying or wanting to be either healthy or unhealthy
is still your choice and that's to be respected. Each one of us holds the
power to choose the lifestyle that honors and enriches our lives.

Surprise—what you don't know MIGHT kill you

You've worked hard, building a career and raising a family. You're
determined; focused on becoming the next entertainment superstar or
business executive. In addition to a successful career, you're looking
forward to a happy, healthy life.

Like many hard working North Americans, you may not make much time for the "E" word (exercise) and an occasional high fat, high calorie meal is not going to kill you. All in all, you feel good and seem to be healthy. You may look or feel a bit over fat (perhaps more over fat than you realized), but you don't feel sick. You have no reason to worry about disease and debilitation for the moment. Life is good and you're productive, progressive and empowered.

Unfortunately, what you are probably not aware of are the chronic, yet preventable diseases linked to excess body fat. This excess of body fat is making a serious dent in the quality of our population's health. According to dozens of reports and studies conducted by various organizations such as the Centers for Disease Control and Prevention (http://www.cdc.gov), obesity is second to cigarette smoking as the leading cause of preventable deaths among North Americans.

Obesity contributes to 300,00 deaths every year in the U.S.

For the first time in history, those who can be described as fit and healthy constitute the minority in the United States, with 80 percent of the adult population over the age of 25 considered moderately overweight to obese. When we initially began writing this book, former Surgeon General David Satcher reported that 61 percent of Americans were overweight, claiming that obesity contributes to 300,000 deaths every year in the U.S. The detrimental medical conditions associated with excess body fat include: cardiovascular disease (i.e. stroke, heart attack), hypertension, Type 2 diabetes, high cholesterol, degenerative joint disease and various types of cancer (i.e. colon, prostate).

Psychological scars

In a recent body image survey, nearly 60 percent of 2,000 over fat women said they would not allow their partner (i.e., spouse, boyfriend, girlfriend) to see them naked. In fact, a survey done by Britain's, *Slimming Magazine*, found that too much body fat has a devastating effect on every aspect of a woman's life. Eighty percent of the women surveyed believed their excess weight was damaging their health, ruining their sex lives and holding back their careers.

It may be image, health or a need for a balance that prompts you to make changes. Regardless of the reasons for seeking alternatives, they are all definitely valid. In this book we will introduce you to information that will help you identify your particular situation, get control of it, and incorporate healthy eating and exercise into your lifestyle.

The truth about genetics

Like many people, you may believe that because your mother and/or father are overweight, you are genetically predisposed to be over fat. In spite of how you view your heredity, keep in mind that genetics may load the gun—but you and your lifestyle squeeze the trigger. You may not be able to change your genes, but you can change your lifestyle and perhaps alter your genetic destiny. The point we're making is that no matter what predicament you find yourself in, if you've got an obesity-related disease or you're over fat, there are things you can do to improve your health.

Nothing is guaranteed

Exercise, of course, is a proven method for releasing body fat and creating health. Equally important is food choice, a necessary component of a healthy lifestyle. Together, exercise and proper nutrition increase your odds of releasing body fat. This combination, when in balance, also reduces your risk of developing a number of diseases. The pursuit of a sustained and healthy lifestyle does not guarantee you will never become ill, but it drastically reduces the risk of being diagnosed with a chronic illness.

We have had many clients and seminar participants ask us, "Why live a life exercising and forever watching what I eat when the future is not guaranteed?" Fortunately, if you choose to eat healthy and exercise regularly, you will quickly experience daily rewards such as positive physical changes in your body, as well as increased energy and improved mood. However, don't assume that nothing will ever go wrong with your body. Disease does not necessarily discriminate.

Stop the disparity

Each year Americans spend more than $40 billion on weight-loss products and services, including drastic stomach-reduction surgeries, a procedure that has nearly doubled since 1998. You don't have to be a rocket scientist to realize the diet industry preys on over fat people as it prospers through the marketing and selling of weight-loss dreams.

According to statistics compiled by the National Eating Disorder Information Center, 70 percent of women and 35 percent of men are dieting at any given time. Unfortunately, says the National Institute of Health, 90 percent of those who actually lose weight on medically supervised diets regain that weight within three years. It has also been reported that 99 percent of those who begin a weight-loss program will not experience long-term success. Actually, more often than not, people who lose weight gain it back within five years, plus an additional five to 10 pounds.

How do we explain this disparity? Well, instead of getting the recommended 60 minutes of exercise five times a week and eating well-balanced and nutritious meals, Americans continue to pursue the quick fix. What many people realize, but don't accept, is that there isn't a quick fix. There is no miracle diet. While many people search worldwide for an answer or wait for the medical industry to come up with a solution, the reality is this: lifestyle determines whether or not you gain or release fat.

We've learned from working with a variety of people who released 20, 30 and 50 pounds or more—and kept it off for over five years—that it is a healthy lifestyle that proves positive. However, it's easier said than done: it means committing to a combination of cardiovascular and resistance exercise (i.e. lifting weights, strength training) while adhering to a balanced, portion-controlled, low-fat eating lifestyle. Our client Tammy said it best: ***"The mindset I adopted as a result of the Wellness Weight-Loss process has helped me learn to love a healthy lifestyle."*** Through the Wellness Weight-Loss process, we'd like to help you establish a healthier lifestyle, one that evolves over time.

Information age

Our goal is to provide you with accurate information rather than instruction. We don't issue rules or directives, but instead educate you and share our proven principles of creating health and releasing body fat. We don't give you restrictions, but remind you of the power of choice. We want to empower you with action steps that you can implement each and every day and that will help to prevent many diseases associated with an unhealthy lifestyle. Remember, it's all about becoming knowledgeable and passionate about living a life of quality.

Reality

Cigarette smoking has been proven to shorten people's lifespan and promote respiratory diseases such as lung cancer. Despite this widespread knowledge, as we stated early on, a reported 25 percent of the adult population continues to smoke. Similar to the pathos of smoking, people continue to eat in excess, remain sedentary, and fall prey to the myriad of diet fads and gimmicks publicized through television, magazines and radio.

As sad as it is to have millions of people fall victim to the quick-fix diet disasters, the reality is that no one wants to be over fat. No one wants to feel tired all the time. No one wants to be a customer of the $1.4 trillion healthcare industry. Wouldn't you rather be a customer of the wellness business, which helps ***create*** health?

If you'd like to establish a lifestyle that supports your health and beauty from the inside out, this book may be your defining experience for no longer battling the bulge. In fact, it may be just a matter of time before you rarely, if ever, think about diets—instead making your lifestyle your weapon in the fight against fat.

It's no secret that healthy habits may be the deciding factor in disease prevention.

Prevention versus screening

With 50 percent of the mortality rate attributed to lifestyle-related diseases, it's no secret that healthy habits may be the deciding factor in disease prevention. What do we mean by prevention, and what's its connection with weight loss? In short, we believe in going directly to the root of the problem; looking at the cause rather than simply treating the symptoms. Once you become aware of what causes the effect of excess body fat, it's just a matter of reversing the cause.

Many people think of health prevention in the same way they think of maintaining their cars—if you follow a regular schedule, all will go well. Just as we change the oil in our cars or have the tires rotated, we get annual prostate check-ups, gynecological exams and routine mammograms. While these exams are important and valuable, they are disease screenings; not sources of prevention. These screenings often confirm a disease—much like a mechanic telling you about a worn-out brake pad or faulty alternator—but they do nothing to prevent the disease from happening in the first place.

With Wellness Weight-Loss, we see the process of prevention as creating health daily. That doesn't mean you disregard the importance of disease screening, but that you begin to see the difference between disease screening and creating health. That's why we want you to think of the Wellness Weight-Loss process as a lifestyle opportunity and valued source of prevention—not a diet.

We encourage you to broaden your definition of health to include the thoughts you think, the relationships you engage in, the food that you eat, and the activities you participate in every day. Dr. Michael Klaper, a pioneer of good health and well being, says, "Health is not something the doctor can apply to you like calamine lotion. Health is something you do on a daily basis, and making wise decisions at the dinner table is one of the best things you can do to assure your health." Consider these words as you embark on your journey toward healthy living.

Wellness Weight-Loss

In our survey of more than 5,000 people, we asked what were the biggest concerns in their life. Overwhelmingly, we learned that health and weight management tipped the scales as the major challenges facing adults in North America. Finances were mentioned, but ranked lower simply because people have learned that working harder and longer is what it takes to earn more. Somehow, most people have found a way to reach their financial goals, while being healthy remains something of a mystery.

Material things can be purchased, however, your health is priceless. If you don't believe this, ask someone who has lost it.

With health and weight management as a major concern, clearly happiness does not come simply by making more money or driving a luxury car. Material things can be purchased, however, your health is priceless. If you don't believe this, ask someone who has lost it.

As we share with you the Wellness Weight-Loss process, please keep an openmind and make this book the foundation to a lifestyle of self-discovery. The Wellness Weight-Loss approach to releasing body fat and keeping it off can help you unlock the keys to the mystery surrounding the obesity epidemic. We want to take you beyond the gimmicks and high-pressured advertising claims, and provide a process-based approach to releasing fat; one that improves your self-esteem, self-worth, confidence and overall well being. No matter where you are in your life, whether you have experienced dozens of diets or you just want to improve your health, Wellness Weight-Loss provides the answers you deserve.

We've become experts in helping people overcome "self-sabotage," and we can help you increase your awareness and finally take control of your weight and health. As you begin to pave the road to a healthier lifestyle, you will learn about the dangers surrounding fad diets, an unbalanced lifestyle and gimmicks that promise a quick fix. You will become educated about how to improve the long-term quality of your life. You will embark on an adventure that will affect the rest of your life.

The numbers don't lie:

- For the first time in history, those who can be described as fit and healthy constitute the minority in the U.S., with 80 percent of the adult population over the age of 25 considered moderately overweight to obese.
- Nearly 60 percent of 2,000 over fat women said they would not allow their partner (i.e., spouse, boyfriend, girlfriend) to see them naked.
- Each year Americans spend more than $40 billion on weight-loss products and services, including drastic stomach-reduction surgeries, a procedure that has nearly doubled since 1998.
- Reports show that 99 percent of those who begin a weight-loss program will not experience long-term success.
- Fifty percent of the mortality rate is due to lifestyle diseases.

Points to remember:

- You have the power to choose a lifestyle that honors and enriches your life.
- If you choose to eat healthy and exercise regularly, you will instantly experience daily rewards such as positive changes in your body, increased energy and improved mood.
- Obesity in North America is the second leading cause of preventable deaths behind cigarette smoking.
- As you evolve with your lifestyle, it is just a matter of time before you rarely, if ever, think about diets again.
- Once you become aware of what causes the effect of excess body fat, it's just a matter of reversing the cause.
- Think of health as a combination of the thoughts you think, the relationships you engage in, the food that you eat, and the activities you participate in, all on a daily basis.
- Health and weight management tipped the scales as the major challenges facing adults in North America.
- The Wellness Weight-Loss process is not about temporary success, but about long-term health.
- You can create health daily.

5

Prevention Is the Best Defense

"The time to repair the roof is when the sun is shinning."
—John F. Kennedy

Do you want to reduce your body fat? Would you like to slow down the process of aging? Does the idea of preventing lifestyle diseases interest you? Whether you want to reverse aging, release fat or live longer, taking a closer look at your current lifestyle is the first step toward preventing chronic illness and improving your overall fitness and health.

To help you take a closer look at your lifestyle, consider the following car metaphor: do you squeal around corners, zip through yellow lights, slam on the brakes at stop signs and change the oil every 15,000 miles? If you do, how long do you think this car is going to last? What condition is this car going to be in 5, 10 or 20 years?

As a friend of ours once said, "Look at my Lexus—one of the finest cars I have ever owned. Do you think I would put soda in the gas tank? But think about the junk I have put into my body over the years—deep fried foods and refined and processed white flour and sugar. There's little difference between using soda for fuel and eating such unhealthy foods." These statements reflect an improved awareness of healthy living, one made possible by the Wellness Weight-Loss process.

Some of us never learned about the role of nutrition and how exercise helps to prevent chronic illness. Many of us look at exercise as a means to be able to eat whatever we want. Diets have taught us that exercise is an option. Some people don't exercise, but eat whatever they want and never seem to gain weight. Others ignore exercise altogether and invest far more time and energy into their careers. Regardless of the route you've taken up to this point, it is important to acknowledge both exercise and nutrition as being critical in preventing lifestyle diseases and keeping the fat you release from coming back. The sooner you grasp and accept this fact, the sooner you can implement it into your lifestyle. The truth is: disease and deterioration do not suddenly start after 40, but at infancy.

The reality

Given everything that we know about eating and exercise, why do you think 40 million Americans have elevated cholesterol levels, 60 million have high blood pressure and 175 million are classified as either over-weight or obese? The answer to this question is not as simple as you would think. First of all, knowing what to do and doing what you know are two different things. Second, as a society we often focus on fixing the symptoms of problems. But unless we learn to identify and reverse the cause of such ailments, we will continue to suffer from their effects.

Unhealthy direction

According to the American Council on Exercise and the National Sporting Goods Association, U.S. residents (with the exception of Alaska and Hawaii) went from spending $2.9 billion on home fitness equipment in 1995 to $3.6 billion in 2000—spending a majority of that money, $2.1 billion, to buy 3.6 million treadmills. Along with exercise equipment, don't forget, Americans continue to spend well over $40 billion on weight-loss products and programs; yet, we are not making visible head-way in reducing the occurrence of lifestyle diseases and obesity in this country.

As mind-boggling as all this may appear, you haven't seen anything yet. Take a look at our healthcare industry. In the U.S., the cost of health-care has skyrocketed from $700 billion in 1990 to well over $1.3 trillion as of 2001. This has taken place despite the landmark U.S. Surgeon General's 1996 Report on Physical Activity and Health, which concluded that a modest amount of moderate exercise could reduce the risk of numerous chronic diseases including heart disease, Type 2 diabetes, hypertension and some cancers.

Despite the urgency of illness prevention, it is quite evident that we continue to move in an unhealthy direction. John Foreyt, director of the behavioral medicine research center at The Baylor College of Medicine in Houston made it clear that if current trends continue, everyone in America will be obese by 2230. Twenty years ago a statement like this would have been hard to conceive. But today, the constant increase in mortality and its link to obesity and lifestyle diseases make it clear that we must stop talking about what we need to do, and instead take control of our destiny and begin reversing the cause.

Cause and effect

*Each and every day you can take action steps
that improve your health and energy.*

Why wait for your lifestyle to catch up with you? Take control now, and learn what actions you can take on a daily basis to prevent common lifestyle diseases. Each and every day you can take action steps that improve your health and energy. Once again, back to the car metaphor; by simply changing the oil every 3,000 miles and investing care into its maintenance, you may be able to keep that car going strong for well over 100,000 miles.

Being proactive means creating health daily. If you are over fat, recently diagnosed with Type 2 diabetes or are a current victim of high cholesterol, you can begin the process of making life better today. If you consider yourself fit and you don't have a lifestyle disease, you can be even more proactive now in order to prevent future happenings.

Let's take a look at our client Pamela. She is 5'5" and used to weigh 174 pounds. Pamela's body-fat percentage was 33.7 at 46 years of age. In order to help Pamela, we had to first find out the cause of her excess body fat. We began with a current lifestyle evaluation (i.e., eating habits, work schedule, stressors, priorities) and then worked backward to discover the circumstances that led up to such a high percentage of body fat.

Taking this approach does increase the likelihood of long-term success, unlike most diets and commercial weight-loss programs that merely treat the symptom of being over fat and not the individual. It is very important to begin with a substantial amount of background information about the person. From there, we help him or her add education and motivation to the process of reversing the cause of excess body fat.

ACTION STEP: Take a few moments right now and write down your typical breakfast, lunch and dinner in a personal journal or diary. If you snack, write down the things you typically snack on throughout the day and then answer the following questions:

1. How much water do you drink per day?
2. Do you eat sweets and junk food? If so, what type, how much and how often?
3. Do you drink alcoholic beverages? If so, what type, how much and how often?
4. Do you eat candy? If so, what type, how much and how often?

5. Do you drink caffeine (i.e. coffee, soda)? If so, what type, how much and how often?
6. Are you currently exercising? If so, what type of physical activities are you involved in?

Reversing the cause

As we explained to Pamela, in treating excess body fat, the first step is identifying the cause; then and only then can you begin to reverse the process. Otherwise, you're going to be continually battling the effects. For instance, the reversal of high cholesterol calls for increased physical activity and healthy eating. The reversal of osteoporosis calls for weight-bearing exercise and resistance training combined with a balanced diet. The reversal of excess body fat calls for cardiovascular and resistance exercise combined with healthy nutrition.

As you begin the process of reversing the cause, the most important thing you can do is find out what the circumstances were that preceded the fat gain or lifestyle disease. If you choose to skip this process and not identify and reverse the cause, you'll find yourself trapped in a cycle of chasing the effects, or what many recognize as yo-yo dieting and denial.

Reinforcement

After two years of consistent reinforcement and follow-through, Pamela reduced her body fat to 19 percent and released a total of 40 pounds of fat. Now at a fit 135 pounds, Pamela continues to invest in her lifestyle by exercising three to four hours per week and sticks to a healthy, yet tasty eating philosophy.

Like Pamela, everyone has a story, however, she proved to be a great example of someone who came to the realization that her health was more important than her outward appearance. For more than 20 years, Pamela sought the perfect body. She was motivated to lose weight and get in shape so that she would look good in certain outfits and hopefully meet someone special and fall in love. There were other external rewards to being fit, however, these were at the top of her list when we first met Pamela.

Like many who enrolled in Wellness Weight-Loss before her, Pamela wanted to look a certain way within a specific amount of time. It was apparent that Pamela was inspired by external incentives, so we used an extrinsic approach to motivate her. However, it is always our goal to help each client make an internal shift—making a healthy lifestyle of eating and exercise rewarding in itself. This shift becomes most noticeable when the client is motivated by intrinsic reinforcement.

What's the difference between intrinsic and extrinsic reinforcement? Intrinsic reinforcement is exemplified when a person exercises and eats healthy for the sole reason that it feels good and is rewarding in and of itself. Extrinsic reinforcement is when a person is motivated to exercise and eat healthy for external incentives—maybe to get ready for a special event, or achieve a certain look, or fit into a certain size.

Intrinsic and extrinsic reinforcement are neither good nor bad. It doesn't matter what motivates a person to make a change, it just matters that they're making progress. However, the fact remains that most people want to lose weight for aesthetic reasons. Since we don't offer the quick-fix to weight loss, more often than not, we attract clientele into our office who are seeking inner fulfillment and with that comes a sincere desire to release body fat and get control over their eating habits.

Now that you know people are typically motivated by either intrinsic or extrinsic reinforcement, don't overlook the mother of weight-loss success—consistency. Consistent reinforcement of either an intrinsic or extrinsic approach is what assures people and keeps them on track. This consistency is what increases the likelihood of permanent fat loss. This process of helping you get to where you want to be involves constant reinforcement that is tailored around what stimulates you most.

Going from fad diet disasters to a lifestyle based on creating health and not dieting again is what the Wellness Weight-Loss process is all about.

Making the shift

The idea of getting in shape for your two-week vacation may be the initial spark that ignites the desire to eat healthy and begin exercising. Entering a challenge or contest for the sake of getting in the best shape of your life may prove to be your foundation of support. However, make it a goal to educate yourself on the prevention of lifestyle diseases and the role exercise and proper nutrition plays, and in no time you may make the shift from extrinsic to intrinsic methods of motivation and reinforcement.

Going from fad diet disasters to a lifestyle based on creating health and not dieting again is what the Wellness Weight-Loss process is all about. Specializing in helping people just like you internalize the reward of taking care of your body and create overall health has taught us many things. Unless you make the shift from extrinsic to intrinsic, your progress is more likely to prove only temporary.

Case in point: Pamela made it clear that she wanted to lose weight and look good by summer. Though, she was on a quest to improve her body, somewhere in the process she made a paradigm shift—changed her worldview of why healthy eating and regular exercise were important to her. No longer did we encourage and motivate Pamela with external rewards. She internalized the experience and came to the realization that her health was at the core of what she now values as quality of life.

What happened?

Pamela, at the age of 46, became empowered with a new knowledge of eating and exercise. Her passion to evolve through life blossomed and she began to exude vitality. Part of what helped her shift was learning about how her lifestyle could either lead to or away from chronic illnesses such as Type 2 diabetes.

Since you are reading this book and "going for fit" you're on the healthy path.

When Pamela began the Wellness Weight-Loss process, she experienced increased energy, released body fat and acquired a new sense of freedom. Her clothes began to fit better and she felt empowered. Pamela's focus shifted from releasing fat and looking good to accepting a lifestyle that put her health as a priority.

Each person has a value system that is uniquely their own. Prior to the Wellness Weight-Loss process, Pamela valued looking a certain way as a priority in her life. However, as she powered through the process, she altered her living condition and changed her way of thinking. "Prior to Wellness Weight-Loss, I valued pork, roast beef and heavily buttered and fried foods, but my value system has changed," says Pamela. "Those foods don't benefit my health, and since I have 'made the shift'—as Krista and Robert always say—I feel and look better than I ever have."

Pamela can't explain exactly when she made the shift; it just seemed to happen. She found herself passing up some of her former favorite dishes and noticed that she was choosing baked and broiled food over fried. But, who's to say when you will make the shift. It may happen now, in 20 years or when you find yourself the victim of high blood pressure, Type 2 diabetes or some other lifestyle disease. Regardless, since you are reading this book and "going for fit," you're on the healthy path. The most important thing is that you are doing something; you're taking a step in a positive direction.

Facing the challenge

Have you ever heard the saying, "If you want to learn the true value of good health, ask someone who has lost it?" Losing your health is not something you would wish on anyone, however, being diagnosed with a life-threatening illness is sometimes what sparks people to make a change. It certainly has a way of getting your attention.

All too often we will have someone enroll in the Wellness Weight-Loss process as a result of a doctor urging him or her to make change (i.e., eat healthy and begin exercising). For instance, a doctor will inform the person whose cholesterol is at 350 that a change in eating habits (along with medications) may prove to be the difference between life and death. No matter what the illness, discovering that you have a life-limiting disease can motivate you to eat healthier and begin exercising. Nonetheless, the challenge remains; in order to release body fat and prevent lifestyle diseases, it helps to bridge the gap between knowing and doing.

We know that carrying extra body fat means extra challenges. We know that millions of North Americans struggle daily with excess pounds and the social stigma attached to it. We know that obesity has reached epidemic proportions worldwide with the number of obese people equaling the number of starving for the first time in history. We also know that both populations suffer from malnourishment, and that means increased illness.

With an estimated 12 percent of the population adhering to a healthy approach to eating, reversing the cause and getting more people to eat differently is not going to be an easy task. Case in point: healthy nutrition is very difficult to come by in a land where 70 percent of all meals are eaten outside the home, 25 percent of the population buys fast food everyday, and the average child consumes 30 pounds of french fries each year. Numbers don't lie. When you consider the fact that $93 billion is spent annually on fast food, getting people to make a shift and seek health is not an easy task.

The future

Entertainment superstar and singer Whitney Houston said it best in her song, "Greatest Love Of All." In short, the lyrics read, "I believe that children are our future, teach them well and let them lead the way." Children are the future, and moving toward the root of change means going to the children and looking out for their best interest. This action step is needed more now than ever because childhood obesity is the major nutritional disorder affecting American children today. It is also the underlying cause of many of the illnesses we're beginning to see in children today. Not surprisingly, the longer a child is over fat the more likely he or she will struggle with weight as an adult.

For the most part, Type 2 diabetes was not seen in children until 1994. Today, we have an epidemic. We are also beginning to see children developing early stages of coronary artery disease and a variety of other lifestyle diseases. All this is related to an increase in excess body fat, a result of a deadly combination—the over-consumption of fast food and decrease in physical activity. Current lifestyle trends among both the adult population and their children may be contributing more to America's rising healthcare and drug costs than the better-known evils of smoking and alcohol abuse. Therefore, let's get empowered and begin preventing the rising rate of obesity among our children.

The U.S. Centers for Disease Control and Prevention predicted that one in three Americans born in 2000 will develop diabetes during his or her lifetime—a forecast that envisions 29 million Americans will be diagnosed, and a further 10 million undiagnosed cases will develop, by 2050.

The first step in preventing excess body fat and its link to lifestyle disease is accepting and recognizing obesity as a disease.

Prevention: the most powerful tool

While surgery and intensive diet and fitness programs have proven successful for many extreme cases of obesity, there is only one surefire way to combat fat among adults and children. The number one approach is prevention.

The first step in preventing excess body fat and its link to lifestyle disease is accepting and recognizing obesity as a disease. It is important however, not to confuse prevention as a method to cure. Being cured of a disease means you are totally free from it. You're no longer predisposed to it, and a need to worry about it is eliminated. Clearly, when it comes to getting rid of excess body fat, there is no cure. Once you get rid of the excess body fat and become fit, the price to staying fit is nothing short of constant vigilance and/or a lifestyle that is forever evolving. Releasing body fat can be hard work and comes with a responsibility of adhering to a balanced nutrition plan and increased activity or regular exercise. Incorporating these healthy habits into your lifestyle on a consistent basis is how you are going to reinforce the progress you make—releasing fat that doesn't come back.

The disease

Many people have a difficult time digesting our claim that excess body fat is a disease. However, when something kills as many as 300,000 Americans a year—more than the number who die from breast, lung, colon and prostate cancers combined, that is a disease. In our view, obesity is insidious, comparable to other widespread epidemics such as AIDS, claiming its victims after decades of weakening their hearts, blowing holes in their arteries, suffocating their organs and grinding down their joints.

Now, imagine that you have a one-in-three chance of developing this disease, and your doctor doesn't know how to treat you. Scary isn't it? As a matter of fact, something like 28 percent of all physicians advise patients to become more physically active. Although studies show that even a small loss in body fat can prevent a lifestyle disease, most doctors don't urge patients to reduce their body fat. And for the doctors that do, there is little he or she may feel qualified to do aside from prescribing some controversial weight-loss drug. Why? Believe it or not, most doctors really don't know how to help you reduce your body fat. Only about a third of U.S. medical schools require separate nutrition courses; even fewer teach the basics of fat loss. If doctors are fortunate enough to have the training, they often don't have the time to spend with you. It is far easier to prescribe some type of medication.

When you cut the fat out of the confusion, you will find very little profit for doctors and insurers when it comes to helping people release body fat and preventing obesity and lifestyle disease. In short, there is little if any financial incentive for doctors to help you release fat. For this reason alone, it is in your best interest to take responsibility for your health. That means educating yourself and establishing a lifestyle that evolves.

This is where we come in—to help you begin integrating what you already know and what you're going to learn from this book. We are aware that you may be quite informed and knowledgeable about the varying types and categories of diets, weight-loss and nutrition programs. However, even if you've already heard much of the information we will share with you, the tools, skills and methods we introduce you to will forever empower you to keep on course.

The course of prevention

In order to empower you in preventing and releasing excess body fat, we want you to picture yourself sailing from Los Angeles to the Hawaiian Islands. You begin your voyage, however, you find yourself one degree off course. This minute degree of deviation may not seem like much at the moment, but as time goes by, you drift farther and farther off course. Eventually, you may find yourself in a place that is not at all where you wanted to end up.

As time goes on, we all want to experience a life that's rich and full of quality. No one wants to find themselves 20 years from now asking, "Where is it?" To find yourself really lost and not aware that you lived a life one degree off course can plague your mind with hundreds of thousands of "what ifs."

If you value the quality of your health now and in the future, begin implementing little modifications until they become habits. These little corrective actions are going to put you more and more on course, headed where you want to be. If this idea of integrating corrective actions sounds too simplistic; consider that this is the primary reason people miss it. Prevention, to us, is sharing information and coaching you in adopting a sustainable lifestyle that creates health daily and releases body fat that doesn't come back. This is why we believe that lifestyle training and psychological support are key factors in your continued success.

Points to remember:

- Disease and deterioration do not suddenly start after 40, but at infancy.
- Each and everyday you can take steps that empower your health and energy.
- You treat excess body fat by identifying the cause and reversing the process.
- Consistent reinforcement of either an intrinsic or extrinsic approach is what ensures your ultimate success.
- A paradigm shift is changing your worldview.
- Children who are over fat are more likely to struggle with weight as an adult.
- Lifestyle training and psychological support are key factors in your continued success.
- Obesity kills 300,000 Americans each year.

6

Quality of Life

"Live as if you were to die tomorrow. Learn as if you were to live forever."
—Mahatma Gandhi

Living a life devoid of aches and pains is of great value. Waking up each day with energy is also a quality component that seems to become more valuable with age. Experiencing a life full of inner peace is a form of quality that is widely sought. You'd probably agree that good health is essential for quality of life. If not, it is our goal to help you discover the connection between quality of life and improved health.

Almost everyone you talk with has an opinion about what makes for quality of life. You've probably heard, "If I win the lottery I will have it all" or "Once I drop this excess body fat I will meet 'Mr. Right' and life will be good." The thought of getting more money, taking long vacations and having a more expensive home and car tends to rank high on the "Quality of Life" list. Consider the following statement made by one of our clients: "It's not so much what you do or what you have that makes for quality of life. Quality of life is, for the most part, discovered in those things in life that are more often than not taken away from you." A brilliant statement in our opinion. This concept definitely rings true when it comes to our own health.

Meet Jeff

At 43 years young and 31 percent body fat, Jeff went to the gym two to four times a month and didn't consider himself overweight. He went golfing on occasion and played with his two little girls on a regular basis. Jeff was happily married to Sharon and considered himself very successful as both a family man and a professional. In Jeff's words, "Life is good and I've worked hard to get where I am." Now that you've met Jeff, we'd like to share with you his story in hopes of putting "Quality of Life" into perspective.

One typical day after work, Jeff arrived home and suddenly suffered a stroke. This stroke was massive and in colloquial terms, it fried Jeff's brain. He lost practically all movement in his body and is now wheelchair bound for the remainder of his life.

If you were to ever meet Jeff, your heart would go out to him. All he does is sit motionless and occasionally screams for no apparent reason. No longer can he play with his children. No longer can he provide for his family. No longer can he play golf or go to the gym. Jeff's quality of life has been severely affected. Frankly put, Jeff has no quality of life.

Silvia's story

The daughter of a multi-millionaire, Silvia was raised in private schools and given a beautiful sports car on her sixteenth birthday. She wore name brand clothing and got everything she wanted. Life was good and Silvia appreciated it.

After graduating college, Silvia returned home to discover her parents had lost everything. The recession forced her parents to claim bankruptcy and sell all their possessions. They had to move into the city and set up residence in a two-bedroom apartment. This abrupt change in lifestyle devastated Silvia's family. Her mother became distraught as a result and turned to alcohol and painkillers to help deal with the sudden hardships. When they didn't think things could get worse, Silvia's father committed suicide.

Ten years later, Silvia's mother is 58 years of age, still drinking alcohol in excess, and looks and feels more like 100 years old. Silvia continues to support her mother financially but has decided not to follow in her footsteps. Silvia is healthy, happily married and the mother of a beautiful little girl. She works as a registered nurse and couldn't be happier. In Silvia's words, "I am very fortunate to have the quality of life I am currently experiencing."

Maintaining perspective

Silvia is not filthy rich, but she is experiencing quality of life. Jeff on the other hand has enough money set aside to pay for three lifetimes, but he has no quality of life. It's apparent to us that quality of life is not measured by the amount of money or possessions we have, but rather in the quality of our overall health.

It's true that worrying about bills and having a relationship go sour can make life unpleasant and stressful at times. No one wants to be in an unhealthy relationship. No one wants to live from paycheck to paycheck. However, part of life is learning to respond, adapt and accept the ups and downs that come with the reality of living on this earth.

Consider the story of Mindy and Ted, deeply in love with each other, financially secure and both in their mid-sixties. It wasn't always this way. While in their fifties and living high and healthy on the beach in sunny California, they lost everything as a result of the recession. Their beach house was repossessed, the government took their yacht, they returned their matching Mercedes to the dealer and all their valuable possessions were auctioned. They even sold their wedding rings to help pay for groceries. They literally had no money; nevertheless, they were able to maintain quality of life.

You may ask, "How is this so?" Simply put, instead of sailing in their yacht, they called friends and went on short voyages with them. They were still very much in love with each other. They weren't able to dine in some of the restaurants they came to enjoy, however, they were still able to go out on occasion. The quality of their life was never affected as they went without the toys and pleasures that financial freedom had previously provided them. To put it in perspective, neither became ill nor suffered a life threatening assault on their body during the course of their financial troubles.

Now, short of five years later, their hard work has paid off once again. They lived on a tight budget, rebuilt their house and reestablished their fortune. They used to own a 42-foot yacht, and now enjoy a 56-foot vessel. "Life has been great and we appreciate each and everyday the good Lord gives us," says Mindy.

Though no one definition is better than the next, the one thing that practically everyone considers essential for quality of life is good health.

The definition

You will soon learn that each person you meet defines quality of life differently. Though no one definition is better than the next, the one thing that practically everyone considers essential for quality of life is good health. Once your health is lost, your basic need to feel good is impaired. The definitions listed below were randomly selected from more than 70 people. Please take the time to contemplate these to help bring clarity to "quality of life:"

Lisa, age 31: "Quality of life means a level of enjoyment, happiness both in personal matters and business. It also means being healthy enough to enjoy the things you like to do. Obviously the healthier a person is, the better his or her quality of life is going to be."

Michael, age 61: "Quality of life to me is having a loving relationship with my wife, children and relatives. Having good health is important and without it I wouldn't be able to experience life pain free, but the love I share with my family makes each day I breathe a blessing."

Nina, age 39: "Quality of life is a true balance of work, family, maintenance of health; inclusive of mental, physical and spiritual. Quality time spent and a healthy prioritization of all elements listed above."

Coleen, age 44: "Quality of life to me means having the energy, time and opportunity to do the things that I love and am passionate about. I love music, intimate moments with loved ones, being healthy, exploring the beauty of the earth that God created, and making a difference on this planet."

David, age 37: "Quality of life is being content and joyful for where you are in life. It is also the willingness to improve in all areas of life; spirituality, physically, mentally, socially and emotionally. Good health is the foundation for quality of life, and having a constant appreciation for life is what gives merit to the word quality."

Gerald, age 54: "Quality of life is the ability to fully enjoy life and participate in daily activities without pain, discomfort, anxiety, hesitation, nervousness, or any other factor that may take away from the pleasure of the activity."

What it's not

You've taken a look at how others define quality of life—and now would be a great time to write down what it means to you. After you have thought about and written down your definition, we would like to share with you not what we believe "quality of life" is, but what we know it isn't.

While learning, appreciating and respecting the fact that each person has a unique and personalized meaning of quality of life, it didn't take long for us to realize how easy it is to misinterpret its true essence. For instance, a onetime client of ours, Susan, believes quality of life is maintaining a 10 in her physical appearance. If she gains a few extra pounds, she feels that her quality of life is hampered. Another client, Barry, feels that quality of life is having the right relationship. Until he is in what he terms the right relationship, Barry does not feel as though he has achieved quality of life. Finally, Tammie believes that as long as she is happy (i.e., not feeling anger, sadness or guilt) she has quality of life.

Quality of life is not winning the lottery, having the perfect body or being the person that everyone agrees with and understands all the time.

Quality of life is realistic; therefore, it does not and cannot co-exist with unrealistic expectations. For example, if you were to get your body into perfect shape, at that moment you would feel great and experience an elevated sense of self. However, it is unrealistic to think you can maintain the perfect body 24-hours a day, seven days a week.

The basic need to feel good is often confused as being synonymous with quality of life; a big mistake. Feeling good for most people means achieving financial success, driving a luxury car and living in a glamorous home. Take those things away, and most people are likely to believe that they're experiencing a decline in quality of life. For clarity, consider the following: One of the most famous entrepreneurs and financial giants of the 20th century, Howard Hughes said in his final days, "I would give everything I have for one day of inner peace." As you can see from Mr. Hughes' avowal, quality of life is more than having and doing more. Quality of life is here and now, and it is up to each and every one of us to tap into its source.

What it is

Regardless of how you define "quality of life," we would like to explore its connection with releasing fat and creating health—mainly because of the relationship between being moderately over fat to obese and the prevalence of lifestyle diseases.

How you've treated your body in the past and how you treat your body today and the days to follow are the major predictors of quality of life.

Have you ever been sick and unable to care for yourself? Have you ever been seriously ill or diagnosed with a life-threatening disease? Unless this has happened to you, you may find it very difficult to see the value and importance in prioritizing your health over your career and relationships. You may find it difficult to choose health over wealth.

We meet people each month who have been diagnosed with lifestyle diseases, but choose to continue their unhealthy eating habits even though this lifestyle has been proven to shorten one's lifespan. This type of behavior is very common among smokers. They'll often continue to smoke even though they know the reality. Until they are on their deathbed or sitting in a doctor's office hearing the words, "You have lung cancer," they will continue to smoke. It is not uncommon for a smoker to get a second, third or fourth opinion before they finally accept the reality that the smoking must stop or they're going to die.

How you've treated your body in the past and how you treat your body today and the days to follow are the major predictors of quality of life. Becoming over fat does not happen with one piece of candy. Having a total cholesterol level of 345 doesn't come about by eating one egg yolk. Lifestyle diseases occur through consistent behavior and conditioning. However, no one is exempt from disease and eating healthy doesn't mean you're going to live without disease and hardships.

We live in a Western culture where time is measured in a linear fashion. Therefore, most people believe quality of life is defined as: The more the better. In contrast, many indigenous cultures from around the world measure time or life in terms of a circle. Time is not seen as linear, but rather as the circle of one's life. In their view, quality of life is captured in that paradigm of a circle. The circle is not a measurement of how long you lived, but instead, **how** you lived.

For instance, just because you exercise regularly, eat healthy and live a life with little stress does not mean you are guaranteed to live to be a centenarian (someone who is 100 years or older). The realistic expectation is living the optimum length of time for you. However, it helps to understand that your optimal lifespan, for reasons that we will never know while on this earth, may be 45 years. But if you are sedentary and have followed an unhealthy eating regimen, instead of living to be 45, you may live to be 28; you may live to be 120 or you may live to be 40 years of age. No one can predict how long you are going to live. However, what is important is living a life of quality that includes a healthy body and mind.

Invest in health daily—don't mortgage it

We recommend that you live each day as though it is your masterpiece.

While quality of life means different things to different people, one thing is for sure—when we invest in our health, quality of life increases; when we neglect our health, quality of life decreases. To improve your quality of life from this day forward, we recommend that you live each day as though it is your masterpiece. We recommend investing in your health daily, not mortgaging it. Trust that if you "pay your dues now" and begin making healthier choices, soon those choices will not feel like "paying your dues" at all. They'll add to your quality of life. Trust that if you can come into a healthy relationship with yourself—your body will live the optimal length of time for you.

Points to remember:

- Good health is essential for quality of life.
- If you want to know the true value of good health,
  ask someone who has lost it.
- Quality of life is not measured by the amount of money or
  possessions one has, but in the quality of their overall health.
- Quality of life does not and cannot co-exist with unrealistic
  expectations.
- Quality of life is not necessarily measured by how long
  you lived, but by how you lived.
- Live each day as though it is your masterpiece.

Wᴇʟʟɴᴇss Wᴇɪɢʜᴛ-Loss ˢᴹ

It's a lifestyle
...not a diet!

PART THREE

Removing Roadblocks

7

Six Reasons Why People Don't Succeed

"The wise man learns from experience.
The very wise man learns from the experience of others."
—Herbert Hoover

Have you ever met a person who needs or wants to lose weight, but for some reason or another, they never seem to take action and do anything about it? In fact, doesn't it seem like most people you meet are either on a diet or looking for a way to improve their overall health and fitness?

We meet people everyday who have spent years waging a war against fat. Many of these people are losing battle after battle to fads, gimmicks and unhealthy alternatives that promise weight-loss secrets. We are happy to tell you that there are no secrets. All it takes is a willingness to change and stay on course.

It is also important for you to understand that for every person who is not successful at weight loss, there are a thousand more people who are. In this chapter we would like to share with you the six most common reasons why people don't succeed in attaining and maintaining their desired body-fat percentage. These stories are real and are provided to give you a point of reference to reflect on so that you can be successful and avoid the pitfalls to which so many people fall victim.

Before you read these stories, please take time to applaud yourself for reading this book. Having the willingness to change and improve the quality of your life is half the battle, and you've taken a major step.

All talk, no action

Let's talk about Gary, age 43, a professional business consultant. Gary is over fat, married and the father of two beautiful children. He carries excess abdominal fat (commonly referred to as beer belly) but talks about changing his habits and losing 50 pounds all the time. Week in, week out, Gary shared his story with anyone willing to listen.

One evening when Gary came to one of our seminars, to his surprise he won a raffle to work with us and begin the Wellness Weight-Loss process. Gary was excited about the opportunity and he announced to everyone how appreciative and grateful he was to finally begin a process that would help him lose the weight he always dreamed about.

Excited, we looked forward to the opportunity to work with Gary. Once the seminar ended, we scheduled his first coaching session. Unfortunately, Gary called us and cancelled his appointment and rescheduled. The next time, Gary didn't make his appointment, and made no attempt to reschedule. Gary didn't call us to cancel nor did he show up. We called him, but he never returned our call.

One week went by, then two, then three. Six weeks later we ran into Gary at a local grocery store. Gary was quick to share with us that he was eating healthy and that he had been exercising. He said he was in a hurry and would give us a call. We found Gary's actions odd and called him a couple of days later. He never returned our calls and finally we moved on and wished him well.

We've discovered after working with hundreds of male clients that more than 80 percent are unwilling to change their eating habits unless something drastic happens.

Gary, like many people, was unwilling to change. The first and most important factor needed to change is willingness. Gary enjoyed the attention he got from talking about losing weight and eating healthy, but he had no intentions of changing. Gary was content with his lifestyle and unwilling to take action and improve his situation.

We've discovered after working with hundreds of male clients that more than 80 percent are unwilling to change their eating habits unless something drastic happens like coronary heart disease, stroke or diabetes.

They said this...they said that

Sharon, age 29, is a legal secretary who is single with no children. Sharon enrolled in Wellness Weight-Loss after 10 years of experiencing fad-diet disasters. Sharon weighed in at 155 pounds, and stood 5'5". Sharon carried her weight well, but was uncomfortable with the added bulge on her hips and thighs.

We enrolled Sharon on a Saturday and one week from the day she walked into our office, she decided to stop and renounce her decision to complete the Wellness Weight-Loss process. Concerned, startled and curious, we asked Sharon why she decided not to continue. Sharon informed us that her cousin's neighbor has a brother who knows this guy at his work who trains with this guy that had a friend that said the Wellness Weight-Loss process was not going to work.

We sat down with Sharon and provided her with a synopsis of our process and why it works. We also shared with her many of our success stories. Sharon even knew a couple of people who completed Wellness Weight-Loss and have testified to others how it improved the quality of their life. Sharon then allowed us to conduct a body composition analysis. We provided her with a grocery list, menu plan and exercise prescription. However, Sharon continued to tell us about how her girl-friend started a diet something like ours and she only lost five pounds. We asked Sharon if her girlfriend went through our process and she said no. We also asked Sharon what her girlfriend has to do with her success!

In short, Sharon is an example of someone who fell victim to acquiring the doubts of others. She succumbed to the doubts of other people, some she didn't even know. Sharon said our process makes sense and she could see how it would help her attain her desired weight and improve her health, but the doubts of her friends and people she didn't know out-weighed the truth that she experienced firsthand and with her own eyes.

Believe it or not, this happens all too often. We encourage you to trust in what you know for yourself to be true. If you do not want to miss out on opportunities like Sharon, choose not to acquire the doubts of others and accept your reality as your own.

Doing what is best for you

Brenda, age 54, has been married for 20 years and works as a registered nurse. On her way home from work one afternoon, Brenda noticed our sign and decided to visit and pick up some information about Wellness Weight-Loss. Fortunately, we didn't have any clients meeting with us at the time and offered Brenda a free body composition analysis on the spot.

Brenda was no rookie to weight loss. She started and experienced over a dozen diets and three commercial weight-loss programs over the last 20 years. She succeeded at losing weight on a couple occurrences, but like many others, she gained the weight back and then some. This time was going to be different for Brenda because she was tired of the start-stop programs and wanted something different—more permanent— a lifestyle change.

Brenda liked our approach and enrolled. We initially provided Brenda with some homework and scheduled her to come in for her first official coaching session. Brenda returned three days later ready to get started with the 21-day induction where we encourage alternatives in place of white or enriched flour, fried and breaded foods, candy, sugar and alcohol.

As each week passed, Brenda appeared to be on course and at the completion of her third week she released 10 pounds—and eight of those pounds came from fat. She was excited about her results and we still had nine weeks to go. Brenda shared with us that her husband was taking her out to celebrate and the next day they had a family celebration for her niece's wedding.

After two weeks Brenda came in for her scheduled appointment. Her energy was down and she seemed sad. We asked Brenda what happened and she informed us that she had been binging for two weeks. Her husband told her that he was proud of her and that he liked her the way she is, and that she proved to him that she could change if she wanted. Members of her family had convinced her that Wellness Weight-Loss was culturally biased and it was a shame that we encouraged her to choose grilled, baked or broiled food over deep fried options and one hundred percent whole grain bread over white. Relatives heard about Brenda eating differently and questioned her loyalty to her culture.

Brenda had lived most of her life allowing people to influence her. She never realized that she accepted restrictions on her life that other people set for her. Brenda's family, culture and tradition set restrictions on her that kept her from being successful at creating health and releasing fat. Brenda wants success, but she is not likely to succeed because she allows others to decide what is best for her. You may have people close to you say things like, "You can't do it" or "You shouldn't be in that program." But who is to say that you can't experience success? You can and you will.

Brenda didn't drop out of Wellness Weight-Loss. She continued to complete a 12-week cycle and at the end she released a total of five pounds of fat and four inches. Initially, Brenda was on pace to release 30 pounds, but she allowed the restriction of others to limit her success. Accepting restrictions on your life that other people have set for you is the third reason why people are not successful in changing their habits long-term.

Procrastination is an excuse

Denise, age 37, is unemployed, twice divorced and the mother of one teenage son. In between jobs, Denise weighed in at 235 pounds. At 5'3" and a body-fat percentage of 44 percent, she is a prime candidate for Type 2 diabetes, a stroke and cardiovascular disease.

We met Denise at a health fair and she scheduled a consultation with our office because she was contemplating the idea of starting a new diet. When Denise arrived for her consultation, she brought with her every excuse in the book.

Denise was taking care of her aunt who recently had a stroke. She was not in a loving relationship and felt lonely. Denise wanted a job, but if she were offered one she would have to turn it down because of her new responsibility of caring for her aunt. She was scheduled for an operation to heal carpal tunnel syndrome and she was having problems with her knees. She couldn't exercise because of her physical limitations, and she didn't have any time to prepare a nutritious meal.

Denise enrolled into Wellness Weight-Loss and before she made it to the four-week mark, she came to the office and asked us to put her coaching sessions on hold. Because she couldn't go for long walks, exercise and take time to prepare her meals, she felt it would be best to take a break and pick back up once she was more prepared.

Sadly, Denise never came back to our office. She threw in the towel because she allowed dilemmas and problems in her life to become an excuse to do nothing. This is the fourth reason why most people fail to succeed at improving the quality of their life through improved eating and exercise habits.

For every person who has a dilemma or problem and uses it as an excuse, there are thousands of people who have the same dilemmas and problems who still succeed.

Please understand that everyone has dilemmas and problems, some bigger than others. There is a good chance you have more difficult challenges than we do. We can't imagine the hardships you may have in your life right now. As we have no idea what you are going through. However, we can encourage you to not allow your dilemmas and problems to become an excuse to do nothing; for every person who has a dilemma or problem and uses it as an excuse, there are thousands of people who have the same dilemmas and problems who still succeed.

Change is part of success

Michael, age 32, is a computer programmer and married with three children. He was given a gift certificate from his spouse to enroll into Wellness Weight-Loss. Michael weighed in at 230 pounds. He was somewhat over fat, but not obese. Michael's challenge was his unhealthy food choices, infrequent meals and stressful lifestyle. His cholesterol was high—290—and he was often stressed to the max.

Reluctantly, Michael walked into our office with all the answers. He quickly shared with us that he already knew how to eat right and which exercises worked best for him. He knew everything about cholesterol and how to lose weight. It was apparent that Michael felt he didn't need us, however, his body and cholesterol levels confirmed that he did, and that maybe he didn't know everything he thought he knew.

We enrolled Michael into the Wellness Weight-Loss process and each time he visited our office for a coaching session, he seemed more and more uptight. As skilled coaches, we specialize in guiding our clients to answering questions in ways that are empowering and geared toward constantly improving. Michael did not like our questions and about halfway through the Wellness Weight-Loss process, he got offended and dropped out.

Michael is a perfect example of the fifth reason why people do not succeed in releasing body fat and improving their health—somewhere along the line people may get offended. People who get offended say things like, "Why do I have to eat that?" or "I have been eating this way all my life," and "It is part of my culture to eat this way." The statements and questions are endless: "They didn't return my call, they didn't do this, and they didn't do that. I don't need a coach, I can do it on my own."

When you make a decision to begin changing your ways and establishing new healthy habits, you may get uncomfortable and offended at one point or another. Change can be difficult, and you may feel as though our suggestions are personal attacks on your values or way of life. For this reason, we can promise you this: As you read this book and we suggest you implement certain action steps, you will have at least one opportunity to get offended.

Avoid becoming offended

Becoming offended is not the first step in the process of being offended. After first being displeased for six weeks, Michael soon became resentful and felt he did not need our help. You see, if displeasure festers long enough, it usually turns to resentment. Soon thereafter, if you are holding resentment you are one step away from being offended.

Michael became offended and estranged himself from the Wellness Weight-Loss process and decided he could lower his cholesterol and reduce the stress in his life on his own. Obviously, we would love to see Michael succeed in improving the quality of his life with proper nutrition, exercise and less stress. But, unfortunately, if you are resentful long enough, the next thing you realize is you're offended and back to your old habits.

Michael left our office and we hoped that he would succeed and not allow his resentment to worsen. After a few months went by, this principle was validated as we ran into Michael coming out of a donut and coffee shop holding a bagel with cream cheese dripping off the sides and a large cup of coffee. Not only was he back to his old habits, he was approximately 10 pounds heavier.

In order to be successful in the Wellness Weight-Loss process it helps to expect to be displeased at one point or another. The reason for this is simple: your body/mind wants to reject new behaviors and hang on to what it is used to. It's human nature.

The key to dealing with being displeased is not allowing it to fester into a feeling of being offended. One way to conquer the dilemma of becoming resentful is to learn to be forgiving to others as well as yourself. Forgiveness is your secret weapon in combating the human trait of becoming offended.

Lying is denying

Nichole, age 27, works in a fast food restaurant and recently lost 85 pounds. She went from 305 to 220 pounds in about two years. She had a positive experience of losing weight, but had grown stagnant for the last six months.

It seemed like in the beginning the weight just melted off like wax from a candle. But, like most dieters, eventually Nichole hit a plateau. After another three months went by, Nichole realized she couldn't lose any more weight doing what she was doing. In her words, "I was doing everything I did before, but the fat continued to stay on my body." During this same time, Nicole started adding pounds back on. She couldn't understand what was going on because she was constantly in the gym pumping weights and enjoying aerobic group classes.

This is how we met Nicole. She was ready for more improvements and enrolled into Wellness Weight-Loss. Week after week, Nicole's attitude and commitment were energizing. We looked forward to reviewing her food journal. It was precise. Her exercise was ideal. Her attitude was spot on. She was bound to not only succeed, but we had plans for her to become a Wellness Weight-Loss coach and begin working for us.

The only concerns with Nicole were her measurements and body composition. She did every thing we suggested, and her weight didn't go down, but up, and her measurements stayed the same. We could not understand why she wasn't releasing body fat. We have had clients who didn't begin releasing body fat until their sixth week, but we were coming close to the end of the 12-week cycle and still, no change for the better.

The truth comes out

In our outreach efforts, we provide community service seminars and we invite many of our clients to attend. These seminars are great sources of support and the topics change each week. It just so happens that Nicole had never attended one of our seminars, because of her schedule. But, fortunately, she was able to attend a seminar we term the T-FACTOR.

If you have been convinced your lifestyle cannot improve, you have been misled. Your life can improve.

This seminar is very motivating. A big part of its focus is to share with those in attendance the realization that truth is the foundation of change. In this seminar we spend a significant amount of time explaining the commonalities of those who succeed in establishing healthy habits, as well as what causes people to fail. In the end, our message is to motivate those in attendance to avoid the pitfalls of the failures.

In this seminar Nicole laughed and testified to things she never wrote down in her food journal. She became an open book at this seminar and acknowledged how she lied and avoided telling the truth in all aspects of the Wellness Weight-Loss process. Nicole shared with us after the seminar that unless she was coming in for a coaching session and body composition analysis, she continued doing what she was doing and did not stick to the process.

We never saw Nicole again after that seminar. She had one more coaching session, which she did not attend. She never returned our calls. We are not sure what happened with Nicole. However, we learned many things from working with her, mainly that Nicole did not believe she deserved more and conditioned herself to accept her life the way it was. Accepting your current situation as being your final situation is the sixth reason why people are not successful at releasing body fat for the last time.

If you have been convinced your lifestyle cannot improve, you have been misled. Your life can improve. Many of us experience difficult times, however, your dreams and goals do not have to come to an end. Negative moments in your life do not have to define who you are.

Nicole could change her life, but she decided long ago that her situation was final. However, her limited beliefs can be removed, and we have coached many people through this type of mindset. The key is to make progressive change—baby steps—that lead to a lifestyle that evolves and not merely exists.

There are going to be things that we may encourage, however, if you reply with, "Well, I don't think, I don't know, I don't feel and I don't feel led." Guess what? You better get the lead out, because in order for you to succeed, it is necessary to go deep and demand of yourself to stay on course.

While keeping your ship on course, you are going to have family, friends—maybe even your own psychological "baggage"—attempting to pull you off target and take you away from the opportunity to make permanent change and establish healthy habits. So, be careful and remain focused if you want to remain on course.

You are not reading this book by accident or by chance. You are reading this book because of a choice you made to educate yourself and improve your health. This is your opportunity. This is the last stop for fat loss. The only thing needed now is for you to seize this moment, decide now and begin implementing change.

Points to remember:

- People don't succeed because they may be unwilling to change.
- People don't succeed because they may acquire the doubts of others.
- People don't succeed because they may accept restrictions on their life that other people have set for them.
- People don't succeed because they may allow dilemmas and problems in their life to become an excuse to do nothing.
- People don't succeed because they may get offended.
- People don't succeed because they may accept their current situation as being their final situation.
- It doesn't have to be this way! You have the power to seize the moment, decide now and begin implementing change.

8

Accept or Resist

"You are where you are because you want to be there.
If you want to be somewhere else, you'll change."
—Jack Canfield

Most of the knowledge and many methodologies used to promote weight loss can be likened to that of late 19th century medical practices. In the late 1800s and early 1900s, doctors did the best job possible based on what they knew at the time. If you had a symptom, the doctor gave you a pill. More than 100 years ago doctors didn't know much about infections, viruses, bacteria and inoculation. Doctors were experts in "trial and error" and did what they believed was best.

The trial and error process stood a long time. By the time a doctor acquired an adequate amount of experience and learned how to take care of his patients, some lived, some died, and then the doctor died before he could transfer his knowledge to others. Today we are very fortunate; we have proven, universal medical information that's widely available to both doctors and patients.

Unfortunately, weight loss has not followed the same progression. As a result, there are countless messages in the media trying to convince you of which approach to weight loss is most effective. Turn on your television and you will be bombarded with 30-minute infomercials that feature people just like you testifying to the world that they have finally won the battle with their weight. We say "hogwash" to most of these advertisements.

As the manufacturing and marketing of these products and programs continues to expand, it is realistic to say, "So will the waist of the average American." As a country, despite a decrease in overall fat intake, we are gaining a substantial amount of body fat. People are becoming even more confused as a result. The abundance of information available in books and on the Internet has caused weight loss to become the most perplexing riddle of all time. Fortunately, in this book and specifically in this chapter, you will come face to face with the real secret to releasing fat and creating health.

The solution

We won't keep you waiting. Here's the secret: exercise and eating healthy are the two major factors in releasing fat and increasing energy. No surprise, right? Almost everyone will agree with that. Why is it then that a large majority of the population continues to flock to weight-loss programs that promise the most unrealistic results? We know that exercise is beneficial to weight loss and your overall health. For the most part, we know the difference between healthy and unhealthy food. So why is it that most of us go for the fads, the gimmicks, the unrealistic promises?

The idea that you can eat anything you want and release fat is outright ridiculous.

Believe it or not, making the transition to a healthy lifestyle after spending most of our lives eating garbage and never really exercising on a regular basis can appear out of reach. It seems so far away that the idea of purchasing supplements (i.e., pills, powders) that produce weight loss appears to be a great idea. You are approached from every angle; even the disk jockey you listen to as you drive home is promoting some commercial diet in hopes of drawing you into the marketing nightmare of weight-loss products. At first you doubt the claims that you can eat whatever you want and still lose weight. After hearing the disk jockey, evening after evening, attest to the magic of this diet, you decide, "What have I got to lose?" If that's not enough, you return home and click on the television and guess what? On every other channel people are preaching to you about how their program is the most sensible for losing weight the right way.

Enough is enough. Choose not to be taken in by such gimmicks and fads. The idea that you can eat anything you want and release fat is outright ridiculous. Truth is: if you have been the victim of such approaches you can almost guarantee that you have compromised your health in one form or another. You may think that you benefited aesthetically. You have lost weight, but it may be primarily muscle. If this is the case, you have just moved one step closer to a slower metabolism. Once you resume eating what many people consider a normal amount of calories, you are likely to gain all your weight back in the form of fat—plus an additional five to 10 pounds.

She didn't know

Patricia at the age of 27 visited our office for a complimentary body composition analysis. At 5'7" and 171 pounds, Patricia's body fat was 33.7 percent. One of the nicest women we have ever met, Patricia decided that the Wellness Weight-Loss process was not what she wanted. She wanted a program with more structure. She didn't want to think about what she was going to eat. She was hoping that we would govern and dictate to her. She didn't like the fact that our approach was an information-based process. Patricia couldn't see far enough ahead that it would be more empowering for her to forge her own path to success.

About four months passed and we received an unexpected phone call from Patricia. She wanted to come in and meet with us again. When she walked into our office we were impressed and it was obvious that she had lost quite a bit of weight. When we compared her new weight to four months earlier, she had lost 17 pounds.

Patricia had gone through a low-calorie commercial weight-loss program that was largely based on prepackaged foods. Although convenient in the beginning, Patricia soon became tired of eating prepackaged foods. When we asked her what she was hoping to gain from Wellness Weight-Loss, she was quick to share with us how the idea of establishing a healthy lifestyle seemed to be best for her at this time. She realized how beneficial it would be to take control of her life and no longer remain co-dependent on some commercial weight-loss program. The idea of learning how to grocery shop, dine out, and not feel deprived was exciting. Tired of not being in control and being co-dependent, Patricia was ready to evolve with her lifestyle.

At this point we decided to move forward and complete her body composition analysis. In our first meeting with Patricia she didn't quite understand the importance of defining her total body weight by pounds of fat and lean body mass. Fortunately, we had Patricia's previous file, therefore we could confirm just how much of her weight loss was lean body mass and how much was fat. Unfortunately, Patricia's weight loss consisted of lean body mass. She had not lost one ounce of fat. The reality is that Patricia lost a significant amount of muscle. This loss in muscle caused Patricia's body-fat percentage to go from 33.7 to 38 percent. Patricia is a great example of why we do not endorse scale use or most commercial weight-loss programs. As we said in the first chapter, the scale is definitely a thing of the past.

Today we are proud to say that Patricia has successfully reached her goal of 140 pounds. She is no longer at 33.7 percent body fat, but a fit 21 percent. Through the Wellness Weight-Loss process she has learned a lot about herself and the importance of investing in her health instead of mortgaging it.

Public acceptance

With thousands of books being published annually on weight loss, wouldn't you hope that some of these authors actually knew what they were talking about? Yes, of course. There are many experts, books, magazine articles and theories on television that endorse a healthy approach to losing weight. However, the majority of weight-loss theories that get widespread exposure and achieve public acceptance are those that are somewhat unique in how they're marketed. This by no way suggests they are healthy—it just means people connect with how they are packaged. It is a matter of strategy, not substance.

Imagine for a moment you are sitting at home one Saturday morning flipping through the channels. You happen upon a weight-loss infomercial that tells you that you can eat as much cheese and fried food as you want and successfully lose weight or your money back. Through our research and experience with thousands of people, we have learned that most people will watch this sort of program and consider such an approach. They will not turn the channel because this type of weight-loss program is pleasing to the eye and ear.

On the flip side, let's say your current lifestyle consists of an occasional pizza, french Fries and food that's covered or sprinkled with cheese. Imagine the same scenario: you are sitting at home flipping through the channels. You turn to a weight-loss infomercial and begin to focus in on the program and product they are selling. The celebrity hosting the infomercial explains how cheese and fried food can lead to heart disease and if you want to lose weight and increase your energy, it is imperative that you choose healthier food. By this time, most people come to the conclusion that this guy is crazy and what they're selling is unrealistic.

If the host is not saying something you want to hear, guess what? You are most likely going to change the channel. Believe it or not, folks, most people turn the channel because they have no interest in sitting through a program that challenges their current lifestyle. Keep in mind that each one of us wants to feel good, and in order to feel good that often translates into remaining in the dark when it comes to the way we treat our body. It is easier to change the channel than become aware of how our daily habits affect our current and future health and weight issues.

Resistance

When it comes to weight loss, more often than not, improved health comes in a distant second to the quick fix. Let's face it: most people don't want to wait 12 weeks or six months before they rid their body of unwanted fat. For the most part, people who want to lose weight want it gone now.

Unfortunately, like any business, supply and demand is what drives the weight-loss industry. Most people aren't concerned about how their approach to weight loss may destroy their health. They just want the weight off now. If the leaders of the weight-loss industry want to be successful, which they naturally do, they must provide the public with what it wants. Consequently, in addition to providing what people want, the weight-loss service or product must do so in a way that paints the picture of not having to give up the food the consumer enjoys most. Infomercial after infomercial advertises that you don't have to give up the food you love. This approach is much more appealing to the public than some weight-loss program that comes with a change in lifestyle.

Meet Sheila

Sheila, 33, has yo-yo dieted for 15 years. Sheila had lost weight in the past, but like many others she regained her weight and at times found herself heavier than when she first enrolled in a weight-loss program. When we first met Sheila she had participated in MD Weight Control, Atkins' Diet, the Zone, Weight Watchers, Cabbage Soup, Sugar Busters, and Suzanne Somers.

We presented the Wellness Weight-Loss process to Sheila and explained how creating health was important to us and how it serves as the foundation for our approach to helping people release fat for the last time. Without hesitation, Sheila was quick to say, "I don't care about my health right now, I am more interested in losing the weight. Once the weight is gone, then we can talk about my health." Sheila enrolled in Wellness Weight-Loss and we wholeheartedly felt we could help her. But as each coaching session passed, Sheila grew in resistance. It didn't take long before Sheila started to take shortcuts and estrange herself from us. There is no doubt that Sheila wanted to lose weight, however, she was not willing to accept the action steps necessary to produce the outcome of releasing fat that doesn't come back.

When we recommended exercise to Sheila, it was as though she were at home watching a television program that went against her beliefs. Mentally, she turned the channel, and she evaded our approach to helping her release fat.

There was no doubt that Sheila was resistant. She was not interested in eating protein that was low in saturated fat. That was not "living" for her. According to Sheila that was like being forced to eat liver with onions. The idea of drinking more water was like being punished. The thought of baking French fries instead of deep-frying them was ridiculous to her, but she maintained her desire to lose weight.

Sheila didn't realize it at the time, but she was in denial. She refused to believe or accept the reality that her inactivity and the food she chose and enjoyed most were what caused her to gain fat in the first place. That lifestyle is what has blocked her from releasing excess body fat. As long as Sheila continues to resist the unwanted reality, the dilemma of losing weight will remain unresolved and the situation will persist.

Acceptance

Acceptance is coming to grips with what is real. Please understand that acceptance does not have to mean that you like or enjoy something. Being able to come into a healthy relationship with one's self is learning to accept what we refer to as unwanted realities. For instance, you grow up wanting, liking and enjoying French fries. However, as an adult you have decided to release fat and begin a lifestyle of creating health and keeping the fat off for good. An unwanted reality is that French fries are high in calories, full of trans fatty acids, and scientifically proven to hinder your ability to release fat, but you continue to eat them expecting to release fat. In this scenario, acceptance would sound something like this, "I accept that French fries are unhealthy, therefore I choose not to eat them."

The unwanted reality of not eating French fries may at first appear unrealistic, however, accepting the reality that French fries may delay your fat-loss goals is a great example of acceptance. Another great example of accepting an unwanted reality for many is the role of exercise. For example, if you resist the role exercise plays in releasing fat and creating health, the excess body fat will persist. This makes true the saying, "If you resist, it persists."

Further, to clarify what we mean by acceptance, consider another scenario: a father who is homophobic has a son that is homosexual. Although the father is homophobic, he still has two choices in this situation. He can resist this unwanted reality and maintain his position that his son is not homosexual. He may say, "My son is not homosexual. Not my son...no way." The second route the father can take is to accept the reality that his son is homosexual. Acceptance in this scenario does not mean the father condones or likes his son's sexual preference. Acceptance in this scenario is merely accepting the reality that his son is homosexual—nothing more, nothing less. Allowing what is to be what it is equals acceptance.

When it comes to fat loss, instead of going from one diet to another and then back to the first one, learn instead to ask yourself this question: "Is there anything I can do or say differently that will bring me closer to my fat-loss goal?" Your creative answer will position you to either strive for a new result or continue resisting—remaining stuck.

The choice is yours

As your coaches, one of the things we recommend is that you choose to eat 100 percent stone ground whole wheat flour instead of white flour (the flour that comes in most crackers, muffins, bread, tortillas and pastries) for instance. Let's say you truly enjoy food that consists of white flour. Many commercial weight-loss programs encourage you to eat foods made with white flour as long as you do so in moderation and stay within your daily points.

It's no secret that food with white flour lack nutrients and may cause a rapid rise in your blood sugar in addition to being high in calories.

Your unwanted reality may be that you do not favor the idea that white flour causes fat gain and may hinder your fat loss. Even though it is scientifically proven, you may begin to question this reality. Why? Because many of these commercial weight-loss programs have clients that lose weight while still consuming food made with white flour. Although this may be true, our question is, "What weight did they lose (i.e. muscle, fat)?"

It's no secret that food with white flour lack nutrients and may cause a rapid rise in your blood sugar in addition to being high in calories. However, you may decide to continue with the white flour, lose weight and prove us wrong. Or, you can accept the reality that white flour is unhealthy and choose to avoid it the majority of the time. Regardless of which direction you choose—resistance or acceptance—the choice is yours.

Palm pushing

To help many of our clients better understand the difference between resistance and acceptance we utilize a palm pushing exercise. We have them bring their hands together, palms pressed tightly against one another and push with all their might. Once they get a feel for the palm pushing, we then demonstrate what it looks like to raise your arms up as though you've won the heavyweight championship of the world.

Now here is the exercise. We want you to palm push with all your might and on cue, we want you to raise both your arms up and apart over your head, without stopping the palm pushing! If you haven't realized it yet, it's not realistic to raise your arms up and apart while continuing to palm push.

Palm pushing is our analogy of someone being resistant. Arms up and apart are symbolic to acceptance. What do you think happens to your body when you palm push? It becomes tense. While pursuing your fat-loss goal, what do you think happens to your body when you resist something that you are not willing to change? Your body becomes tense and you can't move. You get stuck right where you are and continued progress is out of the question.

One of the greatest benefits associated with acceptance is that you experience increased awareness of choices.

We recommend that our clients ask themselves the question, "What am I attempting to control?" when they feel stuck and are no longer making progress. Ultimately, you come to the realization that in order to move forward, to continue to progress, accepting change is your magic wand. When you find yourself no longer attempting to control what is out of your control—in other words accept reality—you begin to experience much more energy in addition to moving toward your fat-loss goals.

When you are resistant (palm pushing) you learn in no time that there is no real benefit. On the other hand, there is an immense benefit ascribed to acceptance. If you resist while pursuing your fat-loss goals you may sabotage your initial goal, and quite often that results in a compromise of your health. One of the greatest benefits associated with acceptance is that you experience increased awareness of choices. You shift your focus toward long-term results and success and away from the short-term promises and fads.

As a result of acceptance, you tap into your creative juices and learn methods of creating health that come with long-lasting, optimum results. So the next time you feel stuck, angry or frustrated, ask yourself, "What am I palm pushing?" or "What am I attempting to control?" When you search for the answer you will be granted a choice. Once you have choices, it is totally up to you—continue to resist or accept.

Points to remember:

- Acceptance is coming to grips with what is real.
- Resistance is not believing or accepting what is real.
- You may not be able to change your genes, but you can change your lifestyle.
- The abundance of information that is available in books and on the Internet has caused weight loss to become the most perplexing health riddle of our time.
- The idea that you can eat anything you want and lose weight is outright ridiculous.
- Resistance for many people is refusing to believe or accept the reality that a sedentary lifestyle and most processed food are the cause of fat gain.

9

Friend or Foe?

"Remember, happiness doesn't depend upon who you are or what you have.
It depends solely on what you think."
—Dale Carnegie

Have you ever had friends that said they would do something for you, but then they didn't? If you haven't experienced such a situation, then imagine having a friend who promises to do something for you but consistently fails to follow through. Keep in mind that this doesn't happen once, but repeatedly. Could you honestly say you could trust someone who is that unreliable? Better yet, do you think you would remain friends with someone who constantly lets you down?

If you have a friend who develops a pattern of disrespecting you, it is very likely that in time you will discontinue the friendship. Friends are precious and hard to come by for the sole reason that trust and respect must be present in order for the friendship to last. We have all heard someone say, "You really find out who your friends are in moments of need." The reason this statement sounds familiar is because we have all had someone we consider to be our friend disappoint and frustrate us when we needed them most.

Thinking you can count on someone and having them let you down hurts and often makes us angry. This anger and displeasure festers and ultimately positions us to make a choice between experiencing ongoing emotional pain by keeping this so-called friend, or cutting ties and moving on. Some of us may decide to maintain the friendship until the emotional pain rises so high that we can't bear it any longer and feel forced to end the friendship.

You may be thinking you could never leave your friend simply because of these shortcomings; however, the reality is that you can and more often than not, you will. The only friend you cannot deny is yourself; nevertheless we tend to fall short on our self-promises. Time and again we make a self-promise, and time and again we let ourselves down. Imagine having a best friend you must count on everyday and watching that person never follow through. If there were no option to end such a friendship, how would you feel having to befriend someone on a daily basis you didn't trust? As hard as it may be to believe, this is exactly what we are up against when it comes to doing for ourselves what no body else can do—fulfilling our self-promises.

The self

Before we begin to clarify methods of follow-through—fulfilling our self-promises—let's take a closer look at the meaning, role and value of self. As defined by Webster's New World Dictionary, self is one's own person as distinct from all others. Self may have a particular meaning to you while someone else may define it another way; however, when it comes to the reality of self, it can either be enlightening or destructive. The reason for this is because self is responsible for what opens up the different facets of your personality and explains the reasons for your behavior.

Self may promote a sense of optimism to include feelings of being self-reliant, self-sufficient and self-confident. Self may also encourage one to be self-centered, self-destructive or self-indulgent. Your self is the foundation of your habits of thought—often referred to as your belief system. Your habits of thought are your perception of where you stand in the world and what you are willing to accept for your life.

Have you been asking yourself lately why you're not as positive as you used to be? Have you failed to meet many of your life's expectations? Have you compromised yourself so much that you don't even recognize it any longer? If you feel you have lost your sense of self or you believe you have never had it, don't worry. Not only can you establish and rediscover yourself, we believe with daily practice you can keep it.

It begins with you caring for and nurturing yourself.

Where do you begin? It all begins with you caring for and nurturing yourself. Make a decision right now to invest time, energy and love into yourself and almost instantaneously you will benefit physically, mentally, spiritually and emotionally. Taking the time to invest in you helps to develop and maintain a positive sense of self. When this happens you are better able to give love and esteem to those that mean the most to you. If you haven't noticed, when we refer to "yourself" we literally mean your self.

The power of self-promise

Would you treat your best friend the same way you treat yourself? Do you follow through with your self-promises to begin exercising and eating healthy? Do you fulfill the promises you make to yourself? Would you like to learn how to fulfill your self-promises?

People promise themselves every day that they are going to lose weight for the last time. Whether you are conscious of it or not, when you consistently fall short of fulfilling your self-promise, you unconsciously damage your inner-self. You lower your self-esteem and this may hinder your ability to evolve and to get control of your weight.

It's true that nutrition is a major determinant in how we feel and how we age. Equally, efficient exercise gives you a leg up when it comes to releasing body fat and increasing energy. However, it's the first-class treatment of you that makes the biggest impact—mentally, physically, spiritually and emotionally. As you come into a healthy relationship with yourself, you may naturally find yourself not truly wanting, liking or enjoying regular exercise and healthy eating, but choosing to fulfill your self-promise.

Habits of thought

In our experience we have discovered that long-term success with releasing fat and creating health daily is heavily dependent upon one's habits of thought. The reason your habits of thoughts are relevant to this chapter is because unless they are addressed properly, the fulfillment of your self-promise may prove temporary or, in a worse case scenario, may not happen at all. When you fall short of your self-promise you become more like your own foe than your best friend. Simply put, we aim to help you become your best friend rather than your own worst enemy.

So what exactly is a habit of thought? It is your beliefs—how and what you think about most. It is apparent that beliefs are what separate someone like Ghandi from Saddam Hussein. We know habits of thought cause some people to succeed and others to fail. Habits of thought may destroy our health or motivate us to create it. In short, habits of thought are rules (i.e. religious practice) we live by, backed by feelings of certainty. Habits of thought are nothing more than ideas that have been reinforced via references (i.e., data, information, personal experiences).

Your habits of thought basically define the roles you accept and play in life. Healthy or unhealthy, your habits of thought influence every value you have, every mannerism you foster, each rule you live by, and all of the many characteristics you display. Customarily, our habits of thought are what cause us to judge others as well as ourselves. If you didn't have habits of thought (beliefs) you would lack substance and simply believe in nothing. Your beliefs are very important, and it's helpful to understand how these habits of thought are formed.

Beliefs were ideas first

What type of person holds a belief that is not supported by references? Someone who is quick to leap from one idea to the next. Take, for example, an analogy of a tripod that has no legs. No matter how hard you try, you cannot imagine a tripod unless it has three legs that are all of the proper and equal length. If one leg were to be shorter than the others or missing altogether, the tripod would thus be rendered useless. However, once you have all three legs, the tripod is complete—the idea is supported and then transformed into a belief.

Now keep in mind that you can develop a belief about practically anything as long as you can find enough legs (references) to support it. In the same way that you can establish a new belief, you can reinforce an unhealthy one. For example, you may witness someone losing weight on a high protein/low carbohydrate diet and allow his or her experiences to support the idea that this may be the diet for you. Watching that person drop weight may prove to be the only leg you need to establish certainty that a high protein/low carbohydrate diet is the way to go. Or, you may view yourself as a failure, because you attempted to lose weight in the past but lacked the discipline to succeed. Such a belief will rule your behavior and allow you to manifest exactly what you predict for yourself—failure.

You may have a friend that took up smoking because his or her favorite entertainer was a smoker. Seeing that celebrity on the big screen earning large amounts of money and appearing happy and healthy may have planted the idea that smoking is cool. Once the idea is formed, the process of supporting it with legs becomes as plain as the nose on your face. For instance, your friend meets someone who has smoked for 60 years but appears to be in good health. Many of his or her friends begin to take up smoking and it becomes the "cool" thing to do. Time moves on as your friend's environment continues to support the idea of smoking. Soon, enough references have developed to create a belief that smoking doesn't necessarily lead to poor health. Or maybe your friend thinks, "I will stop before any major damage takes place." Unfortunately, some 20, 30, or 40 years may go by before your friend is faced with the FACT that smoking is harmful and it does speed up the aging process, diminish health and increase the odds of attracting a chronic illness.

Changing beliefs

How do we change our beliefs? How do we develop habits of thought that make healthy eating and exercise a top priority? Better yet, how do we establish beliefs that empower our behavior to fulfill self-promises?

Again, remember that you can find references for just about anything you consider worthwhile. Case in point, if you want to continue eating foods that are high in saturated fat (i.e. cheese and sausage) you may use the *Atkins' Diet* as your main reference. When it is all said and done, you can believe whatever it is you want to believe. As the old adage goes, "One man's truth is another man's illusion." Each one of us decides what is true and what is an illusion.

Making the change

When you are ready to change a belief, begin asking yourself a series of questions that will eventually create doubt in the belief you wish to modify. As with anything—healthy or unhealthy—if you question or re-examine it long enough, you will eventually come to doubt it. Once this happens you can begin creating new references for your new set of beliefs.

One of our clients, Rachel, had a belief that not eating was the most effective method for ensuring weight loss. We asked her if she had experience with eating practically nothing and she said yes. We asked her if she had lost weight and she said yes. We asked her if she had gained the weight back and she said yes. We asked her if she was interested in not only releasing fat, but also in keeping it off for the rest of her life and she said yes. We then asked her if she had any friends or relatives who ate little to nothing and lost weight but gained it back and she said yes.

After this series of questions, Rachel started to doubt the belief that eating little was the solution to permanent fat loss. As this discussion took place, we began to ask her a second set of questions that created the opportunity for Rachel to establish a new belief. We asked her if she was aware that weight loss was not synonymous with fat loss and she said no. We then explained the science of burning fat and how muscle and frequent eating increases metabolism. We helped her understand that building lean muscle tissue and focusing on burning fat is how you keep fat from coming back. By the end of our session, Rachel had developed a new understanding of releasing fat and how eating little to nothing was absolutely ridiculous if long-term health and fat loss were important to her.

The questions we asked Rachel are the same questions she would eventually ask herself. Fortunately, we were able to help Rachel create doubt in eating next to nothing. Once Rachel understood the science of releasing body fat, we helped her establish new legs (references) to support her new habits of thought. And we are proud to say that Rachel has reached her goal and maintained her fat loss for over three years.

Now when Rachel finds herself not eating or exercising regularly, she goes to that voice inside her head. Continue to ask herself questions or make statements like, "Is eating breakfast helping me keep the fat off?" and "I love the benefits of exercise." The question about breakfast causes Rachel to answer yes in her head and then take action by eating a well-balanced breakfast. In Rachel's words, "Learning to ask myself empowering questions has increased my self-esteem and willingness to remain fit and healthy. These tools have literally saved my life and helped me keep control of my weight."

You are truly your own best friend and you communicate with yourself more than anyone else.

Internal dialogue

Did you know it's been estimated that 85 percent of the conversations you hear everyday are you talking to yourself? You are truly your own best friend and you communicate with yourself more than anyone else. Because of this overwhelming amount of dialogue, the words you use and the questions you ask yourself are to help you, not stop you from moving in a direction that supports your desired outcome. You may have heard motivational speakers in the past recommend the use of self-affirmations and positive self-talk. As silly as it may sound or feel when you first implement such tools, we can't recommend this approach enough. It works!

The major difference between those who fulfill or come short on their self-promise is internal dialogue—that constant voice you hear in your head. What is internal dialogue? It is the conversation you have with yourself regarding everything that is going on in your life. The conversation that takes place in your head can be loud and aggressive, however, it is forever constant and in real time—meaning it is communicated at the same speed as if you were saying it aloud. Internal dialogue can be divided into three classes:

1) Statements you make about yourself.
2) Questions and answers that are exchanged with yourself.
3) Labels you place on yourself.

With each statement you make, every question and answer you process, and for each label you place on yourself—internally—there is a physiological change that takes place. For example, if you conjure up thoughts of being embarrassed or nervous, you will experience sweaty palms. If you concentrate and think about eating a sour lemon, your mouth will respond with increased saliva. Therefore, it makes a lot of sense that your present thinking may very well determine your future circumstances. Be it fat loss, follow through or giving up, your thoughts play a major role in what you experience and how you treat yourself.

The following self-defeating questions are prime examples of what our internal voices may ask:

- What if I lose motivation?
- What if I can't stick to the Wellness Weight-Loss process?
- What happens when I get too busy to eat?
- What do I do about my vacation coming up?
- Why can't I seem to follow through?

In addition to these kinds of questions, many of our clients have admitted to internalizing the following negative statements:

- When I lift weights I get too big.
- Intellectually I understand what to do,
  but emotionally it doesn't sit well with me.
- I hate to exercise.
- I don't have time to eat healthy.

If the self-limiting questions and statements aren't enough, we tend to apply labels to our self. These labels have a powerful influence on our perception of self:

- I'm fat.
- I'm helpless.
- I'm undisciplined.
- I'm a loser.

Feelings follow thoughts

What if I forget what I am supposed to do? What if I don't follow through? Exercise is boring. I don't have time to maintain a healthy diet. When you ask self-limiting questions or make self-defeating statements like these, you create reasons to doubt yourself. Remember, whether it's a question, statement or label, we encourage you to make it your personal mission to choose to empower yourself.

Whether it is one you ask yourself or someone else, questions determine much of how we feel; what decisions we make and how we think—our habits of thought. Whatever you ask yourself, you will always come up with an answer. So, what determines your questions? It is your thoughts that manufacture your questions; thinking is nothing more than a relationship between questions and answers. Contemplate this concept for a moment. What kind of questions and statements are going on in your mind right now?

*Contemplate this concept for a moment.
What kind of questions and statements are going on
in your mind right now?*

If you want to learn more about the questions you are asking yourself, take five minutes a few times per day and write down some of the questions you hear yourself pondering. You may hear yourself asking, "What if I don't reach my goal?" or "Why do I give up all the time?" Such questions will cause you to back them up with what may be defined as excuses.

Remember, continue to question the things you want to change. At the same time, ask yourself quality questions that will build up evidence to support the things you want to keep. By changing your questions, you alter your experience. Whatever you ask for, you will get an answer to—whether your belief is true or not. If you ask, "What's wrong in my life?" or "How come I can never keep the fat off?" you will get an answer. Rephrase self-limiting questions into a positive such as, "How can I keep the fat off?"

By posing quality questions like, "What can I do to eat breakfast everyday?" you are more likely to think proactively and arrive at an answer that moves you toward your desired goal. The quality questions you ask yourself will cause you to respond and not react; therefore positioning you to choose what is in your best interest.

Another example would be reinforcing the idea of training with weights three times per week and eating healthy. If this were your goal, you would ask yourself questions that would support these actions, such as, "How can I increase my lean body mass and bone density?" and "What food do I eat to remain fit and healthy?" When you ask yourself such questions you will come up with answers—references that reinforce your beliefs or habits of thought.

Time to practice

Instead of saying...	Say...
I don't have time to exercise.	How can I make time for exercise?
I always give up.	What can I do to stay motivated?
I hate to exercise.	I love the benefits of exercise.
I am predispositioned to be fat—it's my genetics.	Genetics play a role, but I am in control of my lifestyle.
I have tried to lose weight before.	I have experience with weight-loss programs.

Friend or foe?

What would happen if you labeled your friend a loser? What would happen if you told your friend that his exercise approach is boring? What would happen if you informed your friend she isn't going to stay motivated? If your friend continues to be your friend, you can count on the fact that he or she would be hurt, maybe even angered by your statements. This is why the questions you ask yourself, the statements you make internally to yourself and the labels you place on yourself need to be helpful, not hurtful. Once more, if you talked to your best friend the way you talk to yourself, would you have a best friend?

Points to remember:

- Fulfill your self-promise by doing for yourself what nobody else can do for you.
- A low self-esteem may hinder your ability to resolve to evolve and get control of your weight.
- Long-term success with fat loss and creating health daily is determined heavily by one's beliefs—habits of thought.
- You can find references that support just about any belief that you consider worthwhile.
- Self is one's own person as distinct from all others.
- When you are ready to change a belief, begin asking yourself a series of questions that will eventually create doubt in the belief you want to change.
- The major difference between those who fulfill or flake on their self-promise is the internal dialogue that takes place in their head.
- Feelings follow thoughts.
- Ask yourself quality questions that will enable you to build up evidence to empower your new belief.
- If you talked to your best friend in the same way you talk to yourself, would you have a best friend?

10

Change of Habits

"The greatest thing in this world is not so much where we are,
but in what direction we are moving."
—Oliver Wendell Holmes

We'd like to think of ourselves as two people with very healthy lifestyles: we eat a balanced diet and exercise regularly. So when we began writing this chapter and compiling a list of unhealthy habits, we figured none would pertain to us. TO OUR SURPRISE, when we compared the list to our own habits, we realized it was time to make a few changes.

What is a habit?

A habit is a conditioned action or way of thinking that we have performed so often it becomes almost an involuntary response. Habits require no prior planning. They are automatic, repetitive actions. Habits can be beneficial or detrimental; it all depends on the habit. Some habits—such as eating breakfast or brushing our teeth—are constructive, desirable and healthy. There are other habits, however, that can be self-defeating, stunt our growth or cut years from our life.

One thing is certain; habits are not developed overnight. It takes years for something to become a habitual part of our daily lives to the point where we are not even aware of doing the action. It takes years for it to become embedded into our everyday routine. Because of this, exchanging a habit for a new behavior may take time, sometimes as much time as it took to create the habit in the first place.

The good news is that habits, no matter how long we have held them, are not permanent. We always have the power, the option, the choice and the control to change our habits for the better.

The challenge

People of all ethnicities, cultures and nationalities spend large sums of money and countless hours year after year attempting to break unhealthy habits. Much to their despair, the majority falls short, experiencing little, if any, success. There are many reasons so many people fail in their efforts to change their habits, but two tend to stand out above the rest.

First, the desire and belief to change is not strong enough. Many people who fail in creating healthier lifestyles fall short even though they can see the benefit. There may be other people in their lives insisting that they lose weight or eat healthier. These people may encourage or even nag the person, but unless the individual is ready, willing and able, creating health is unlikely to be met. Second is a lack of knowledge. Many people want to change their habits, but simply do not know how to do it properly. They lack the knowledge necessary to make their dreams a reality.

Identifying and acknowledging your strong points is crucial when it comes to altering your undesirable behaviors.

The first step

First and foremost, it helps to praise ourselves for all the healthy habits we have, including brushing our teeth, working hard, being kind and generous to others, taking the garbage out and paying our bills. Too many times, people focus on the things they do that are considered unhealthy. The truth is that you probably have more healthy habits than unhealthy ones, but because current habits are automatic and don't require conscious thought, you may not be aware of them.

Identifying and acknowledging your strong points is crucial when it comes to altering your undesirable behaviors. At times of change, it's important to boost our self-esteem. Heightening self-esteem is crucial, as is paying attention to the positives that will help us follow through with our change of habits.

What makes a habit unhealthy?

Whether a habit is healthy or unhealthy depends on the effects it produces in your life. If it helps you to achieve your goals, improves your health, adds meaning to your life, and makes you more effective, then it's probably a healthy habit. If, however, it impedes your effectiveness, wastes your time, or decreases your life expectancy, it's very likely an unhealthy habit.

Let's look at some examples; many people binge on junk food and do not exercise. Why are these habits considered unhealthy?

As research has shown, a non-active lifestyle and poor eating habits often result in fat-gain and obesity. We know that being over fat increases one's risk of acquiring numerous chronic illnesses. For this reason alone, we feel confident labeling a sedentary lifestyle and binging on junk food as unhealthy habits. Furthermore, any eating routine that does not improve our health and help us reach our fat-loss goals is not a healthy habit.

Identify your unhealthy habits

In order to change your unhealthy habits and replace them with healthy ones, it helps to first identify what they are. Take a few minutes to write down the unhealthy habits that you would like to change.

This step is important because it raises your awareness of your current habits. Writing your intentions down on paper helps you visualize your transformation, allowing you to forecast the benefits of exchanging a destructive habit for a healthy one. To help you understand the formula of how to change an unwanted habit, we will share with you one of the most common and unhealthy habits we've come across in working with our clients: skipping breakfast.

Skipping breakfast is an example of an unhealthy action we want to replace. Most of our clients say they don't have the time to eat breakfast in the morning; others say they're not hungry. "I do not have the time. When I wake up I am showered and out the door, taking the kids to school and then on the freeway to work," says Laura. What Laura and many others don't realize is how not eating breakfast compromises their success in releasing fat.

Not eating breakfast is a sure-fire way to slow down your metabolism and increase the likelihood of an oversized lunch. Not being hungry in the morning is the first sign of a slow metabolism. By simply eating a well-balanced breakfast you will not only jump-start your body's ability to burn additional calories, you also position yourself to maintain more energy throughout the day, and you're better prepared to not fall victim to unhealthy splurges and binges.

Clearly identifying which of your habits are healthy and unhealthy is the first step in helping you to make changes for the better.

Filling the need

There is no magic pill or potion for changing habits. Habits, whether healthy or unhealthy do serve a purpose. That's right! Even the unhealthiest habits serve a purpose. The habit may help you relieve stress or allow you to let off steam and feel a little better, for the moment at least. This is the major reason why once you identify the habit you want to change, it is critical that you replace it with a behavior that serves the same purpose. For instance, if you tend to binge whenever you are stressed, find a healthier substitution for this habit.

The sole reason we form habits in the first place
is to fill a desire.

The sole reason we form habits in the first place is to fill a desire. As you break the unhealthy habits it is to your benefit to find a way to fulfill these desires. They don't go away. Making the choice to no longer follow through with the unhealthy habit means performing an alternative action in its place.

Instead of drinking a beer every time you come home after a stressful day at work you might opt instead to go for a 30-minute walk. Instead of purchasing chips, cookies and ice cream when grocery shopping you may decide to skip those aisles all together. What you substitute in place of your unhealthy habit isn't as important as whether you feel good about the choice you make. (As long as you are moving forward.) After all, the reason you consider it unhealthy is because it leaves you feeling guilty or bad about yourself.

What's the benefit?

In the beginning, one of the most important steps in breaking an unhealthy habit is to look at why you find this action (behavior) so compelling. In other words, what's the benefit for doing this seemingly negative thing? Since you've already classified this as an "unhealthy" habit you may be tempted to say there isn't one. Look closer, there is always a benefit.

Let's say your unhealthy habit is eating fried donuts. (Yes, most donuts are fried or deep-fried). What's in it for you? You fulfill your hunger and craving, and feel a sense of enjoyment, for the moment. What if you have an unhealthy habit of drinking alcohol in excess? The benefit could be that your mood is altered, you relieve some stress and escape from the pressures of life for a while. Whether the habit does you service or harm, there is always a benefit associated with it or else we wouldn't engage in that behavior.

By identifying the benefits behind each habit as the above examples show, you will be able to find another way to achieve or receive the positive benefits.

What's the compromise?

Next, take a look at the compromise. What is it that you are losing by keeping your habit? This step may prove to be easier. Why is it that you consider it an unhealthy habit in the first place? Eating a deep fried donut is an unhealthy habit because it doesn't create health and it interferes with your goal to release fat, right? Right. When you eat a deep fried donut you are trading the benefit of a temporary satisfaction of your craving for your health and success of your goal.

Drinking alcohol in excess after a stressful day at work is an unhealthy habit because you're sabotaging your fat-loss goal and taxing the health of your liver. When you alter your mood with alcohol you are compromising your commitment to your personal success and self-worth. When you drink in excess you are sabotaging the promise you made to yourself to succeed. When you look at it that way, most unhealthy habits don't seem to make much sense, do they?

Breaking the habit

Now that you've weighed both sides of the issue—your benefit (why this habit is so compelling to you) and your compromise (what you are losing by keeping this habit)—it's time to move toward change. Fortunately, because you have taken the time to identify your habits with their associated benefits and compromises, you are now more aware of these actions. Now, every time you perform one of these habits, you will be aware that you are making a choice. You are choosing what you value more: the benefit or the compromise.

Each time you start to engage in an unhealthy habit, you're actively choosing to participate in a behavior that you know compromises your goals and standards of success. Which do you value more? Do you value the relief you get from drinking alcohol in excess or do you value the promise you made to yourself? Do you value having a deep fried donut (or any other temporary craving for something sweet) or do you value success in creating health and releasing fat that doesn't come back?

Making your list

Once you have made your list of unhealthy habits, pick one to work on first. Too much of a change too soon can be overwhelming, so take it gradually. Just make sure you enjoy the healthy alternative you choose to replace the unhealthy habit. Remember; this exercise won't be effective if you choose an alternative that doesn't fill the desire or benefit.

Brainstorming the alternative

Now it's time to think of an alternative to each unhealthy habit, and write those alternatives down. Taking the time to make this important list will keep you from floundering for something to do when you're tempted to revert to your unhealthy habits. This list will provide you with an instant replacement activity.

For instance, if you're not eating breakfast because you're either not hungry or too rushed, it's time to reorganize your morning routine to include a quick breakfast. Focus on the benefits of eating breakfast and how skipping it compromises your success.

To help you change this unwanted habit, write down some of the food you like. Keep in mind that the meals you write down meet your time frame and do not require a lot of effort to prepare. You may want to start with something quick, like a bowl of cereal (i.e. Optimum Power Breakfast or Kashi). Be patient. New habits take a conscious effort to implement and are often uncomfortable in the beginning stages. However, with effort, time and consistency, these once foreign actions will soon become part of your everyday life.

Below is a brief view of what your list might look like.

Old Habit	Alternative Habit
1. Not eating breakfast.	1. Eat a bowl of cereal.
2. Late evening snacking.	2. Brush your teeth, get in bed and read.
3. Extra serving of food at dinner.	3. Go for an evening walk.
4. Eating junk food at movie theater.	4. Eat before you go. Take water and a healthy snack with you.

Exercise

Exercise is a great tool to help you break unhealthy habits. Exercise relieves stress, increases your energy and makes you feel better about yourself, all of which reinforce the benefits and inspire you to want to do it again. As you become healthier and more fit and firm, you'll also become more productive, better able to deal with stress, and less likely to participate in unhealthy habits.

Adding exercise and its benefits to our lives is easier than most people think. For example, instead of spending your lunch hour at some fast food drive-through, make and bring your own lunch to work and use the extra time to go for a short walk. It can be much healthier, can save you money (those daily lunches do add up), you'll get a second wind of energy for the afternoon, and best of all, it puts a healthy spin on your entire day.

Adding a walk at lunch is only one idea. For every situation, for every unhealthy habit, there is a healthy alternative. If you crave a donut every time you pass the reception desk at your work, take another route. If you finish the entire can of peanuts every time you buy them, buy something with fewer calories to snack on. If you stop and chat too long with people at the gym, wear headphones, wave and keep moving through your workout.

The power to choose

By now you may have come to realize that the only way to continue with an unhealthy habit for very long is to deny its existence. If you've gone through the steps in this chapter honestly, then you have a clearer under- standing of what your healthy and unhealthy habits are. From now on, when you find yourself resorting to old behaviors, the thought will pass through your mind that you are trading X for Y each time you carry out that action. When you put your health, energy and overall well-being at the top of your priority list, you will find that you are less likely to trade anything for it.

Be gentle with yourself and if you slip back into your old routine, just pick up right where you left off, using a healthy alternative the next time.

A powerful method for avoiding relapse is remembering that we have a choice about continuing habits or making a change for the better. When we choose to break promises we have made to ourselves, we actively lower our self-esteem. So, what choice will you make? The one that makes you feel down about yourself or the one that makes you feel empowered? The choice is yours.

Making small changes in your life is a step-by-step process. So be gentle with yourself and if you slip back into your old routine, just pick up right where you left off, using a healthy alternative the next time. The first few times you choose the alternative habit it may feel foreign and seem challenging and unnatural, but soon, with your heightened sense of awareness you'll see that it gets easier and it will become a part of who you are.

Points to remember:

- Praise yourself for the healthy habits you have.
- Confirm which habits are healthy or unhealthy.
- Identify and confirm your unhealthy habits and choose one you want to change.
- Recognize how the habit benefits you and causes you to compromise your personal success.
- Find an alternative behavior that fills the same desire.
- Repeat the alternative action until it becomes your new habit.

PART FOUR

Defining Your Destination

11

Clear Vision

"The future you see defines the person you'll be."
—Jim Cathcart

Have you ever wanted something so bad that you thought about it each moment of every day? Imagine thinking about something so frequently that you enable yourself to turn that idea into a reality. As hard as it may be to conceive, your thoughts do determine your future circumstances. Learning to visualize the things you want to be, have and do is without question a sure predictor of your future happenings, so make sure your vision is clear.

After you have made the decision to release fat, take time to establish a vision of where you want to be. Once your vision is clear—no fuzzy pictures—your decision to succeed will be anchored. As this happens your habits of thoughts (beliefs) and attitude will become congruent with your vision. Your vision is your personalized blueprint of the future.

Carmen's story

In the early spring of 2000, Carmen walked into our office determined and eager to get started. She wanted to trim down her 247-pound frame. Standing 5'3", Carmen was confident, but unsure of which approach she wanted to take. One thing was sure—she was weighing all her options.

We embraced Carmen's energy and shared with her how weight loss is not synonymous with fat loss and assured her that our approach would get her where she wanted to be. At the same time, we made it clear that Wellness Weight-Loss was not a diet and we did not promote or endorse shortcuts. Carmen loved the idea of never gaining the fat back. More importantly, Carmen favored the idea of establishing new habits to ensure long-term success.

Off to a great start and five months later, Carmen was down from 42 percent body fat to 30 percent and she released 43 pounds of fat from her frame. Carmen's ultimate goal at the time was to get down to 125 pounds with 18 percent body fat. At 31 years of age, this goal was attainable, however, Carmen's vision was a little fuzzy. She was having a difficult time imagining what she would look and feel like.

To capture a new cycle of motivation and take advantage of the current momentum, we asked Carmen, "On a scale of 1 to 10 with 10 being the highest level of intention, what is your level of intention for weighing 125 pounds and being at 18 percent body fat?" Carmen blurted out that she was a 10. With no apparent lack of motivation, Carmen was committed to move forward and to realize her dream.

During this time we asked Carmen to browse through some magazines and find a picture of someone with a similar body type, but at the weight and shape she wants to ultimately be. After going through magazines and searching on the Internet, Carmen came to her next coaching session excited and ready. She had found the picture of where she was going. And for the next 17 months there was not a day that went by without Carmen looking at this picture and visualizing her future accomplishment.

Amazingly, Carmen reached her goal of 125 pounds and 18 percent body fat. It took nearly three years to accomplish this transformation, however; Carmen believes she is forever a work in process. As typical as it is to lose weight and gain it back, Carmen is not concerned with relapsing. She is committed to a lifestyle of habits that reinforce where she is physically, intellectually and emotionally.

When looking at the picture Carmen brought in nearly three years ago and comparing it with where Carmen is today—you can see an amazing resemblance. The power of a clear vision has proven itself once again.

Once you know what you want,
you can easily become the architect of the future YOU.

Your vision

Now it's time for you to bring your vision into focus. It's time to get a clear mental picture of yourself living and experiencing what you foresee as the future you. If you are 50 pounds over fat, begin seeing yourself 50 pounds lighter than where you are today. Albert Einstein said it best, "You're imagination is your preview of life's coming attractions."

Begin forming the image of where you are headed. Once formed, take what you have only imagined and make it your vision. To do this, ask yourself where you want to be. What is your ideal body-fat percentage? How fit and healthy would you like to feel? The answers to these questions will help you describe in detail the outcome you are seeking. Once you know what you want, you can easily become the architect of the future YOU. For instance, you may currently weigh 300 pounds and find yourself doing everything for everyone else except yourself. Your vision may be to bring balance into your life and weigh 150 pounds at 18 percent body fat. If you want it, you can achieve it. That "it" we are talking about is what makes up your vision.

Establishing the vision

There was an old sculptor in Mexico who had a large piece of granite sitting in his back yard. Everyday the young schoolboys and girls would walk by this large stone and never think twice about it. After a couple of months they noticed the elderly man chiseling and grinding away at this huge piece of granite. They had no idea what he was doing. At the end of four months when he had completed his project, here stood the thing he had visualized for well over six months—a lovely lion made of granite. As the school children passed by they were shocked. One of the children commented to the old sculptor, "I didn't know there was a lion hidden in the granite." The sculptor had used his imagination and had visualized the lion, which in turn made his dream come true.

Now is time for you to decide what's hidden in your piece of granite. To aide you in this process, complete this statement, "My personal vision is..."

Where you are and what you want will ultimately determine what your personal vision is going to be. Your vision can be situated three months from now or three years from now. Whatever it is, write it down and hold it high on your priority list. If you need an example of what some of our clients have stated in their personal vision statements, consider the following:

- "My personal vision is *to live my life at 150 pounds and 18 percent body fat.*"
- "My personal vision is *to exercise three days per week and eat healthy ninety-percent of the time.*"
- "My personal vision is *to fit into a size six and be a healthy role mode for my children.*"
- "My personal vision is *to read one book a month.*"

Fortunately, when we go for inner growth and are proactive in our approach, our desired result will eventually materialize as outer growth

Obstacles

Ever hear someone say they were doing great, but then somehow got distracted? Let's face it, things that delay our desired outcome are inevitable during the journey. Fortunately, when we go for inner growth and are proactive in our approach, our desired result will eventually materialize as outer growth—similar to the process of harvesting crops. This is the reality of adhering to a process, and learning to delay instant gratification.

In the meantime, and aside from learning to delay instant gratification, there are a few things you can do to proactively prepare for potential setbacks. To help you better establish your vision and prepare for likely obstacles, we encourage you to ask yourself the following question: "What do I think might get in my way or limit me from experiencing my vision?" Before you answer this question, please take time and put some serious thought into how you answer. How you answer this question may prove fundamental in ensuring your success.

The answer to this question houses a predetermined setback that can be anticipated and confronted in advance: for example, we have had client's answer this question as follows: "My self-sabotaging behavior is what stops me from succeeding," "I never seem to plan my food," and "The lack of family support is what estranges me from my vision." Knowing these obstacles may arise makes it possible to develop a plan to counteract these potential setbacks. In one case we addressed the issue of self-sabotage by going straight to its cause. In the other scenario we designed a strategy for overcoming procrastination when it came to grocery shopping and weekly planning. In regard to the case of lacking family support, we looked at esteem issues and acquiring outside support systems.

Where there is a will, there is a way!

Intention

How committed are you to releasing the fat? Are you dedicated to reversing the cause of excess body fat? Setting goals, creating your vision and moving toward your desired outcome is easier said than done.

However, we believe you are destined to experience your vision if your intention is clear and meaningful to you.

The next step in creating a clear vision of where you are going is to assess your level of intention. Assigning a value to your level of intention, as Carmen did, helps you gauge how important and meaningful your vision is to you; it helps clarify your level of commitment. So on a scale of 1 to 10 (10 being the highest), what is your level of intention? If your intention level is a seven or lower, we believe it is necessary for you to take more time to yourself and reevaluate your life's priorities.

What we have learned is that there's a lot of energy surrounding the highest numbers, and unless you are answering an eight or higher, your energy is questionable. For instance, when we ask a newly married couple what their level of intention is in making their marriage work, we consistently get a 10. If you are going into the process of releasing fat and your intention level is a six, guess what? You have lost before you've begun.

Intention is a very powerful component in moving toward your vision. Though everyone has good intentions, in our practice we do not work with anyone who has an intention level of seven or lower. For those who have a low intention level, we encourage them to begin journaling their thoughts on paper. Sooner or later, these people come to the realization that releasing fat and creating health is a priority in their lives and they intend to succeed. At this point, people return to our office with an intention level off the scale.

Execution

Before you can begin pursuing the vision of your mind's eye, ask yourself, "Beginning today, what is the first action step I can take that will bring me closer to my vision?" With your intention level being an eight or higher, there is no doubt you will execute and follow through.

As your momentum naturally matures, you want to ask yourself the daily question, "What is a tangible next step I can take to manifest my vision?" Ask this question everyday. Repeating this question and answering it everyday will bring you closer to your vision. Why? Because in every answer is an embedded action step that you can put into practice.

Live your vision today

In our past professional careers, we both taught martial arts. During this time we would explain to our students that the only difference between a student wearing a white belt and those who had been awarded their black belt is the technical knowledge and personal experience of going through the process.

It wasn't necessary for our white belts to earn a black belt before they carried themselves as a black belt. A white belt who aspires to one day earn a black belt can acquire the attitude that resonates from a black belt prior to experiencing the process. In short, our white belt students were empowered to train and act as if they were already at the black belt level. We referred to this philosophy as having a "black belt attitude."

If your goal is to live your life at 150 pounds and you currently weigh 230 pounds, beginning today, you can live your life as though you are already at your ideal body weight. There is no need to delay until tomorrow what you can begin experiencing today—you can live your vision now!

By beginning the process of creating health today and for the rest of your life, you bring the future into the present. When you're going to release fat permanently, it is only fitting to see yourself adhering to a lifestyle that is congruent with your vision. Live your vision by seeing and performing optimally from this day forth.

Points to remember:

- Your habits of thought (beliefs) and attitude will become congruent with your vision.
- Write your vision down and hold it high on your priority list.
- When we go for inner growth and are proactive in our approach, our desired result will eventually materialize as outer growth.
- You are destined to experience your vision if your intention is true in meaning and high in number.
- There is no need to delay until tomorrow what you can begin experiencing today—live your vision now!

12

Master Your Motivation

"Any definite chief aim that is deliberately fixed in the mind and held there, with determination to realize it, finally saturates the entire subconscious mind until it automatically influences the physical action of the body toward the attainment of that purpose."
—Napoleon Hill

How many times have you started an exercise program or made a commitment to improve your eating habits? You probably started off with tremendous enthusiasm and determination to succeed. Then, after a few weeks, the enthusiasm wore off and you went back to your old ways of inactivity and unhealthy eating. This common scenario happens all too often. But the truth is, it doesn't have to be this way.

When we ask people what they believe stops them from following through with their goals, most say that it's simply lack of motivation. We've had clients say to us on countless occasions, "I am motivated in the beginning and then I lose it." As you may have experienced or may soon come to learn, motivation is important not only in getting started, but in following through, remaining on course, and getting back on course if you fall off.

There is much to say about mastering motivation, and for this reason we have dedicated an entire chapter to its understanding. Obviously many people face a challenge when it comes to motivating themselves. High achievers say it takes motivation to reach goals. We know motivation is not some secret formula sold exclusively to professional athletes and motivational speakers. Instead, motivation is a mental strategy—a skill—that anyone can learn to use. It is something that you have in reserve for whenever you need it. (Different extremes for different people, depending on how it has been fostered. We all have it!) Motivation is that very thing that helps you do what is necessary when you really don't feel like it.

So, as you learn what motivates you best, we encourage you to tap into the underlining principles that make motivation the powerhouse that it is. This means learning how it works and taking a closer look at how you can empower your attitude, take control of your environment and model someone whom you see as a prime example.

What is motivation?

Motivation is derived from the word "motive." Webster's New World Dictionary defines motive as an inner drive or impulse that causes one to act; incentive. Motivation comes from knowing what you want and why you want it. To properly benefit and prolong motivation, it helps to write down your goal along with the reasons why it is important to you.

The stronger one's motive, the greater the chance is of achieving the goal.

The stronger one's motive, the greater the chance is of achieving the goal. Your motive, or reasons why, are upheld when they are in alignment with your mission, passion and values. You want your motive so strong that if someone woke you up in the middle of the night and asked you why you are pursuing your goal, you would be able to answer them without a moment's hesitation. The secret to success is discovering your true reason for wanting to make change.

Regardless of what your goal is, the second you uncover the center of your motive is when motivation becomes a burning desire from deep within your soul. Pursuing a goal is easily summarized in the two directions of motivation: toward and away.

First, you have the people who are motivated to move toward their goal. For example, if you were asked why you want to lose weight and you answer, "I want to have more energy and be able to keep up with my children," or "I am getting married in three months and I want to wear this beautiful dress," then you are most likely a "toward" person when it comes to motivation. You work toward goals—you are goal oriented.

The second direction of motivation is defined as "away." For example, if you were asked why you want to lose weight and you answer, "I feel terrible and it is time for change," or "I don't like this cellulite on my legs and I want it gone," or "I had triple bypass surgery and I don't want to experience that again," you work from an "away" direction of motivation. You like to get away from discomforts and the things that don't feel good.

Which one is better?

Having "toward" motivational tendencies is more accepted in our culture. People admire those who are goal driven and motivated. However, don't disregard the people with "away" motivational tendencies. This group tends to be comprised of problem solvers who work best under pressure and during moments of discomfort or even fear. The only major concern is the further they get from the problem (dilemma), the less serious it seems and the less motivated they become. (Until being faced with the problem or threat when it arises again.)

It is equally important to watch out for anxiety stress. People who are motivated away from things often experience a lot of pain and worry before they take action. Having "away" motivational tendencies can be positive, but be aware that away motivation runs hot and cold. When you are moving away from things, you're not sure where you're going to end up. Your attention is on what you don't want and not what you do want. This is what unhealthy consciousness and healthy consciousness is all about. What is your attention focused on? Not being unhealthy or becoming healthy? As you can see, there's a big difference.

Act as if

Have you ever heard the saying "fake it until you make it?" Well, if you want to live a healthy lifestyle, begin acting as though you are currently a healthy person. Your thoughts are very important when it comes to maintaining motivation. As you act as a result of your motivation, don't forget to constantly remind yourself why you wish to succeed. Your reasons establish a strong motive.

Motivation is needed when we don't feel like eating healthy or when we don't want to go for a walk. When you are unmotivated to do the things you know are necessary, do them and your actions will alter your mood for the better. Remember, actions are a great source for out-witting your thoughts and getting them to stimulate motivation.

Proper planning

Once you have a strong motive, it helps to have a proper plan. A plan provides you with assurance, belief and direction. Notice that we said, "proper planning," because not just any plan is going to work. A proper plan allows you to determine the cause of the effect so you can reverse it. Simply put, the cause for becoming over fat is easily reversed by eating healthy and exercising regularly. If you don't reverse the cause, you will only be chasing the effects.

First, take a serious look at what caused the initial fat gain. Are you less active than you used to be? Is your life out of balance? Are you always on the run and eating fast food or not eating at all?

It is no secret that we just can't get away with the things that we used to do when we were younger. The older we get, the more effort it takes to keep the fat off. There is no quick fix to health and fitness. It takes a clear and specific goal, a strong desire, the proper plan, lots of action and most importantly, consistency.

Remember to always dig deep; get to the heart of why you want to accomplish your goal. Memorize the reasons why it is important to you, then, act as if you are already there. If you live your life with courage, you will eventually become courageous. The mind is a powerful tool—use it to your full advantage. The old "fake it until you make it" saying actually works!

Develop a plan for success and take action steps everyday toward the accomplishment of your goal. Remember that each action you take brings you one step closer to personal victory. Praise yourself for every progression you make no matter how small it may seem at the time. Remind yourself daily that you have made this choice. This is your life and you are in control of how you want to live it!

Now that you have a better understanding of motivation, it is time to become familiar with the underlining principles that empower your motive. Knowing which direction of motivation works best for you is essential. However, developing a positive attitude and being aware of your environment is of equal importance. Motivation is a day-to-day process that's fueled by three factors—attitude, environment and the modeling principle.

The positive attitude

With a positive attitude you can do, have and be everything you want in life! If motivation had a best friend it would be a positive attitude. Having a motive for why you are doing what you are doing is intensified with a positive attitude. If you're focused on releasing fat and creating health daily, change your attitude and we assure you that you'll change your life. The late Dr. Albert Schweitzer said it best; "The greatest discovery of any generation is that human beings can alter their lives by altering the attitudes of their minds."

Get excited about your goal and the journey! A positive attitude or outlook on life can lead to constructive behavior and create success. Motivation will help to push you, but your attitude is what will lead you to success. Consider the following tips for maintaining a positive attitude:

- Think of yourself as a success.
- Remind yourself of past achievements.
- Choose not to dwell on failures, evaluate what happened and adjust future actions to get the desired result.
- Surround yourself with positive people and ideas.

The positive environment

An upbeat, positive person draws other people like a magnet. After all, who would you rather be around—someone who is strong and motivated, with the confidence to keep moving forward? Or, someone who stays stuck in one place, thinking of reasons why things don't seem to happen? No contest!

Take a hard look at your environment and decide right now how you are going to allow it to affect you.

Take a hard look at your environment and decide right now how you are going to allow it to affect you. Being motivated is a plus in your efforts to release fat and create health, however, your environment may be the very thing that causes you to deviate from achieving success.

All too often we will have a client who has a positive attitude, but his or her work environment is the exact opposite of the life he or she wants to lead. For example, Darla explained to us that at her work, everyone is stressed. Each day that Darla arrives at work she is welcomed by either a dozen donuts or bagels with cream cheese. When she passes them up, not an hour goes by before one of her co-workers offers her a tasty treat that's full of fat and processed sugar. This continues for most of the day.

It is apparent that Darla's work environment does not support her goal to release fat and to eat healthy. Her lack of support doesn't disappear when she leaves work. When Darla arrives home, her sister and parents eat foods that are high in calories and unhealthy. Her family teases Darla by making negative comments about what she eats, and no one in her family supports her endeavor to lose weight.

We expressed our concern to Darla, for what she is up against is no easy task. It is our belief that either her family and/or co-workers will influence her or she will influence them. Recovering alcoholics face this issue too, and in the early stages of recovery, they often alter their environment with people who will support their goal to stop drinking. Many refrain from bars and parties until they have control of their new lifestyle.

Until you are strong enough internally and your lifestyle reinforces the progress you make, we suggest you keep your guard up in varying environments and stick to your guns. Remember, it is your decision to succeed that counts. You are in charge of your life—not your environment. Choose to influence others and be a positive role model of health and wellness.

The modeling principle

We are big believers that if you want to succeed at something, find people who are walking the walk and model their actions. Think the way they are thinking, act the way they are acting and do what they have done to get where they are. Please note that we are not saying to become a stool pigeon; we are simply promoting the concept that having a mentor can prove extremely beneficial.

We are big believers that if you want to succeed at something, find people who are walking the walk and model their actions. Think the way they are thinking, act the way they are acting and do what they have done to get where they are.

It is important that you avoid modeling someone who merely talks the talk, but doesn't walk the walk. There are many people walking the earth who fit this mode. For example, there are personal trainers who will tell you what to eat and how to exercise, but they're either over fat or not in shape, and most likely eating the same food they told you to avoid. Choose your mentor carefully.

There isn't a week that goes by when we go grocery shopping that we don't run into one of our clients. The first thing they do is scan our shopping cart. The same thing happens when we exercise at the local health club or when we dine at a nearby restaurant. It is reassuring for our clients to witness us eating healthy and exercising regularly.

We take our responsibility as role models seriously. Everything in this book is being lived and experienced daily. As you adhere to the Wellness Weight-Loss process in this book and begin creating health daily, you are modeling a lifestyle that reinforces improved health and zest for life. Now, move on to the next chapter and get some goals!

Points to remember:

- Motivation is derived from the word "motive." Webster's New World Dictionary defines motive as an inner drive or impulse that causes one to act; incentive.
- Motivation comes from knowing what you want and why you want it.
- If you want to live a healthy lifestyle, begin acting as though you are currently a healthy person.
- Fake it until you make it.
- The actions we take determine the results we make.
- Communication with yourself encourages commitment, energy and overall self-esteem.
- With a positive attitude you can do, have and be everything you want in life!
- Take a hard look at your environment and decide right now how you are going to allow it to affect you.
- We are big believers that if you want to succeed at something, find someone who is walking the walk and model their actions.

13

Goal Getting

"If you don't know where you are going,
how will you know when you get there?"
—Anonymous

In 1953, as the story goes, a questionnaire was circulated among the graduating seniors at Yale University. They were asked the question, "Do you have clear, specific, written goals, and have you developed complete plans for their accomplishment after you leave this university?" The outcome of the survey was surprising. Only three percent of the seniors had clear written goals for what they wanted to do after they graduated. Thirteen percent had goals, but had not written them down. The other 84 percent had no goals at all, except to graduate and enjoy the summer. Twenty years later, in 1973, the surviving members of that Yale graduating class were surveyed again. Among other questions, they were asked, "What is your net worth today?"

Clearly planned out goals are like gold

When they totaled and averaged the results of this survey, they established that the three percent who had clear, written goals when they left the university 20 years earlier were worth more financially than the other 97 percent put together! And goal setting was the only characteristic that the top three percent had in common. Some had attained excellent grades and some had poor grades. Some had worked in one industry and some in another. Some had moved from one side of the country to the other, and some had stayed in the same city. The one common denominator of the most successful graduates was that they had been intensely goal-oriented from the very beginning.

Goal getting

At Wellness Weight-Loss, we know the value of having a clear, specific, written goal and plan for releasing fat. A significant component of our success with clients is writing out—specifically, what is to be accomplished and how it's going to happen. During this part of the Wellness Weight-Loss process we use the term "goal getting" instead of "goal setting," simply because the word "getting" illustrates action whereas "setting" suggests a more passive approach.

Despite difficulties and opposition that may arise, the goals you set are without a doubt the goals you'll get if you follow through with the plan.

We also keep in mind the ironies of life and how in the real world few things come easy, and goals are rarely achieved without having to overcome obstacles. Despite difficulties and opposition that may arise, the goals you set are without a doubt the goals you'll get if you follow through with the plan. We have experienced the pleasure and power of goal getting and have witnessed firsthand how it has helped hundreds of our clients become more confident, motivated and successful, enabling them to follow through and experience lasting success.

Denise's story

Each year Denise would make a New Year's Resolution to finally lose 30 pounds. Year after year, resolution after resolution, Denise set her sights on losing weight for the last time. This cycle of setting a goal to lose weight continued for more than 20 years. Over the past two decades Denise experienced temporary successes, losing 10 and 20 pounds here and there, but by the age of 47 she found herself 65 pounds over her preferred weight.

Feeling unsatisfied about her weight, life suddenly took a turn for the worse when she was called in to see her family doctor a week after her annual screening. Her doctor informed her that she was now diabetic and mere points away from being diagnosed with hypertension (high blood pressure). Stunned, saddened, but ready to do something about her situation, Denise was quick to take action and therefore was able to avoid having to take blood pressure medicine. She was also adamant about preventing the many hardships (i.e. amputation) that typically stem from Type 2 diabetes by losing weight, changing her eating habits and increasing her physical activity.

Denise went on a mission to learn as much as possible about her new disease and sought our expertise. Eight months later Denise was 55 pounds lower in fat and her blood pressure was a solid 110 over 70. Denise was fit and firm and radiated health.

It has been over two years since Denise was diagnosed with Type 2 diabetes. However, she is now in the best shape of her life. Her blood pressure remains that of an athletic teenager and her 130-pound frame measures in at 22 percent body fat. It has become quite obvious to those close to Denise that her new lifestyle will prevent her from ever seeing 185 pounds again.

Denise has inspired many around her to make positive changes in their lives. Denise has become a role model to close friends, co-workers and relatives, as her diagnosis with Type 2 diabetes has changed her life for the better. "It took being diagnosed with diabetes to change my life. My experience with this disease has helped those closest to me improve their habits. In many ways my challenge with diabetes has helped others. It is a sad thing to have to learn the hard way, but thank God I had the courage to improve the quality of my life," says Denise.

Lucky to be alive

We have had clients like Denise and some as young as 18 years of age walk into our office wanting to improve the quality of their lives. Regardless of the initial reason for walking through our door, all of these clients now share the belief that they are fortunate enough to be alive. This type of belief or wisdom, if you will, is a powerful tool—one that can motivate you to rise above the pitfalls of excess body fat, low energy and diseases related to poor health.

The perfect time to get started is today!

The perfect time

Before you move on to the eight-step process, it is important that you understand that not everything is within your control. What we mean by this is, life can be very unpredictable. There is never a perfect time to set a goal—life will always throw you curve balls. If you are waiting for the perfect time to get started, you may fall into Denise's New Years Resolution trap. There are many things you simply have no control over. So don't let these distractions or the thought of waiting for the perfect time pull you down or away from your goal of attaining a lifestyle that evolves. The perfect time to get started is today.

Ready...Set...Goal!

You're ready and eager to get started and begin the process of creating a more fit, firm and fabulous you. However, before we get into the nitty-gritty of goal getting, let's discuss four reasons why everyone can benefit from setting and getting goals.

1) Goals help to establish a vision of where you want to be.
2) Goals are like road maps and serve as a guide, helping you to stay on course.
3) Goals that are clear, specific and realistic put you in a position to experience small successes on your way to larger ones; the result being a boost in self-confidence and self-esteem.
4) Setting and moving toward a goal means following a plan that will empower you to live life to the fullest.

Now that we have a better understanding of what goals are, let's move on to the process of not only setting them, but also getting your personal goals to become a living reality.

STEP 1: The first thing you want to do in this eight-step process is, ask and answer the following question. Before you write your answer down, keep in mind that a safe and healthy approach to releasing fat is one to three pounds per week. However, in our experience it is more realistic for a client over 200 pounds to expect to lose up to three pounds and those under 200 pounds to aim for a release of one to two pounds every seven days. With this range in mind, fill in your response.

"In one year how much do you want to weigh?"

Your Answer: _____

In step one, your goal may or may not be what we consider realistic. However, as we proceed with this process and work our way backward, reality will naturally surface. Clarity will be accomplished through the establishment of benchmarks (i.e. six month, three month and weekly goals) that will serve as markers along your way to the one-year goal. Note: This eight-step process considers your total body weight—not your percentage of body fat. So, as you learn what your body-fat percentage is, specifically your lean body mass (LBM), make it your goal to maintain and build your LBM and reduce your body fat.

STEP 2: To establish this benchmark: take your current weight and add it to how much you want to weight in one-year, then divide by two. For instance, if you currently weigh 250 and your 12-month goal is to weigh 180 pounds—do the math: 250 + 180 = 430. Now divide 430 by 2 and your six-month benchmark is 215 pounds.

"At the six month mark how much are you going to weigh in order to be half way to your one year goal weight?"

Your Answer: _____

STEP 3: Now it is time to figure out your three month benchmark to ensure you're on pace to succeed at accomplishing your sixth month and one year goal. During this step, the reality of where you want to be in one year may change because taking a healthy approach to releasing fat means releasing no more than two to three pounds every seven days. In a three-month period you can safely release 12 to 36 pounds. However, not everyone can release three pounds per week. To help you come to a realistic answer, use the following formula.

What is your current weight? _____ lbs.

Multiply your weight by 10%: _____ x .10

Your Answer: _____ lbs.

Example: You weigh 250 pounds. Multiply 250 by 10 percent and your answer is 25 pounds. Now subtract this number from your total body weight. In this example you would weigh 225 pounds in three months.

"In three months how much are you going to weigh?"

My Realistic Answer: _____ lbs.

"In order to accomplish your three-month (12-week)goal, how much fat do you need to release each week in order to be on pace to succeed?"

Your Answer: _____ lbs.

Example: Like the above example, to release 25 pounds of fat in 12 weeks you are going to release two pounds per week. To figure this out, you simply take the number of pounds you are going to release over 12 weeks and divide by 12 to get your weekly answer.

STEP 4: To make your goal realistic and to begin moving toward its accomplishment, it is time to establish a target date. A target date is the difference between a dream and a goal. Determining a date is how you solidify where you're going. Your three-month target date will be 84 days after your start date.

"**What is your start date?**"

Your Answer: _____

"**What is your target date?**"

Your Answer: _____

STEP 5: Before moving on in this process, it's important that you can answer "yes" to the following two questions. If not, it is strongly recommended that you sit down with someone you trust and examine these questions and your answers.

"**Is your three-month goal realistic and specific?**"

Circle Your Answer: Yes   or   No

"**Is your three-month goal challenging?**"

Circle Your Answer: Yes   or   No

By sincerely answering "yes" to these two questions, you're ready to move on to step six. If you answered "no" to either question, take time and evaluate the reasons for your answers and move toward doing what you believe is necessary to change your answer of NO to YES.

STEP 6: The "how" part of the goal getting equation is learning how to structure your three-month goal by devising a strategy for optimum and efficient use of your time and energy. To begin with—it helps to break your three-month goal down into weekly and daily "action" and "result" portions.

To begin with, we would like to explain what we mean by action and result portions.

a. The "action" portion of your weekly and daily breakdown is what we define as the incremental steps necessary to get you from point "A" to your desired result.

b. The "result" portion of your weekly and daily breakdown is what we define as the specific objective and its target date. Simply put, the RESULT is the outcome of your actions.

How do you implement the action and result formula of this process? Proper planning is the secret ingredient to setting yourself up for success and implementing these two components. For instance, we recommend that you choose one day each week to sit down and do your planning. To keep things consistent, this could be the same day and time each week, such as every Monday morning, every Wednesday evening, every Sunday afternoon, etc. During your planning session, you will identify daily actions along with their corresponding results, providing you with a daily structure and reminder of how to keep your goal in focus.

DAILY EXAMPLE

ACTION	RESULT
1. Eat every two to three hours.	1. Stabilize energy and blood sugar, while keeping metabolism in high gear.
2. Grocery shop!	2. You'll have the food on hand which will keep you honest with yourself. Promise to eat well and consume healthy food that serve to empower your goal completion.
3. Exercise Monday, Wednesday and Friday.	3. Exercising is going to increase your energy level and cause your body to burn excess calories that will greatly help you move toward your goal achievement.

STEP 7: Eighty-five percent of all communication that we engage in is with ourselves—through internal thoughts, images and conversations. Use the power of this medium to help you reach your goals. Write down on paper or in your journal and say out loud to yourself three self-affirmations. This communication with yourself empowers you as a person, reinforces your commitment and reaffirms your goal.

Express and utilize positive affirmations that are personal and in present tense. Consider the following examples: "I am having a great day," "I am focused and moving toward my goal," and "I am proud of myself for following through with my self-promises." The more you tell yourself that you're doing well, the better you're going to feel. Following through with the commitment to yourself is a way to honor your self-promises while increasing self-value, self-esteem and a creating true inner confidence.

STEP 8: Review your goals daily and keep the subjectivity out of your personal evaluations. If and when you fall off or deviate from the plan, identify what happened and get back on course. This contingency method is easy when you are evaluating your progress from a neutral position. Objective evaluation means no self-judgment. Knowing where you are and where you are going is very powerful; now it is even more powerful because you have established your vision and broken your goal down to the required action and result steps necessary to succeed.

Once you come to the end of your three months, continue repeating the eight-step process to ensure continued success and your well-deserved wellness.

Points to remember:

- Wisdom comes from learned experiences and through others.
- Not everything is within your control.
- Goals help establish direction.
- Goals must be clear, specific and realistic.
- Communication with yourself empowers your commitment, energy and overall self-esteem.
- Proper planning is the secret ingredient to implementing the "how" part of the goal getting process.
- Review your goals daily and keep the subjectivity out of your personal progress evaluations.

PART FIVE

Nutrition 101

14

Carbohydrate Confusion

"Exercise is king and nutrition is queen.
Put them together, and you have a kingdom."
—Jack Lalanne

You want a lifestyle that evolves. You're motivated. You have a vision and a clear and specific goal. And now you are ready to learn more about food. First up on this list of macronutrients is the one—the only—carbohydrates (carbs). Seen as the bad boy of food, carbs have received negative attention and we aim to bring clarity to the confusion surrounding this all-important source of fuel.

Have you ever wondered why so many people think carbs make you fat?

Why the confusion?

It's no wonder that people are completely confused about the role of carbs in their diet. While some endorse carbs and others insist on avoiding them at all costs, Americans remain skeptical about which path to take. Fortunately, in this chapter we put to rest the confusion surrounding carbs—explaining in plain English what they are, why they're important and how their consumption doesn't necessarily lead to excess body fat. We hope that, by the end of this chapter, you will be fully aware of the consequences of avoiding carbohydrates.

Have you ever wondered why so many people think carbs make you fat? To bring clarity to this mess, let's go back to the early 1980s where America as a country was under the spell that eating fat is how you get fat. During this time the food industry was quick to capitalize on the no-fat revolution by offering a variety of low-fat and reduced-fat food. Unfortunately, avoiding fat didn't equal a leaner country: Americans continued to get fatter. Recently, the blame shifted to the consumption of carbs; therefore, igniting the confusion surrounding carbs.

> *The U.S. Department of Agriculture reports that over the past 40 years, per capita consumption of sugars has increased an astonishing 32 percent from 115 pounds of sugar per year in 1966 to 152 pounds in 2000.*

Carbohydrate confusion

Confused about carbs? Not sure of how many to eat? Not even sure you know what foods they're found in? You're not alone; there isn't a week that goes by without someone inquiring with surprise, "Vegetables are carbs?"

There are millions of people who don't know which foods are considered carbs. To help you become more aware of which foods contain carbs, it's easier to list the food that doesn't contain carbs: fats and meat (protein)! Every other food has some amount of carbs because it was originally derived from a plant source. The reason that every food that comes from a plant contains carbs is that carbs function as the plant's own source of energy. There's only one major exception to this rule: milk and yogurt also contain carbs.

Carbs 101

Carbs are your body's number one source of energy. They fuel your muscles and brain, and supply the energy for essential body functions like breathing and organ function. Without adequate carbs in your nutrition habits, your body has to rely on alternate, less efficient energy pathways that ultimately leave you weak, tired and light-headed. Besides providing energy, food containing carbs are typically packed with vitamins, minerals, fiber and phytochemicals.

The name carbohydrate is derived from the fact that they are made of three elements: carbon, hydrogen and oxygen. "Carbo" refers to carbon, and "hydrate" to water, a combination of hydrogen and oxygen. Carbs are one of three macronutrients that provide calories; the other two are protein and fat. Each gram of carbohydrate by weight provides four calories of energy.

There are three main types of carbohydrates: simple or monosaccharides (i.e. fruit) and disaccharides (i.e. milk) and complex or polysaccharides (i.e. pasta). The primary difference between these carbs is in their chemical structure. To form different types of carbs, the elements are arranged in a different order. Simple carbs have a very simple chemical structure, while complex carbs are, well, more complex!

Basically, simple carbs (monosaccharides and disaccharides) are easier to breakdown than complex carbs (polysaccharides). Think of the difference between a straight line (simple carbs) and a road map with many branches (complex carbs). Since they're both made of the same elements, the big difference can be found in how they're digested. This isn't rocket science: simple carbs are digested more quickly, and complex carbs take longer because of their more complex structure.

Regardless of which type of carbs you eat, all are broken down into the simplest denominator—glucose (sugar). When you eat carbs, they are broken down into glucose, and then absorbed into the bloodstream through the small intestine and transported to the liver where they are either re-released into the bloodstream or converted into glycogen and stored in the liver and/or muscle cells.

Slower is healthier

When you eat carbs, your blood sugar increases because glucose is released into your bloodstream. Upon being introduced to your bloodstream, glucose becomes blood sugar. How quickly your blood sugar rises depends largely on the type of carb you eat, the amount, the combination of other foods (i.e., fat, protein) and your own personal physiology. As a response to the increase in blood sugar, your body responds by secreting the hormone insulin, which in turn helps "escort" that sugar out of your bloodstream and into your cells—preferably into your muscle cells.

Our bodies are amazingly miraculous—designed to protect us even when we abuse them.

Why is it important that insulin removes the sugar out of your bloodstream? First of all, if your body doesn't remove sugar from your blood stream, your arteries will basically corrode and you will be prone to various chronic diseases like Type 2 diabetes.

Our bodies are amazingly miraculous—designed to protect us even when we abuse them. For instance, when you eat a high-sugar meal and it causes your blood sugar to rise quickly and is elevated for long periods of time, your body secretes more and more insulin to bring it down. Over time, however, the body becomes less sensitive to the insulin, requiring even greater amounts to get the job done. The result is high circulating levels of insulin, blood-sugar roller coasters, cravings, mood swings and a tremendous difficulty in releasing fat. The muscle cells become more and more resistant to the effects of insulin, and the body becomes more efficient at storing that sugar in the fat cells.

It is to your benefit that you choose food that isn't made primarily from sugar.

What can you do to reduce the amount of stored blood glucose (sugar) in your fat cells? Choose alternatives to simple carbs like white sugar, brown sugar, confectioner's sugar, corn syrup, honey, maple syrup, high-fructose corn syrup, and alcohol. It is to your benefit, both in overall health and in releasing fat, that you choose food that isn't made primarily from sugar: candy, cookies and pastries. The reason? They cause an accelerated rise in your blood sugar, increase your risk of developing Type 2 diabetes and they can either prevent you from releasing fat or cause you to gain fat.

Introducing the glycemic index

Have you ever heard someone say carrots are high in sugar? Maybe you've heard others recommend avoiding corn and potatoes because they will make you fat. Before you avoid such delicious, nutritious foods packed with health-protective substances, it's time you become familiar with how these carbs got a bad rap.

Since the 1970s, there has been a lot of research on carbs and their immediate effect on blood glucose—or blood sugar—levels. However, not until 1981 did a team of scientists led by Dr. David Jenkins, a professor of nutrition at the University of Toronto, Canada, introduce the concept of the Glycemic Index to help determine which foods were best for people with diabetes. Developed and promoted for its ability to better prepare people striving to win the battle of the bulge and control fluctuations in blood sugar, the glycemic index has proven quite effective.

"Glycemic" (pronounced gly-SEEM-mic) refers to "blood sugar" and "index" is the number that measures the effect a particular food has on your blood sugar. Tested by real people and with real food, the Glycemic Index is simply a ranking of food based on their immediate effect on blood sugar levels. With the use of 50 grams of pure glucose powder, the Glycemic Index is set at 100, and every other food is compared to and ranked according to its actual effect on blood sugar levels. For instance, to test bread, the person would be given 100 grams of bread (about 3 slices of sandwich bread) because it contains 50 grams of carbs. Over the next two hours—sometimes three hours if they're diabetic—a sample of blood is taken every 15 minutes during the first hour and thereafter every 30 minutes. On a separate occasion, the same person will go through the process again, but this time they will consume 50 grams of carbs in the form of pure glucose (three tablespoons).

Once the referenced food is compared to pure glucose and an average value is calculated, computer programs are used to plot blood sugar levels on graphs. The process to establishing a food's ranking is not based solely on the response of one person or the result of one testing. The reference food is tested on two or three separate occasions on as many as 8 to 10 different people.

Make sense so far? The glycemic index is great for heightening your awareness about certain food and how they may cause your blood sugar to rise quickly, however, it may give certain carbs a bad rap and influence you to avoid them. When we look at the positives and negatives of the glycemic index, we feel it is our responsibility to share with you that the glycemic index is best utilized as a research tool and not for your daily selection of food.

Instead of recommending that you avoid the Glycemic Index alto-gether, we want to share with you how to benefit from using it. However, nothing is more valuable than your common sense to eat plenty of fruits, vegetables, whole grains, beans and other seeds.

We have provided you with a small Glycemic Index Table to give you a closer look as to how certain food rank in comparison to others. Measured by how fast a particular food converts to glucose and enters the bloodstream, causing your blood sugar to increase in two or three hours after eating, is the basis for the number given to each particular food. The lower the number the longer it takes for the referenced food to convert to sugar.

Remember, glucose is given the value of 100 and is the base for which these foods were measured. We share this with you because there are Glycemic Indexes that are based on white bread being valued at 100. However, to simplify the Glycemic Index Values it is helpful to think in terms of percentages. Fifty grams of glucose raises a person's blood sugar by 100 percent while 50 grams of corn raises blood sugar by 54 percent. Also notice that foods high in fiber are listed lower on the Glycemic Index. This is because fibrous carbs help to stabilize blood sugar levels. This will be discussed in greater detail in the next chapter.

Foods with a glycemic value of 70 or more are considered high, a value of 56 to 69 inclusive is considered moderate, and a value of 55 or less is considered low.

GLYCEMIC INDEX

FOOD	VALUE
Maltose (as in beer)	105
Glucose	100
White rice (instant)	90
Baked potato (Russet)	85
Cornflakes	81
Pretzels	81
Rice cakes	77
Donuts	76
French fries	75
Cheerios	74
Popcorn	72
White bread	70
Soft drinks	68
Grape nuts	67
Couscous	65
Sweet potato	61
Wild rice	57
New potato (Red)	57
Corn	54
Yams	51
Oatmeal	49
Carrots	47
Oranges	42
Peaches	42
Strawberries	40
Apples	38
Pears	38
Soy milk	30
Black beans	30
Garbanzo beans	28
Grapefruit	25
Tomatoes	15
Apricots	10

It is important to note that the glycemic index can be very confusing. With most of the testing taking place outside of the United States, the manufacturing and processing of certain foods that are tested have a different index number than those available in your local grocery store. The only common denominator is in fact the number of grams (50)used to compare its effect on your body to that of glucose. For this reason we encourage you to consider the glycemic index and not live by it. Eating foods that are high in fiber, vibrant in color and not quick to cook is in our opinion the truest determining factor for whether it is low in its effect on your blood sugar.

To learn more about the glycemic index and acquire the index number of hundreds of food, visit www.mendosa.com in addition to our web site for updates.

Back to blood sugar

When carbs (i.e., glucose, sugar) are absorbed into your bloodstream, cell receptors tell your brain when there is too much sugar in the blood. The brain signals the pancreas to release a hormone called insulin. Insulin's job is to decrease the amount of sugar in the liver and blood by opening the door to your cells to let the glucose in. If the storage areas in your muscle cells are full, the sugar can be absorbed in the next available storage area—your adipose tissue—more commonly known as fat cells. Fat cells can stretch to accommodate a large amount of stored energy in the form of fatty acids (fat) or glucose.

On the flip side of insulin and as a result of a surge, you may experience a drop in blood glucose to below-normal levels, and those low levels set off hunger signals. But even after enough carbs are consumed to restore the levels, hunger commonly persists, and you may find yourself overeating.

The foods you eat can cause a rise in blood sugar levels and this can lead to...increased fat retention.

The foods you eat can cause a rise in blood sugar levels and this can lead to unforeseen splurging and increased fat retention. Becoming aware of how certain foods affect your blood sugar may prove useful, therefore the glycemic index is beneficial. However, it does remain true that the glycemic index can mislead you with its food ranking. For instance, even though carrots have an index number of 47 and instant white rice has 70, it would take six or seven servings of carrots to match the blood glucose effect of one cup of rice.

There are a few things you can do, however; a more helpful gauge is a chart such as the glycemic load, which refers to the blood glucose effect of a standard serving of a food rather than a fixed amount of carbs. The glycemic load value for carrots puts them in a far more favorable light, lower than spaghetti, apples and even lentils. Unfortunately, as of now, tables charting the glycemic load are not generally available to the public or to health experts who dispense dietary advice.

The good news about the load

With over 700 foods being calculated for the glycemic index, Jennie Brand-Miller and her associates at the University of Sydney have calculated their glycemic load. Originally published in the July 2002 issue of the American Journal of Clinical Nutrition, a table for the glycemic load is published in the new version of her book, The New Glucose Revolution, (Marlowe, January 2003).

Harvard School of Public Health professor and researcher Walter Willett, M.D., and his associates first published the glycemic load, which is the glycemic index of a food multiplied by its carbohydrate content in grams, in 1997. Since the genesis of the glycemic load, Dr. Willett has published a few foods that have been calculated for the glycemic load in journal articles. This is why we recommend reading The New Glucose Revolution if you want further explanation and the glycemic load for a variety of foods.

Breaking down the glycemic load

Common sense tells you that an apple is healthier than a can of soda. However, as we exposed with rice when compared to carrots, the glycemic load takes into consideration a food's glycemic index as well as the amount of carbs per serving.

As with a carrot, it only has four grams of carbs. To get 50 grams, you'd have to eat about a pound and a half of them. The glycemic load takes the glycemic index value and multiplies it by the actual number of carbs in a serving.

For instance, the glycemic index for carrots is 47. Convert this number to a percentage and multiply by four and you get the glycemic load. A glycemic load under 10 is low, 11 to 19 is moderate, and 20 or more is high.

$$47\% \times 4 = 1.08$$

By contrast, a half-cup of cooked oatmeal has a glycemic index of 49 and 27 grams of carbs giving it a glycemic load of 13.

As you can see, the mathematics of calculating the glycemic index, the glycemic load and accounting for the carbs in grams that make up a serving can become complicated. Again, we stress and encourage you to choose a wide variety of low-glycemic vegetables (i.e., broccoli, asparagus), replace refined food with whole grain products, and eat plenty of fibrous fruits (i.e., berries, apples).

A simple, scientific solution

Carbs are an essential macronutrient, however, not all carbs are created equal when it comes to lowering your body-fat percentage and creating health. What we have discovered is that low-calorie foods—even carbs—that are packed with vitamins, minerals, phytochemicals and fiber are not going to hinder your efforts to release fat.

In addition to reducing carbs that are highly processed and known to cause a rapid increase in blood sugar, an effective way to control insulin is to eat smaller portions.

In addition to reducing carbs that are highly processed and known to cause a rapid increase in blood sugar, an effective way to control insulin is to eat smaller portions. Eating every two to three hours can significantly help control insulin and burn more body fat. This is based on the idea that eating less often slows the metabolism, and leads to binging. Eating more often can help stabilize blood sugar and control appetite and insulin levels. Lower insulin levels help the body burn fat while higher insulin levels promote fat storage. Essentially, we recommend that you eat a portion (size of the palm of your hand or clinched fist yielding at least 20 grams) of protein and carbs for breakfast, lunch and dinner. In between these meals we encourage you to snack on a fibrous carb or protein portion or a combination of the two (i.e. almonds, yogurt).

The low-carb process

Have you ever heard of the Dr. Atkins' Diet Revolution or Sugar Buster's Diet? If you haven't, millions of people have and to their despair, millions of people have failed. Sure, we've met people who swear by these diets. But in our experience and with most of our clients who have chosen this route in the past—the low-carb approach to fat loss has been nothing short of a nightmare.

When we first meet a potential client, we learn as much as possible about his or her current eating habits and past diet experiences. Peggy, is a very inspirational person and she was quick to inform us that low-carb diets are the worst. Before we even asked her to explain her experience, Peggy didn't miss a beat.

At the recommendation of her best friend who lost 35 pounds, Peggy decided to go with the low-carb approach to weight loss. Peggy was aware that fad diets come and go, but this one was exploding. It was hard to believe that she could lose weight by feasting on beef, eggs and bacon, but the proof was that of her friend: 35 pounds in two months.

Excited, motivated, and ready to go, Peggy jumped in with the perception of attaining the body of her youth. The only requirement was to eat less than 25 grams of carbs per day. Other than that, Peggy could eat whatever she wanted. On day one Peggy would eat steak and eggs for breakfast. Throughout the day she snacked on beef jerky, cheese, sausage, chicken, turkey and anything else that contained little to no carbs. In little time, maybe 10 days, Peggy was in the process of losing weight. Not just a pound or two—the weight seemed to be melting off her body. It was an amazing experience according to Peggy. Eating all the fat and protein she wanted and losing weight was like magic. There was no doubt that in a couple of months Peggy would be a true testament to the low-carb revolution.

What Peggy didn't know

It is true that Peggy was losing weight and she felt great, however, she was not aware of the unhealthy processes taking place within her body. During the first three to five days Peggy was on the low-carb diet, her body began to deplete the glycogen stores in her muscle and liver. Remember, glycogen is a source of energy that is created primarily from the consumption of carbs.

Unfortunately, the dramatic weight loss noticed in the initial stages of the low-carb diet is practically all from glycogen and water loss.

The reason Peggy's glycogen stores were depleted first is due to the fact that they were the most readily available stored source of glucose (energy) for the brain and body. Now keep in mind that during this stage in adhering to the low-carb process, there is very little if any fat burning taking place. Unfortunately, the dramatic weight loss noticed in the initial stages of the low-carb diet is practically all from glycogen and water loss. The water loss is secondary to glycogen loss, because glycogen is stored with three times its own weight in water. And as glycogen is depleted, water is simultaneously released from the body. Peggy also noticed that during the initial stage of the process, she had to urinate more often than usual.

While Peggy began to notice the scale lowering in numbers, she also became aware of a loss of endurance and strength, a significant surge in fatigue and some irritability. The reason behind these physiological changes was the loss of glycogen—her body's number one energy source that had just been severely depleted.

Focused and set on following through with the low-carb diet, Peggy continued to keep her eye on the scale. Now that glycogen was history, Peggy's body began to pull from its fat stores. This is good, right? Well, yes and no. Peggy's body did begin to burn body fat and she did start to lose fat pounds. But, fat is not the ideal source of fuel for your body, if you hope for it to function at an optimal level. Our body is not used to relying on fat exclusively; doing so sends the body into a metabolic tizzy. Here is what happens:

- As the fat is released from its storage sites, muscles burn some of the fat as fuel and some makes its way to the liver.
- With the brain being used to burning glucose for fuel (to the tune of 150 grams per day) and unable to burn fat (it won't cross the blood/brain barrier), fat can't be converted to glucose. The liver soon converts fat to "ketones," creating a state known as "ketosis." Ketones are a secondary fuel source the brain can use. However, the brain can only use ketones for about 50 percent of its energy needs. The other half MUST be glucose.

Some key points to remember when considering the reduction or restriction of carbohydrates in your diet:

a. **Muscles are broken down** to provide proteins to create glucose for the brain, meaning you're losing muscle along with your fat.
b. **Brain function suffers** because ketones are not its preferred fuel source. Research shows that learning, memory, reaction time and mood are all compromised.

Ignorance is not bliss

Peggy was not aware of what was going on inside her body. Her only reference was witnessing her friend losing weight, and now she was experiencing the same thing. In seven short weeks Peggy lost a whopping 40 pounds. We aren't sure how much of her weight loss was fat, however in our experience the majority of her loss was lean muscle tissue. Unfortunately, she gained all the weight back plus an additional five pounds. This relapse not only saddened Peggy, it lowered her self-esteem.

Peggy now knows the truth about low-carb diets. She knows that losing weight on the scale does not equal improved health. Releasing body fat and keeping your valuable muscle is how you lower your body-fat percentage and increase health at the same time.

Peggy no longer avoids carbs. What Peggy has learned is that if reducing your body fat is the goal, it helps to understand how to combine your carbs with protein, be aware of the timing of your meals and understand how some carbs can cause a rapid rise in your blood sugar, which may lead to excess body fat.

Peggy is an advocate of never repeating the same mistake twice. It has been two years since we first met Peggy and at 43 years young, she has acquired the body of her youth: standing 5'5", weighing 135 pounds with a body-fat percentage under 25. Peggy's lifestyle is one that reinforces her desire to maintain permanent fat loss.

Increased risk effects of ketosis (low-carb diets) are:

- Kidney stones
- Gout
- Lightheadedness
- Various cancers
- Poor long-term weight control
- Reduced athletic performance
- Rising blood pressure
- Osteoporosis
- Dehydration
- Headaches
- Keto (bad) breath
- Heart disease

Summary

When someone asks if the low-carb approach is healthy, we are quick to say no. Many of those who ask already know the answer. However, it does help to hear someone explain it again.

It is also helpful to back up our reasons with solid, scientifically proven facts. If this is the case for you, consider this summary: 1) Essential vitamins and nutrients come from a balanced diet, and low-carb diets are certainly not balanced; 2) You can get many essential nutrients from fruit, vegetables and grains. Low-carb diets only allow very small amounts of fruit and vegetables—definitely not enough to give you your recommended daily intake; 3) Low-carb diets claim to clear up all sorts of ailments, but the bottom line is these diets are lacking in the nutrients essential for good health and the high level of protein puts a huge strain on your kidneys.

Despite knowing the risks, people are still attracted to low-carb diets because they enjoy seeing instant results on the scale. In the short-term, most people who go on these diets do lose weight, and they lose it very quickly. However, the majority of weight loss comes from the loss of water and lean muscle tissue, which is what is necessary to keep the fat from coming back. Also, if you're attempting to reduce your fat weight permanently, losing precious lean muscle tissue is like sabotaging your own body. Muscle tissue is metabolically active, and burns calories even when you are at rest. A decrease in the amount of muscle tissue you have will lead to a decrease in the number of calories you use each day to maintain your weight, making it much harder to keep your weight under control when you stop following the low-carb diet.

Choose not to become one of those people who encourage yo-yo dieting and seem to remain stuck in the cycle of losing and regaining weight.

Choose not to be one of those people who encourage yo-yo dieting and seem to remain stuck in the cycle of losing and regaining weight. Low-carb diets attract these types of people. Eat your carbs; just be wise about your choices.

Points to remember:

- Each gram of carbohydrate by weight provides four calories of energy.
- The reason that every food that comes from a plant source contains carbs is that carbs function as the plant's own energy.
- Carbs are your body's number one source of energy. Carbs fuel your muscles and brain, as well as supply the energy for essential body functions like breathing and organ function.
- Simple carbs have a very simple chemical structure, while complex carbs are, well, more complex!
- Regardless of which type of carbs you eat, all are broken down into the simplest denominator—glucose (sugar).
- How quickly your blood sugar rises depends largely on the type of carb you eat, the amount, the combination of other foods (i.e., fat, protein) and your own personal physiology.
- "Glycemic" (pronounced gly-SEEM-mic) refers to "blood sugar" and "index" is the number that measures the effect a particular food has on your blood sugar.
- The foods you eat can cause an increase in blood sugar and this can lead to unforeseen splurging and increased fat retention.
- For a listing of the Glycemic Index, log onto the Internet and visit ***www.mendosa.com.***

15

Fiber-Carb Connection

"Some things you have to do every day. Eating seven apples on Saturday night instead of one a day just isn't going to get the job done."
—Jim Rohn

Throughout human history people have consumed plant-based foods such as whole grains, vegetables and fruits. Even during times when animal-based foods were in short supply, plant-based foods remained plentiful and easily accessible. Proof positive: rice has always been the staple food of Chinese and other Asian cultures. Corn and beans have always been the staple food of the South American peoples. Wheat has been the staple food of the Armenians, Greeks, Romans and the people of the Holy Land for well over 4,000 years. Carbohydrates (carbs) have been the choice of food since the beginning of time. However, in this day and time, many people feel that carbs are bad for them.

We cringe when we hear someone say, "Carbs are bad," because they're not. As we explained in Chapter 14, carbs are the human body's primary source of fuel. The key is to know what type of carbs to eat. But that's easier said than done. With the technological advancement of agriculture and the domestication of cereal plants and the refinement of foods, it can be quite difficult to know the difference between healthy carbs and those that increase body fat and the risk for diseases like Type 2 diabetes. With this said, what is the difference between the carbs of old and those that are readily available in grocery stores in North America?

The curse of modern-day carbs

Before current methods of processing plant-based foods were introduced, carbs would convert slowly into blood sugar when eaten, converting it into a low glycemic product as explained in Chapter 14. However, as a result of technology and the mass production methods, obesity and

Type 2 diabetes have increased among Americans. One of the reasons: mass production methods strip off the fibrous coating of grains and mill other plant-based foods into super fine particles that cause carbs to convert more rapidly to blood sugar.

Take flour for instance, and it doesn't matter if it is whole-wheat or white flour. When you eat products made from flours like breads, crackers, pizza crust, pastries, pretzels and chips, for example, they convert relatively quickly to blood sugar. The speed at which carbs are converted to glucose in the blood has enormous implications on our hormonal and caloric balance, as well as our metabolism in general. The fiber that normally is found in unprocessed food is there to control this speed. But, when that fiber is absent, as it commonly is in processed foods, the carbs we ingest are digested too quickly.

If you are wondering how you can slow the conversion process of a carb source to blood glucose, begin eating carbs that are high in fiber and as close as possible to their natural form.

When you eat a highly refined carb, your blood sugar is affected and your pancreas is called to secrete insulin to clear the sugar from your blood. The reason for this is that sugar is quite toxic when circulating through your bloodstream—it's like a whip or knives slashing the inside of your arteries. It is very important to get glucose out of the bloodstream and into cells where it can be burned for energy, which is exactly what insulin does. For this reason, one of the worst procedures in modern day manufacturing is the denaturing of fibrous carbs through frequent processing and refinement methods. This is what makes dietary fiber an important element in our food supply. When it is lost, we are exposed to increased risks of lifestyle diseases. Our digestive system is not designed to run on highly concentrated carb sources such as white flour and table sugar, which convert quickly to blood glucose.

If you are wondering how you can slow the conversion process of a carb source to blood glucose, begin eating carbs that are high in fiber and as close as possible to their natural form. When consuming carbs in this manner, the process is slowed dramatically and your pancreas is less likely to secrete a vast amount of insulin into your blood. The result: your body is less likely to store glucose in fat cells. Also, when you regularly consume high fiber foods, you lower your risk of becoming insulin resistant and developing Type 2 diabetes.

The fiber-carb connection

When it comes to the type of carbs to eat and those to avoid, we recommend that you choose fibrous carbs that are typically low on the glycemic index. If you don't want to memorize how food measures on the glycemic index, we don't blame you. Simply choose carbs that have color (i.e., yams, bell peppers, broccoli), and you'll soon notice a pattern when compared to other, higher glycemic carbs listed on the index. What we have discovered is that foods higher in fiber also maintain a lower position on the glycemic index. The less fiber and the more refined a carb is (i.e. potato, white rice, rice cakes), the higher it rates on the glycemic index.

Though many scientists do not endorse the glycemic index, practically all recommend the consumption of carbs high in dietary fiber. Part of the rationale behind endorsing high fiber carbs is to control blood sugar. When you control your blood sugar, you lower the risk of becoming insulin resistant, a process where cells become resistant to the affect of insulin, leading to the possible development of Type 2 diabetes. Insulin resistance is also partly responsible for the obesity epidemic, is one of the primary causes of high blood pressure, and is responsible for the high level of unhealthy fats in the blood; all of which have been proven to lead to an increased risk of heart disease.

As you have learned, high-fiber foods can be very beneficial. But many of us aren't sure exactly what fiber is, and which foods contain it. We'll answer these questions, and show you how fiber can help you win the battle of the bulge.

What is dietary fiber?

Dietary fiber is the indigestible portion of plant-based foods, most of which passes through our system unchanged. What this means is fiber can't be broken down by the digestive system nor can in be absorbed into the bloodstream. Simply put, we lack the enzymes to digest fiber. It is for this reason that when people analyze foods high in fiber, they are lower in calories. We can't absorb calories from fiber. Fiber can be divided into two categories, characterized by divergent physical characteristics and dissimilar effects on the body: water-insoluble and water- soluble. Each form functions its own way and each produces different physiological benefits.

Water-insoluble fiber

This form of fiber, including cellulose, hemicellulose and lingnin, does not dissolve in water. The insoluble fibers tend to promote regularity and can be found in such products as wheat bran, seeds, popcorn, brown rice, breads, cereals, pasta, beans and other whole grain products. Insoluble fiber, when combined with fluids, stimulates your colon to keep waste moving out of your bowels. Without fiber, waste moves too slowly, increasing your risk of constipation, diverticulosis, and eventually, colon cancer. It is also thought to be a combatant against a number of gastrointestinal diseases.

Soluble fiber supports the growth of healthy intestinal bacteria, appears to lower blood cholesterol levels, and slows down the rate at which sugar is absorbed from the intestine

---

Water-soluble fiber

The soluble fibers include pectins, gums and mucilages, all of which dissolve in water. These fibers are found in fruits, vegetables, seeds, legumes, dried beans and whole grains, including oats, barley, rye and wild rice. Prunes are also high in soluble fiber. Today's pitted prunes are moist and convenient—an excellent snack and a great way to get more natural fiber into the diet. Soluble fiber supports the growth of healthy intestinal bacteria, appears to lower blood cholesterol levels, and slows down the rate at which sugar is absorbed from the intestine, which may help regulate your blood glucose level.

Lowering cholesterol

When you eat, your body secretes compounds called bile acids into the gastrointestinal tract for the purpose of fat metabolism. Cholesterol is a principal component of bile acids. Researchers believe that soluble fibers bind to cholesterol-rich bile acids and cause them to be excreted from the body when they would otherwise be re-absorbed. As cholesterol from the blood circulates through the liver, it is pulled out to manufacture more bile acids on order to replenish those that have been excreted. With less cholesterol in the blood, less plaque is formed on the walls of the arteries that lead to the heart and the brain.

The trickiest accomplishments of fiber may lie with the stickiest kinds—gums and pectins—as they may keep cholesterol under control by removing bile acids that digest fat. The same types of fiber may also regulate blood sugar. This process is accomplished through a process in which the gut's lining is coated, delaying an emptying of the stomach. As a result, these fibers can slow sugar absorption after a meal and may reduce the amount of insulin needed. This regulation of blood sugar can stabilize your energy levels and prevent Type 2 diabetes.

Fiber brings with it supplementary health benefits in addition to lowering cholesterol. There is plenty of evidence available on how a high-fiber diet can protect you from the following diseases:

- Heart disease. Nurses Health Study data points to a reduction in coronary heart disease in women whose diets contained the highest amounts of fiber. Fiber may lower LDL (unhealthy) cholesterol and blood insulin levels, and may reduce the risk of blood clots. The American Heart Association's most recent dietary guidelines call for eating fiber-rich whole grains, fruits and vegetables.
- Type 2 diabetes. In a Harvard School of Public Health study that looked at more than 65,000 women, those who ate the most fiber had a 30 percent reduced risk of developing Type 2 diabetes, com pared to women who ate the lowest amount of fiber.
- Cancer. High-fiber diets including whole grains contain phytochemicals, selenium and vitamin E, all of which are believed to have anticancer properties. To help reduce your risk of cancer, the American Cancer Society recommends eating five or more servings of fruits and vegetables daily and consuming whole grains rather than refined carbs.

What about releasing fat?

Fiber is a weight watcher's dream, since fibers called cellulose and hemicelluloses take up space in the stomach, making us feel comfortably full and satiated longer—so we consume less food. Eating fibrous foods can also decrease swings in blood sugar that make dieters weak, tired and irritable. Fiber binds with some of the fat that you eat, preventing its absorption by accelerating the foods movement through your body. Focusing on fibrous carbs allows you to eat larger volumes of food and take in more nutrients without taking in excess calories.

How would you like to eat a fibrous carb that, by the time you are done chewing and digesting it, has burned more calories than you ate? When it comes to releasing fat, a fibrous carb such as a stalk of celery comes with only 10 calories; however, you burn more calories eating it. The same goes for a leaf of lettuce, which yields only one or two calories!

When researchers at Tufts University reviewed published studies on the effects of fiber on hunger, they found that people who consumed an additional 14 grams of fiber a day ended up eating 10 percent fewer calories than before. In another study, researchers at University Hospital in London, Ontario, used detailed food diaries to compare the fiber intake of study participants at different weights. They found that those who maintained a healthy weight ate 30 percent more fiber than the overweight participants. Then there are the 25 scientific studies reviewed by Drs. M. Yao and Susan Roberts of Tufts University that showed that people on high-fiber/low-fat diets lost three times as much weight as people who ate only a low-fat diet.

These studies prove that people benefit from increasing daily fiber intake. In addition, we have personally benefited from high-fiber diets, as have our weight-loss clients. Aside from the fact that it provides bulk, which many of our clients contribute to feeling more full, fibrous carbs slow digestion, which makes you feel satisfied longer.

Your common sense may help you determine that dietary fiber is beneficial. However, how much is enough? Contrary to popular belief, increasing your dietary fiber must be approached in a careful manner.

Getting enough fiber

The fifth report in a series of reports published on September 5, 2002 by the Food and Nutrition Board of the National Academy of Sciences on the dietary intake of fiber recommends adults 50 years and younger to consume 38 grams for men and 25 grams for women, while for men and women over 50 it is 30 and 21 grams per day, respectively, due to decreased food consumption. The average American diet barely consumes half of this amount with an intake of 10 to 15 grams daily.

To increase your fiber intake, choose whole grains, beans, fruits and vegetables over refined white flour and processed baked goods.

It is not that Americans are not eating enough carbs. The concern is that most Americans fill up on refined carbs that lack fiber, vitamins, minerals, antioxidants and phytochemicals. These carbs that lack fiber are the same foods that give carbs a bad name. The challenge you are faced with is sorting out the inadequate carbs and increasing your consumption of quality carbs. How do you accomplish this?

To increase your fiber intake, choose whole grains, beans, fruits and vegetables over refined white flour and processed baked goods. Foods labeled "high fiber" contain at least five grams of fiber per serving. Foods that have 2.5 to 4.9 grams of fiber per serving are labeled as "good sources" of fiber. It is important to increase your fiber intake gradually, as a large increase in fiber over a short period of time may result in bloating, diarrhea, gas and general discomfort. Add fiber gradually over a period of time (about three weeks) to avoid abdominal problems, and be sure to increase your water intake as well. Consider the following tips:

- If you have any illnesses, especially intestinal problems, be sure to check with your physician before increasing your fiber intake.
- Increase your intake of water as well. Too little fluid combined with more fiber may cause constipation.
- Increase fiber gradually. If you've been eating only 10 grams of fiber a day for years, it's not a good idea to increase it to 40 grams all at once. This can cause gas, bloating and possibly diarrhea. Instead, raise your intake by a few grams of fiber each week.

Americans are spending over $1.3 million on laxatives each day.

Fiber in, fiber out

Very rarely will you read a weight-loss book that takes time to discuss the importance of dietary fiber and the process of elimination (i.e. defecation or bowel movement). The reason we feel this issue is worth mentioning is simply the fact that Americans are spending over $1.3 million on laxatives each day. Furthermore, the mass production of highly refined carbs is not helping matters.

First of all, our body and digestive system are designed to benefit from the foods we ingest. After our body has captured the nutrients it needs from the foods we eat, it works diligently to eliminate the rest. After we eat a food and it is broken down and enters our small intestine, much of it is absorbed into our blood. However, what the body does not use is then processed by the large intestine (colon) and prepared for elimination from the body.

If your diet is low in fibrous carbs, you may find yourself going days without eliminating waste products. If this is the case, it is apparent that your metabolism is not working at its full potential. When waste sits in your colon longer than it is supposed to, certain toxins can be re-absorbed back into your system—making the job even harder on your liver. This can bring a screeching halt to your fat-loss efforts, not to mention an increase in health problems.

To help you evaluate whether or not you are eliminating wastes properly, look at frequency. How often are you having a bowel movement? Some say with every meal you consume a day, you should have a bowel movement. We believe it is healthy to have two to three bowel movements per day. However, if you are having two bowel movements a day and you want to ensure you are eliminating efficiently, consider testing the transit time—the time it takes once the food enters your mouth to leaving your body. To do this, eat a cup of beets and track the process by noting the day and time they are consumed to the day and time they are eliminated.

It is ideal to notice the red color of beets showing up in 14 to 16 hours (transit time) with the last sign of them in about 55 to 72 hours (retention time). If you are not seeing the red color of beets within these parameters, we encourage you to seek the advice of a medical doctor to rule out digestive problems.

Put fibrous carbs to work for you

Are you ready to begin adding fiber to your diet? You can begin this process by tracking your fiber. As you increase your daily fiber gradually, you will quickly notice an increase in energy and a drop in your waist-line. Begin by limiting highly processed and refined carbs like white flour products, white rice, refined sugar, most frozen dinners and candy. At the same time, begin adding whole grain products, paying particular attention to yellow, orange, blue and red vegetables and fruits.

Remember, carbs are not inherently bad; it is the processes that many carbs go through that are unhealthy.

Remind yourself daily of the type of carbs eaten by our stone-aged ancestors. Carbs eaten in traditional cuisines offer increased health as opposed to the modern-day manufacturing of carbs. Remember, carbs are not inherently bad; it is the processes that many carbs go through that are unhealthy. There are multitudes of carbs available that are not highly processed and refined, and the choice as always is yours to make.

Points to remember:

- Throughout human history, people have consumed plant-based foods such as whole grains, vegetables and fruits.
- When you eat products made from flours such as breads, crackers, pizza crust, pastries, pretzels and chips, for example, they convert relatively quickly to blood sugar.

- Our digestive system is not designed to run on highly concentrated carb sources (i.e. white flour, table sugar) that convert quickly to blood glucose.

- When it comes to the type of carbs to eat, we recommend that you choose fibrous carbs that are typically low on the glycemic index.

- Insoluble fibers tend to promote regularity and are found in wheat bran, seeds, popcorn, brown rice, breads, cereals, pasta, beans and other whole grain.

- Soluble fibers are found in fruits, vegetables, seeds, legumes, dried beans and whole grains, including oats, barley, rye and wild rice.

- Fiber brings with it many health benefits in addition to lowering cholesterol.

- Fiber is a weight watcher's dream.

- Add fiber gradually over a period of time (about three weeks) to avoid abdominal discomfort, and be sure to increase your water intake as well.

- Carbs eaten in traditional menus offer us increased health over carbs processed by modern-day manufacturing methods.

16

Fat Facts

"Success does not consist in never making mistakes but in never making the same one a second time."
—George Bernard Shaw

We have all heard about the importance of eating a well-balanced diet, but what role does dietary fat play in the equation?

Who wants to be fat? No one wants to add to his or her percentage of body fat. However, the theory that "eating fat makes you fat" has encouraged us to avoid fat at all costs. This aggressive campaign began in the 1980s, and people have made great strides in avoiding fat consumption. For this reason, fats have become the enemy, and grocery stores have succumbed to the demand and now stock their shelves with non-fat and low-fat products. The question however still remains: "Does fat make us fat?"

Fat. Fat. *FAT!* The mere sound of the word strikes fear in the hearts of millions. Why? Aside from not wanting to increase the bulge, the threat of heart disease—which is linked to a high-fat diet—is the number one killer in America, claiming thousands of lives each year. However, that isn't the only detrimental health risk linked to fat consumption. Stroke, several types of cancers and even poor eyesight may be caused by the over consumption of fat.

We know that unhealthy fats increase cholesterol levels, which is a known risk factor for heart disease. We are aware that a high intake of dietary fat (fat in food) may slow down our ability to break down and burn existing body fat stores. But we also know that not all fats are created equal. We need certain types of fat to keep in good health, increase energy and maintain healthy skin and hair. Fat is in a sense an oxymoron; it has the ability to induce many health risks, while it still remains an important part of a well-balanced nutrition plan.

There are different kinds of fat, some healthy and some toxic to the human body. It is our goal to provide you with a nutritional breakdown of the good, the bad and the ugly—fats that are readily available, accessible, blatant and camouflaged in thousands of non-fat and low-fat foods. In the end, we hope that you will acquire a broader understanding of the role of dietary fat and increase your awareness of which types hinder or support your well being.

Cholesterol challenge: LDL vs. HDL

Cholesterol is the main villain in the battle of heart health, and dietary fat is directly related to cholesterol levels in the blood. High levels of cholesterol are associated with an increased risk of atherosclerosis and other heart-related diseases. This said, before we introduce you to the three types of fats, we would first like to provide you with a simple but true explanation of what is meant by HDL and LDL cholesterol.

Unhealthy fats are one of the prime culprits that negatively affect your cholesterol levels. Modern-day research has taught us that cholesterol levels are often the predecessors of obesity and coronary heart disease. However, just as in the case of fat, there are healthy and unhealthy types of cholesterol. Low-density lipoprotein, widely known as LDL, is the unhealthy (bad) cholesterol. High-density lipoprotein, or HDL, is the healthy (good) cholesterol. To help better understand LDL, it may be helpful to think of the Ls in LDL as Lousy and Lethal. Think of the H in HDL as Helpful and Healthful.

Cholesterol analogy

Consider the following analogy; the LDLs are the debris (the trash), and the HDLs are the cleaners (the janitors). The bigger the party, that is, the more unhealthy fat you eat, the more trash you have accumulated in the streets, or arteries. The janitors come through and sweep the streets, clearing them to allow transport. Oftentimes, the HDLs are overworked and underpaid, which leads to more clutter in the streets. It may get so clogged that traffic can't get through at all—which is awful news for blood and the vital nutrients it carries.

The good fat

Unsaturated fats are considered "healthy fats." They contain the essential fatty acids that our bodies are unable to produce on their own. They also help lower LDL (unhealthy) cholesterol. As an added bonus, many of these fats are rich in antioxidants, which have been shown to protect against cancer and heart disease. They are derived mainly from plant and some seafood sources, and are liquid at room temperature. Unsaturated fats are broken down into two main categories: monounsaturated and polyunsaturated. Like some proteins, these types of fat are considered essential—meaning they are necessary but our body is unable to produce them. Therefore we need to ingest unsaturated fats through our consumption of food. Like aspirin, healthy fat is a natural anticoagulant that prevents excessive blood clotting that may lead to stroke. It may also keep our arteries flexible and can prevent sticky plaque from forming, which can lower the risk of heart attacks.

We need to ingest unsaturated fats through our consumption of food.

Healthy fat can prevent the over-production of prostaglandin's that can cause excessive joint inflammation. All of our cells are lined with a lipid bi-layer that comes from healthy fat, as well as the myelin sheath that coves our nerves. Healthy fats are vital for the absorption of fat-soluble vitamins A, D, E and K. If you are not getting enough healthy fat, you may have dry skin, dry hair or blurred vision. Healthy unsaturated fat can be found in olive oil, flaxseed oil, soy products, olives, nuts, seeds, natural peanut butter, avocados, and coldwater fish such as salmon, tuna and sardines. Depending on your caloric intake, we suggest 30-50 grams of healthy fat per day.

The omega family

Polyunsaturated fats are of two kinds, omega-3 and omega-6. The omega-3 and omega-6 fatty acids are not inter-convertible in the body and are important components of practically every cell membrane. Although we need to consume both for optimal health, research shows that it is more beneficial to consume twice as much omega-3 as omega-6. The easiest way to get your omega-3s is through ground flaxseeds or flaxseed oil, walnuts and deep-sea, cold-water fish such as salmon, mackerel and tuna. Accordingly, omega-3 fatty acids reduce appetite, elevate mood, decrease inflammation, and increase energy and mental clarity. Fortunately, getting our omega-6 fatty acids is easier. They are abundant in most cooking oils, and therefore, in most of the foods we eat. The bulk of our polyunsaturated fat comes from omega-6 fatty acids.

It is important to note that most fat sources contain a combination of poly- and mono-unsaturated fats. We have found that foods are typically classified based on the highest amount of fat they contain. For example: olive oil is 17 percent saturated fat, 74 percent mono-unsaturated and only nine percent polyunsaturated, therefore it is classified as a monounsaturated fat, even though it consists of three percent omega-3 and six percent omega-6.

The bad fat

Carla is 130 pounds with 20 percent body fat. Three percent of Carla's fat is essential for insulating and cushioning her vital organs. The remaining 17 percent make up her body's fat energy reserve.

She has 77,350 calories of excess fat waiting to be used. However, glucose is the body's preferred fuel source, so she will never break down all of her fat for fuel. With so much extra fat, why would she want to include fat in her diet? It's simple; her body needs dietary fat to survive.

As mentioned earlier, fat consumption is required to maintain healthy organs and arteries. Unfortunately, the body is picky, and it doesn't respond well to all forms of fat. This brings us to saturated fat— the bad (unhealthy) fat. Saturated fat, whose carbon atoms are saturated with hydrogen, are solid at room temperature and negatively affect our arteries. Unlike unsaturated fats, which have spaces available on their carbon atoms making them biologically active and ready to be utilized for your bodily functions, saturated fat is solid and sticky and often ends up clinging to the walls of our arteries and forming plaque.

It's important to note that the body is able to create all other necessary fats by rearranging the bonds of unsaturated fats, so saturated fat is only good for one thing—nothing. The buildup caused by saturated fat and cholesterol is called atherosclerosis (the hardening and narrowing of the arteries). This may result in the leading cause of death in North America—coronary heart disease.

Saturated fat has also been linked to various forms of cancer and obesity.

Once atherosclerosis sets in, arteries lose the flexibility to contract and expand in the same manner that healthy ones do. The long-term effect can be the blockage of oxygen to living tissue. All of our cells need oxygen to survive and when the passage becomes blocked, the cells die. If the arteries to your brain become blocked, you suffer a stroke. If the arteries to your heart become blocked, you will suffer a heart attack. If the arteries to your organs or limbs become blocked (as in peripheral arterial disease), you may lose the use of that area.

Saturated fat has also been linked to various forms of cancer and obesity. Quite often the fat becomes lodged in the folds of our intestine and prevents absorption of vital nutrients. Over time this undigested fat rots in our gut, promoting digestive problems and possibly the development of colon cancer. Ingesting too much saturated fat will result in the deposit of fat in our fat cells. Fat cells continue to stretch to accommodate the fat in our diet. Therefore, as they stretch, our waist and hips continue to expand.

Food sources that are high in saturated fat are pork, beef, dairy products—especially cheese, palm kernel and coconut oils. Simply put, if you're eating an animal that previously walked or flew, you're consuming some if not a lot of saturated fat. If you want to improve your health and trim your waistline, we suggest a maximum of 10 grams or less of saturated fat per day if you eat less than 2,000 calories per day, and a maximum of 20 grams if you eat more than 2,000 calories daily. This is easy to do when you choose egg whites, fish and soy products. If you can't imagine life without animal products, choose low-fat dairy products, and extra lean cuts of red meat, turkey and poultry.

NOTE: One 12-ounce steak comes with a whopping 75 grams of saturated fat, an extra lean (trimmed fat) sirloin steak has approximately nine grams, while a portion of skinless chicken breast has only two grams of saturated fat. One gram of fat is equal to nine calories.

The ugly fat

At this point you probably can't imagine that any fat could be worse than saturated fat. Well, guess again. The worst fat on the market today is often referred to as trans fat or trans fatty acids. Used as a preservative and as a binary agent, manufacturers take a healthy fat (liquid) such as soybean oil and change its chemical composition in order to make it a solid. Basically, they heat oils such as vegetable or soybean and add hydrogen along with a metal catalyst like nickel or cobalt. This process is called hydrogenation and is basically toxic to humans. Taking healthy oil and making it unhealthy via treatments like hydrogenation is not beneficial to the human body. The hydrogenation process alters the oil's chemical structure, making it useless to the human body. This process is so unhealthy that most European countries limit trans fatty acids to four percent in any food—some have banned them altogether.

Gram for gram, trans fats have 15 times more risk for inducing coronary heart disease than saturated fats. Some researchers believe this fat changes how cells process insulin—which can lead to Type 2 diabetes—and have even linked trans fats to cancer. A report released by the National Academy of Science's Institute of Medicine concluded in July, 2002 that the only safe intake of trans fats was "zero"—which is considerably less than the 3.8 grams of trans fats contained in 3.5 ounce serving of French fries.

Although you may get less trans fat in your diet than other fats, even a small amount greatly increases your risk of disease. According to a 2001 study undertaken at Harvard University, the risk of Type 2 diabetes rises by 39 percent when caloric intake of trans fatty acids swells by as little two percent in women. Until recently, another challenge when addressing trans fats is that they are not properly represented on food labels. The good news is that as of July 9, 2003, the FDA issued a regulation that requires manufacturers to list trans fatty acids on the Nutrition Facts panel of food and even some dietary supplements. Food manufacturers have until January 1, 2006 to comply with the new FDA regulations. So, until then, read the ingredient list on the food label—the closer you see the words "shortening," "partially hydrogenated," "hydrogenated" or "fractionated" to the top, the higher the amount of trans fat in the product.

In order to skirt around the red tape, many companies partially hydrogenate the oils—a process that claims to cut the trans fatty acids in half to a level somewhere between 21-24 percent of content, but many researchers say this is a level still too toxic to the body. A Dutch physician, Dr. Martin Katan found that trans fatty acids lower HDL (healthy cholesterol) and raise LDLs (unhealthy cholesterol). This finding is supported by the report released by the National Academy of Science's Institute of Medicine, which states that trans fats promote heart disease by boosting levels of LDL cholesterol and lowering HDL cholesterol.

If trans fats are so toxic then why are so many products utilizing the hydrogenation process?

Hydrogenated and partially hydrogenated oils can be found in deep-fried foods, margarine, cookies, muffins, cakes, and pre-packaged foods like crackers, breads, cereals and most snack foods. During a recent informal survey of 140 varieties of crackers on a typical supermarket shelf, only three brands did not contain partially hydrogenated oil. It can seem very difficult to avoid this toxic process, and even when you think you're succeeding, others may hide it from you. For instance, many fast food chains promote the use of 100 percent vegetable oil...unfortunately, it may be 75 percent hydrogenated!

This information can be very shocking and you may be thinking: if trans fats are so toxic then why are so many products utilizing the hydrogenation process? Simply put, it all boils down to profits. Literally since the days of Napoleon, people have been searching to replace real food with artificial food for the sole purpose of high-profit potential. Consider the savings: when you hydrogenate an oil, you get approximately five times its use and it prolongs the shelf life of a product, which results in increased profits. For obvious reasons, you will not find us endorsing hydrogenated oils in any manner. When we call for oil, we mean one hundred percent unsaturated, non-hydrogenated oil!

In 1999, the U. S. Food and Drug Administration (FDA) proposed that the "Nutrition Facts" labels on foods be required to disclose trans fat content. But the FDA delayed finalizing its regulations until it could consider the Institute of Medicine's report, which wasn't released until July 2002.

Now that new regulations are finally in place, the FDA estimates that by January 1, 2009, trans fat labeling will have prevented from 600 to 1,200 cases of coronary heart disease and 250 to 500 deaths each year.

All about fat

When is comes to fat, plant and cold-water fish sources are the healthiest choice. Keep your fat choices as natural as possible. Below is a list of additional information on fats and oils.

EXTRA VIRGIN OLIVE OIL: high in monounsaturated fat, tasty and readily available worldwide, olive oil is ideal for salad dressings and cooking. Studies have shown that monounsaturated fats like olive oil may reduce the risk of coronary heart disease.

ALMOND: nuts and oils are mainly monounsaturated fats. Almond oil has a high smoke point so it is great for cooking and frying. Almonds can be ground to make almond butter—a great alternative to peanut butter.

AVOCADO: similar to olive oil, avocado oil is high in monounsaturated fat. Although this fruit is full of healthy fat, it is very high in calories so beware!

FLAXSEED: your best choice for alpha-linolenic acid, (a type of omega-3 fatty acid), that is necessary for optimum brain function and elite sports performance.

GRAPE SEED: great cooking oil. Not only tasty, but can withstand more heat before altering its chemical structure. Grape seed oil is ideal for salad dressings, cooking, frying and baking because it has no after taste, a high smoke point so it will not burn or splatter and it is high in omega 3 and 6 fatty acids so it raises HDL and lowers LDL cholesterol. The unique properties of Grape seed oil based on its fatty acid composition and antioxidant content make it an extremely stable, durable oil that has been appreciated for over 100 years.

PEANUT: unrefined peanuts are a great choice. Processed products like peanut butter are not a great choice with their high saturated fat content and trans fatty acids. Use sparingly and choose natural brands like Laura Scudders.

COCONUT: semi-solid at room temperature, even unprocessed, coconut oil is extremely high in saturated fats. Use sparingly, if at all.

HIDDEN FATS: they are everywhere. Choose to eliminate processed foods that are higher than 20 percent fat. To determine the average fat calories add a zero to the weight in grams (15 grams of fat is approximately 150 calories).

MONO- AND POLYUNSATURATED FATS: these are the healthy fats. They do not clog arteries, in moderation; can contribute to a healthy diet. They include olive, flaxseed and walnut oils.

SATURATED FAT: this solid fat, is found in beef, butter, lard, cheese, the skin of chicken, whole milk, whipped cream, egg yolks and other products that come from animals. Coconut and palm oils also are saturated. Too much saturated fat raises the level of artery-clogging cholesterol.

PALM KERNEL AND PALM OIL: differing in their chemical composition, palm oils contain palmitic and oleic acids, which are the two most common fatty acids around. Palm oils are about 50% saturated. Palm kernel oil contains primarily lauric acid and is 80% saturated.

TRANS FAT (TRANS FATTY ACIDS): these are formed when oil is hydrogenated. Some naturally occurring trans fats can be found in small amounts in animal products. Like saturated fat, trans fat raises the level of harmful blood cholesterol (LDL) and lowers the more beneficial HDL cholesterol. Trans fats are found in many processed, convenience and fast foods—French fries, fried chicken, donuts, pastries, cookies, crackers and some breakfast cereals.

PARTIALLY HYDROGENATED OIL: this manufacturing process creates trans fat. A hydrogen atom is mixed with non-saturated liquid oil from plants like corn or soy to make fat such as shortening and margarine that stay solid at room temperature.

FRACTIONATED OIL: a manufacturing process that uses high temperatures or solvents to separate hydrogenated oil into liquid and solid parts creates this type of oil. When listed on food labels, it indicates the presence of trans fat.

Points to remember:

- Fat can be considered an oxymoron, however, it remains an important part of a well-balanced nutrition plan.
- Cholesterol is the main villain in the on-going battle with heart health, and dietary fat is directly related to cholesterol levels in the blood.
- Low-density lipoprotein, widely known as LDL, is the unhealthy (bad) cholesterol. High-density lipoprotein, or HDL is the healthy (good) cholesterol.
- Unsaturated fats are broken down into two categories: mono-unsaturated and polyunsaturated. Called essential fatty acids, they are derived mainly from plant and deep-water fish sources and are liquid at room temperature.
- Polyunsaturated fats are of two main kinds: omega-3 and omega-6 fatty acids. The ideal ratio is to eat twice as many omega-3 fat sources than omega-6 fat sources.
- Saturated fat—the bad (unhealthy) fat, whose carbon atoms are saturated with hydrogen, are solid and negatively affect our arteries.
- One 12-ounce steak comes with a whopping 75 grams of saturated fat, an extra lean (trimmed fat) sirloin steak has approximately nine grams, while a portion of skinless chicken breast has only two grams of saturated fat. One gram of fat equals nine calories.
- The worst fat on the market today is often referred to as trans fat or trans fatty acids.
- Hydrogenated and partially hydrogenated oils can be found in margarine, baked goods, deep-fried and pre-packaged foods.

17

The Protein Puzzle

*"The word protein means **of first importance.**"*
—Hippocrates

The weight-loss industry is chock-full of controversial theories surrounding the consumption of protein. The U.S. government Daily Reference Values state that protein should comprise 10 percent of your daily calories (for adults and children over the age of four). Some authors say to eat carbohydrates (carbs) until noon, followed by only protein the rest of the day. There is also the popular high carb/low protein diet. With all this conflicting information, no wonder the puzzle surrounding protein remains such an enigma.

Instead of climbing aboard the "he said, she said" nutrition bandwagon, we are instead going to go beyond the assumptions printed in biased books and published in outdated research. In this chapter you will be introduced to the proven principles of protein nutrition that reflect the latest research and safest approach to achieving optimum health. From the information provided here you can piece together the importance of protein and how it benefits your health and fat-loss goals.

Protein is arguably the most misunderstood of the three macronutrients. However, with all the mystery encasing protein, one thing we do know for sure is that without its consumption, combined with carbs and fat, life would not be possible. Practically every cell in your body expends considerable time and energy manufacturing various types of proteins. Every imaginable part and function of your body utilizes protein in some way—from the enzymes critical to the digestion of food to the fibers that serve to plug leaky blood vessels.

As children we were raised with this indelible image of protein as something of a nutritional hero. For many of us, the idea of living without protein meant going without fried chicken or barbequed ribs.

As time passed however, the smoke of Sunday BBQs began to clear and the effects related to the over-consumption of animal protein slowly began to emerge. In recent years, researchers have linked a high intake of animal protein to heart disease, osteoporosis and other disorders. Despite these widely publicized findings, most people we talk to and meet in seminars throughout North America still choose high-protein diets when attempting weight loss.

As you begin to process the information provided in this chapter and become more aware of protein, its consumption and purpose, keep in mind that you are likely to hear different philosophies surrounding how it can and cannot benefit you. For example, if you were to walk into a gym and ask a bodybuilder what he thinks of protein, it is almost guaranteed that he would advocate the consumption of 1.5 to 3 grams per pound of body weight daily to acquire and maintain lean muscle tissue. If you talk to a vegetarian you may be instead lectured as to the harmful effects of animal and dairy protein, prompting the likely question, "If I don't eat enough meat, how will I get protein?"

What these examples show is that you are likely to hear different philosophies surrounding protein depending on the source. The debate ranges from which source of protein is the most complete to which type of protein is essential for building muscle. As if that weren't enough, when you add in the media hype and empty promises offered by high-protein advocates and self-anointed "diet gurus," all you end up with is a recipe for confusion.

Our goal is to answer many of your questions about protein. We encourage you to use this information as a foundation, rather than an absolute, and continue to pursue the necessary answers when making decisions regarding your health. The purpose of this chapter is to share with you facts on the following:

- The structure and function of protein
- Typical protein sources
- Common misconceptions about protein
- How much is too much

What is protein?

Proteins are very much like carbs. Both are made up of carbon, hydrogen and oxygen, however, protein is also comprised of nitrogen and occasionally sulphur. It is the presence of nitrogen that sets protein apart from the other macronutrients. As in the case of carbohydrates, each gram of protein, by weight, provides four calories of energy.

Proteins are made up of sub-units called amino acids. According to the University of California, Berkeley, *Wellness Letter Book* there are 22 different kinds of amino acids that are used to make proteins in humans. The body can manufacture 13 amino acids on its own; these are called "nonessential." The other nine amino acids are alternately labeled "essential." The reason an amino acid is considered essential is that the body does not produce it; therefore, it must instead be derived from whole foods. This includes the amino acid, histidine. Adults generally produce adequate amounts of histidine, however, this is not the case when it comes to children. Healthy sources of histidine are drawn from poultry, fish and soy-based food.

With 22 different kinds of amino acids available, every cell in your body can choose from the pool of amino acids in order to construct specific proteins to meet the very diverse needs of human physiology.

When a food contains all of the essential amino acids, it is categorized as a complete protein. If it is missing any of the essential amino acids, it is considered incomplete. All animal proteins—red meats, poultry, fish, and eggs—are complete proteins. For the most part, all plant proteins are incomplete proteins, with the exception of soybeans and soy based foods such as tofu, which are complete.

However, a combination of incomplete protein sources can be made complete by eating them in the same meal or within the same day with another protein. For instance, rice and beans as well as peanut butter and bread are traditional combinations that provide complementary proteins, making them complete. Most incomplete proteins will be burned for energy instead of used to build and repair tissue unless the missing amino acid can be obtained from another food source. Case in point: rice proteins are incomplete because they're missing the amino acid lysine. However, by adding beans to the meal, which are rich in the amino acid lysine, you have a complete protein. As well, bean proteins become complete when a food rich in the amino acid, methionine is added. Guess what contains a lot of methionine? You guessed correct—rice.

With 22 different kinds of amino acids available, every cell in your body can choose from the pool of amino acids in order to construct specific proteins to meet the very diverse needs of human physiology. For example, you have a combination of amino acids (hemoglobin) that make it possible to shuttle oxygen to living tissue. Insulin (responsible for getting glucose into the muscles) is composed of 51 amino acids. Amino acids are responsible for a number of functions involved in maintaining life, from hormone production to immune function.

Protein breakdown

Now that you are aware of what makes up a protein, what exactly are amino acids? The amino group of one amino acid can link with the acid group of another amino acid to form a chain of amino acids. This link is referred to as a peptide bond. When two amino acids are joined together, a di-peptide (di = "two") is formed; when three amino acids are joined together, a tri-peptide (tri = "three") is formed; finally, when four or more amino acids join together, a poly-peptide (poly = "many") is formed. A typical protein may contain 500 or more amino acids, joined together by peptide bonds. Each protein has its own specific number and sequence of amino acids. Other bonds, sometimes containing sulphur, also hold the chains of amino acids making up a protein. The shape of the molecule is important as it often determines the function of the protein. Each species, including man, has its own characteristic proteins. The proteins of human muscle, for instance, are different from those of beef muscle. As we continue to provide you with more pieces of the protein puzzle, consider five of protein's most important functions:

- **Proteins are messengers:** they are involved in the transmission of nerve impulses through our body. They make up substances called neurotransmitters and neuro-peptides that are responsible for sending messages to and from the brain and facilitating communication between cells. Hormones are also made up of proteins. These are essential in maintaining communication and control of the human body. Without certain kinds of protein, we would not be able to send or receive signals to and from our brain or tell our liver to metabolize fats. Therefore, our entire intra-cellular communication is derived from protein.
- **Proteins are transporters:** proteins are involved in the transportation of a variety of particles throughout our bodies, ranging from electrons to macromolecules. For example, a protein that is attached to our red blood cells transports iron; fat is coated in protein in order to be absorbed into the blood stream and transported to the liver to be metabolized.
- **Structural proteins:** proteins are responsible for the contracting and strengthening of muscle tissue. Other organic material such as hair, bone and collagen (found in skin, nails and connective tissue) is also made up of proteins. Without protein, you would not be able to heal a cut on your finger nor mend a broken bone.

- **Proteins fight infection:** protein is responsible for the production of white blood cells (our immune system), and antibodies are proteins that bind to foreign particles such as bacteria and viruses. When you are unable to fight off a virus or infection, your doctor gives you synthetic proteins in the form of antibiotics.
- **Protein can prevent cravings for sweets:** protein aids in the regulation of blood glucose to help stabilize our energy so we don't get those highs and lows during the day. Protein can slow absorption of glucose into the bloodstream so you won't get that insulin surge. When your blood sugar is at a moderate level, you are less likely to crave sweets. We tend to crave sweets when our blood sugar is too low!

Protein can prevent cravings for sweets: protein aids in the regulation of blood glucose to help stabilize our energy so we don't get those highs and lows during the day.

Protein digestion

Regardless of which protein source you choose, immediately following the initial physical breakdown of chewing, the chemical breakdown of protein begins in the stomach. As the food settles in your stomach, a chemical breakdown begins with the secretion of a substance called pepsinogen which, when combined with the hydrochloric acid in our stomach, is converted into an enzyme called pepsin. This enzyme along with rennin found in gastric juice serves as a catalyst causing giant protein molecules to begin breaking down into peptides (amino acids). As they are being broken down, the muscle in your stomach walls then moves these peptides into the duodenum, which is the first part of the small intestine. At this point, and with the help of the enzymes peptidases and trypsin, the duodenum and pancreas work together to complete the digestion of amino acids. Finally, amino acids are absorbed through the wall of the small intestine and are introduced into the bloodstream.

The process of eating a chicken breast (protein source) and then having it breakdown into smaller molecules (amino acids), which the body can absorb and then use to fuel other life processes is simply miraculous. The human "machine" of digestion must work properly in order for this process to produce useful amino acids. Therefore, it is only to our individual benefit that we choose our protein sources carefully. The more concentrated the protein source is with saturated fat and trans fatty acids, the more difficult it is for your machine (body) to complete this process.

Protein sources

When it comes to eating foods that contain primarily protein, there are a wide variety of sources to choose from. You have whole foods like meat, turkey, chicken and fish. There's milk, yogurt, bread, pasta, beans and grain products; even vegetables contain a fair amount of protein. For instance, if your daily calories consisted of no more than broccoli, you'd exceed the Recommended Dietary Allowance (RDA) of protein, however broccoli alone would be incomplete.

When most people think of protein, they automatically generate an image of some kind of animal-based protein (i.e., steak, beef, milk). However, what many people aren't aware of is that you can get all your protein needs from a plant-based diet (i.e., grains, beans, greens). From spinach to asparagus to lemons, most all vegetables, grains and fruit contain some degree of protein (amino acids). This is not to say that we are recommending you give up animal-based protein sources. All we're doing is helping you become aware of how easy it is to consume adequate amounts of protein. Whether it is meat, vegetable or grain, protein is protein. When broken down to a molecular level, it is what it is: a chain of amino acids.

Supplementing protein

If you feel that you are often hurried, not eating enough food or possibly lacking sufficient protein, you may decide it is necessary to supplement your daily protein intake by consuming partially digested proteins called hydrosylates (found primarily in protein powders). You also have free-form amino acids, which are nothing but formulations containing single peptides. Just walk into practically any supplement store and you will be mesmerized and probably overwhelmed by an endless array of protein sources in the form of powders, pills and liquids. However, if you decide to use a protein source outside of whole foods, be sure the amino acids you consume are essential (histidine, isoleucine, leucine, lysine, methionine, phenylalanine, threonine, tryptophan, valine).

If a person can eat broccoli and consume the government's recommended dietary allowance of protein, why the large selection of protein sources over and above real food? This is due partly to our "hurry up and go" society and the constant debate and marketing hype over which protein source is the best for building and maintaining that all-important muscle tissue.

The ever-expanding protein propaganda continues to fuel the misconception that in order to build muscle it is necessary to consume large amounts of protein. The reason for this is that there is some actual truth intertwined with this misconception. As we have mentioned, it is true that protein consumption is essential for building new cells for the purpose of muscle growth and repair. It is also true that the more athletic a person is, the more cell repair is needed. However, protein itself is not a stimulus for muscle growth. The question then that remains is: "How much protein is enough?"

Recommended dietary allowance (RDA)

How much protein is sufficient for sustaining life? What's needed for meeting the demands of resistance (strength) training? These are questions without simple answers. We have learned through our experience that the amount of protein necessary varies from person to person and is dependent on individual physiology and activity level. For this reason, we agree with many sports physiologists and coaches who believe that athletes and bodybuilders require more protein than those who are sedentary. However, we also believe that additional protein intake can be achieved as a result of increasing overall daily calories.

First, let's look at the Food and Nutrition Board of the National Academy of Sciences dietary guidelines for protein, and then explore two extremes: 1) How much is enough? and 2) How low can you go? After that, we believe you'll be able to come to your own conclusion about how much protein is necessary for the lifestyle you want to lead. Now to get the ball rolling, let's take a closer look at the RDA.

The Food and Nutrition Board (FHB) of the National Academy of Sciences (NAS) establish the Recommended Dietary Allowances (RDAs). These numerical values provide nutrition guidance to health professionals and to the general public. RDA is generally accepted throughout the world as a valid source of information. At least 40 different nations and organizations have published standards similar to the RDA.

Up close with the RDA

The RDA was established to address the nutritional needs of the average healthy person living in the United States. With this said, what is the RDA?

First of all, the RDA is the average daily dietary intake of a nutrient that is sufficient to meet the requirement of nearly all (97-98%) healthy persons. When it comes to consumption, the RDA for adults is 0.8 grams of protein for each kilogram (2.2 pounds) of body weight. That adds up to 64 grams of pure protein for a 175-pound man, and 47 grams for a 130-pound woman. If you are curious about how you measure up to the RDA protein guidelines, divide your weight in pounds by 2.2 to get your weight in kilograms. Then simply multiply your kilogram weight by 0.8 to calculate the RDA standard protein requirement for adults. For example, if you weigh 150 pounds and divide it by 2.2, you'll find you weigh 68.18 kilograms. Multiplied by 0.8, you'll come up with 54.54 grams for your daily protein requirement.

To help you better understand where grams of protein come from, consider that milk, chicken, and fish have six to eight grams per ounce. Eating a four-ounce chicken breast yields approximately 24 grams of protein. As well, a one-pound steak can supply 100 grams of protein by itself. For a 175-pound man, eating a fair amount of vegetables along with a one-pound (16 ounce) steak doubles his RDA in one meal.

As you become more aware of which foods do and don't contain protein, you will find it difficult not to meet the RDA. When one cup of milk contains eight grams of protein; yogurt, 10 to 13 grams per cup; an egg, six grams—getting your supply of protein is easily accomplished. For instance, people who track their protein consumption very rarely include a slice of bread or half-cup of pasta, which consist of three grams each, in their calculations. For the most part, people only count foods that are considered "high" in protein (i.e., meat, dairy products), therefore underestimating the amount they are actually consuming.

Consider how much protein is found in foods generally categorized as carbs: Beans have seven grams per half-cup (cooked); nuts, six grams per ounce; and grain products (often overlooked as protein sources) supply 16 to 20 percent of our total protein intake. As mentioned earlier, vegetables contain protein, a half-cup (one serving) of broccoli or asparagus yields two grams.

For most people, four ounces of lean meat, a cup of beans, and a cup each of pasta, yogurt, and milk supply more than enough protein in one day. But, if you were to perform resistance training and exercise regularly, maybe you would benefit from more protein. What then, is the high end of the protein consumption spectrum?

How much is enough?

There are hundreds of thousands of people who have lost weight on high protein diets. In the short term, it is likely that you may lose weight on such a diet, but it may prove dangerous to your health as we discussed in

Chapter 14, *Carbohydrate Confusion*. Let's be clear—a high intake of protein is not the solution for keeping the excess fat off.

"How much protein is enough for exercising bodies who want to be fit and gain and maintain that all-important muscle tissue?"

We agree with the American Heart Association that high protein diets are not healthy, however, larger amounts of protein are necessary for some of us. For instance, children, teenagers, burn victims, people recovering from illness, and pregnant or nursing mothers benefit from a little more protein per kilogram of body weight than the RDA. On top of that, there are additional protein necessities for high intensity athletes and bodybuilders. However, the question that remains is, "How much protein is enough for exercising bodies who want to be fit and gain and maintain that all-important muscle tissue?"

It does appear that both strength and endurance athletes require more cell repair than inactive, healthy people, so it makes sense that an increased consumption of protein is important to highly active people. In our experience, both as athletes and weight-loss, health and fitness specialists, almost all of our clients who perform both resistance training and cardiovascular exercise benefit from more than the RDA—from 125 percent (1.0 g/kg body weight) to about 175 percent (1.5 g/kg body weight). And in cases where the client or athlete is in a caloric deficit, we may recommend up to 35 percent of his or her total daily calories come from protein.

We believe that this amount of increased protein is easy to acquire from a healthy diet, because the more active you are, the higher your energy needs, and thus the more food you eat. For example, we may recommend that a 140-pound long distance runner consume 64 grams of protein per day (using 1.0 g/kg), and a 200-pound wrestler consume 136 grams of protein (using 1.5 g/kg). The bottom line is that for most people who perform high intensity athletics, and partake in resistance training and cardiovascular exercise regularly, there may be a substantial benefit from increased protein beyond the RDA.

In the world of bodybuilding, consuming 1.5 grams per kilogram of body weight is usually not enough. We have met bodybuilders who consume two to three grams per pound of body weight, for instance. At 200 pounds, this means consuming 600 grams of protein per day. Though we believe this is a prime example of excessive protein consumption, many bodybuilders swear by this approach. But according to one of the most notable bodybuilders and action stars of all time, this penchant for protein often is taken too far. In Arnold Schwarzenegger's book, *Arnold's Body Building for Men*, he writes: "Kids nowadays... tend to go overboard when they discover bodybuilding and eat diets consisting of 50 to 70% protein—something I believe to be totally unnecessary...(In) my formula for basic good eating: eat about one gram of protein for every two pounds of body weight." If a 200-pound man where to adhere to Arnold's formula he would consume approximately 100 grams of protein per day.

With the average American consuming more protein than the RDA, some to the extent of 50 percent more, there is no actual evidence that a high intake of protein endangers your health, provided the protein isn't accompanied by much unhealthy fat. Then again, no matter how much you weigh and what activities you take part in, we recommend that you do not consume more than twice the RDA (unless under the supervision and care of a medical doctor, registered dietician or Wellness Weight-Loss Coach). Keeping your protein intake under twice the RDA is in agreement with the National Research Council.

So, if you weigh 200 pounds and are consuming more than 150 grams of protein per day, cut back. Also note that it is important to acquire as much protein as you can from plant-based foods, rather than sources that contain unhealthy fats. Lastly, to help you move into a healthier relationship with your protein consumption, it's time to become familiar with the effect of exceeding your body's protein needs.

Beyond the limits

The question, "How much protein is necessary to gain and maintain lean muscle tissue?" is likely to remain unsolved, forever the fodder of debate. However, with a large majority of people concluding that carbs are bad and protein is good, the American philosophy of more continues to translate into better. With this kind of mindset, a growing number of people now worry about not getting enough protein. What many people don't know is that it's practically impossible in our culture to be protein deficient. But, what happens when you eat over and beyond what is truly necessary?

Some people incorrectly believe that in order to build muscle, consuming more protein is required. Unfortunately, eating more protein will not cause cells to create more body proteins. For this reason and according to current research, we do not recommend protein consumption above 35 percent of your daily calories. Aside from stressing your kidneys, increased protein, by itself, is not a stimulus for muscle growth.

The way you stimulate muscle growth is through exercise, specifically through resistance (strength) training.

> In the fifth report in a series of reports from the FHB presenting Dietary Reference Values for the intake of nutrients by Americans and Canadians, adults are encouraged to get 10 to 35 percent of their daily calories from protein.

To make more sense why more does not equal better in the protein puzzle, take a closer look at what happens when you exceed what you really need. As your body uses broken down proteins (amino acids) to meet cell demands, whatever is left is excess. So what happens inside the cells of people eating more protein than they need to make body proteins? This excess (ketoacids) is either used as a source of energy or is converted to glucose (gluconeogenesis) or body fat.

The reality is that protein is not a clean burning fuel. For one, it contains nitrogen, unlike carbs and fat. Secondly, nitrogen leaves ashes in the body when protein is burned. These ashes are in the form of amino acids, which flood the system and create a large workload for the liver and kidneys, which have to get rid of them. Remember, our body prefers carbs and fat as its primary source of fuel; therefore, consuming excess protein is not an efficient way to energize the body.

We are often asked, "What about repairing and building muscle tissue after breaking it down through resistance training? Isn't it imperative to consume more protein?" It may be hard to believe for those who give all the credit for their lean physique to a high intake of protein, but the aforesaid recommendations are efficient for increasing muscle size as long as you perform resistance training.

According to Dr. Carol Meredith at the University of California at Davis, muscle protein synthesis decreases during exercise and nearly doubles during recovery. Her research demonstrates that additional protein (studies of 1.35 grams of protein per kilogram of body weight per day) does not increase muscle mass or strength. However, resistance training like weight lifting has proven to be a powerful anabolic (building) process that improves protein synthesis (increased muscle tissue).

If you are concerned about whether or not you are consuming too much protein—there is an easy way to tell. When you over consume protein, you will excrete excess nitrogen in the urine, however, some is lost in the feces, sweat, through the skin, fingernails, hair and other bodily excretions. If you are consuming more nitrogen than you are excreting, you're in a positive nitrogen balance, and may store nitrogen in the body. If you are consuming the same amount of nitrogen that you're excreting, you are simply in nitrogen balance. But, if you are excreting more nitrogen than you are consuming, you are in negative nitrogen balance and are losing body protein.

Unless you are going to have your doctor conduct a urinary urea nitrogen test—comparing the amount of nitrogen (from dietary protein) coming into the body versus what is being lost—we recommend that you take notice of the odor of your urine. For instance, if you become aware of a strong odor in the urine (it is usually quite strong and easy to identify), cut back on your protein and increase your water intake. If the condition persists longer than three to five days, consult your doctor to rule out other conditions.

Countries with the highest consumption of animal-based products also have the greatest incidence of osteoporosis, atherosclerosis, heart attacks and strokes.

How low can you go?

Before reading this book, you probably assumed that eating an ample amount of meat meant you were getting plenty of protein. Though most meat products are complete proteins, you probably weren't aware that countries with the highest consumption of animal-based products, such as the United States, Sweden and Finland, also have the greatest incidence of osteoporosis, atherosclerosis, heart attacks and strokes. As well, excess protein, which is linked to diets rich in animal-based foods, have been proven to cause destruction of kidney tissue, progressive deterioration of kidney function and a loss of calcium from your bones.

In response to the question, "How little is too little protein?" first consider the philosophy that if you only eat animal-based protein, you will die; however, on the flip side, if you follow a plant-based diet you will thrive. If you find this difficult to believe, consider the accomplishments of the Olympic Gold Medalist and once-dominant 400-meter hurdler, Edwin Moses. This vegetarian went eight straight years without losing a race. Then you have the vegetarian who captured bodybuilding's 1980 Mr. International title, Andreas Cahling. His physique was so impressive during his competition days that he was often referred to as the next Arnold Schwarzenegger. In addition to these two examples, the list of highly accomplished athletes who acquire their protein solely through a plant-based diet continues to prove its weight in gold.

After finalizing that even the most demanding training methods can be performed without increased protein needs, we decided to venture out and discover what many experts consider low consumption of protein. As we began researching the low end of protein consumption, we discovered a wide spectrum. On the low end of human protein needs, it was reported by the American Journal of Clinical Nutrition that we need only two and a half percent of our daily calories from protein. To our contentment, many populations have lived in excellent health on this amount. In addition, the National Research Council says that just over eight percent of our calories need to be from protein. This figure however, was not based on a minimum, but what is recommended for the majority of the population.

Further studies have shown that most healthy people can stay in nitrogen balance on as little as 20 grams of high-quality protein per day. Less than that, and the body starts breaking down protein structures like internal organs and muscles, which reduces your body's ability to function normally and resist disease. But, what is considered "high-quality" protein?

Animal and plant-based proteins

All animal and plant cells contain some protein, but the amount of protein present in food varies widely. And along with the amount of protein, the quality of protein is also important, and that depends on the amino acids that are present. If a protein contains the essential amino acids in the proportion required by humans, it is said to have a high biological value. If it is comparatively low in one or more of the essential amino acids it is said to have a low biological value.

In general, proteins from animal sources have a higher biological value than protein from plant sources, but this is not to say that you can't acquire your protein needs from plant sources alone.

In 1993 the Protein Digestibility Corrected Amino Acid Score (PDCAAS) was adopted by many health organizations as the method of evaluating protein quality based on human amino acid requirements. The PDCCAS is based on the digestibility, essential amino acid profile and its ability to supply these amino acids to humans. (Past measurement methods were based on the amino acid requirements of rats). According to the PDCAAS rating system, soy protein is equal in quality to that of casein (protein in dairy), and egg whites.

Regardless of whether you decide to increase or decrease your current protein intake, remember that if you are eating high quantities of dairy and animal protein, you are also consuming unhealthy fats, drugs, and hormones. If you have a difficult time envisioning life without animal protein, we encourage you to purchase free-range chicken, turkey, and beef. You may want to experiment with ostrich, bison or wild range meats as an alternative to those found in common grocery stores.

By minimizing the consumption of animal-based proteins such as cured meats (i.e., bacon, salami, hot dogs), you will also avoid chemicals like nitrates and nitrites, which are known to form carcinogens in the stomach. In place of these cured meats we recommend taking baby steps in the direction of products made from turkey or veggie versions made from soy.

According to Dr. John A. McDougall, dairy products like cow's milk, for example, are not only high in saturated fat, but also linked to ear infections, respiratory problems and allergies in children, and even gastrointestinal conditions and osteoporosis in adults. The author of both The McDougall Plan and McDougall's Medicine, he has over 1600 references to back up his work.

Last word

This may be the last word on protein for this chapter, but it's not the final word when it comes to the nutrition science of protein consumption. Despite poorly designed studies of protein needs, and the many different opinions preached in books, magazines and newspaper articles on protein consumption, we strongly believe that as long as nitrogen balance is considered and unhealthy fats are kept to a minimum, most people need not worry about too much or too little protein.

As you are beginning to learn more about your body and how to prioritize your health, we recommend that you begin calculating how much protein you currently consume daily. Once you have an estimate of your daily intake, we encourage you to calculate your protein needs according to the RDA; have your percentage of body fat assessed and adhere to the RDA for two weeks. At the two-week mark, have your body fat assessed again to discover whether you gained or lost body fat and lean body mass. In the meantime, if you feel like you are lacking energy, increase your carb and healthy fat calories. Continue this process until you come into agreement with your body's protein needs.

Keep your protein consumption simple. Entire populations have benefited from avoiding many of the animal-based proteins that run rampant in America and consuming more cold-water fish (i.e., halibut, sea bass) and soy products. Take, for instance, the people that reside in Okinawa. They have the largest population of centenarians in the world and they eat very little animal-based protein. The same goes for those who adhere to the traditional Mediterranean diet, which also is low in saturated fats.

As we conclude this chapter and move toward bringing the how, when and what to eat into focus, we hope that you are more aware of the importance of protein and its recommended ranges. While the protein puzzle remains unsolved, in time and with consistency in your efforts, you will be able to determine what is ideal for you and your activity level. Remember, it is your choice to either create health or diminish it with your protein choices.

Points to remember:

- Without the consumption of protein, life would be impossible.
- Protein is comprised of carbon, hydrogen, oxygen and occasionally sulphur.
- There are 22 different kinds of amino acids that are used to make proteins in humans, according to the University of California, Berkeley, *Wellness Letter Book*.
- We agree with the American Heart Association that very high-protein diets are not healthy. However, it appears that both strength and endurance athletes require more cell repair than inactive, healthy people, so it makes sense that an increased consumption of protein is important to highly active people.
- You can meet all your protein needs with a plant-based diet.
- Protein is not a clean burning fuel. It contains nitrogen (unlike carbs and fat), and nitrogen leaves ashes in the body when protein is burned.
- If you are consuming more nitrogen than you are excreting, you're in a positive nitrogen balance, and are storing nitrogen in the body. If you are consuming the same amount of nitrogen that you're excreting, you are simply in nitrogen balance. But, if you are excreting more nitrogen than you are consuming, you are in negative nitrogen balance and are losing body protein.
- It is your choice to either create health or continue diminishing it with your protein choices.

18

Food for Thought

"Let thy food be thy medicine and thy medicine be thy food."
—Hippocrates

Are you ready to come face to face with one of the most blatant culprits blocking millions of people from releasing fat for the last time? If you think it is lack of exercise—take a second look at the title of this chapter. Although millions of people are exercising at home and in health clubs, most remain stagnant in their attempts to release fat. This doesn't mean exercise is irrelevant, because it's not. Exercise is essential for releasing fat and creating health daily; however, what you put in your mouth is of equal importance.

You could easily argue the fact that nutrition is 80 percent responsible for whether or not you release fat. All the same, nutrition alone, especially in the form of low-calorie diets, does not equate to long-term success. Consider those who remain sedentary, but target weight loss by eating less and less just to lower their total body weight. As a result of this approach, metabolism is often slowed—making weight loss more difficult with age. The good news is—it doesn't have to be this way!

Now that you are more familiar with carbs, fiber, fats and protein consumption, it is time to coach you into a healthy, tight, toned and trim body. In addition to the role of exercise which we explain in the following chapters and Appendix C, this chapter brings food into perspective by helping you better understand what, when, how much and how often to eat. We are not asking you to turn your back on what you may consider part of your cultural beliefs or tradition, but to consider the principle of adaptation: health is created and fat is released through the process of adjusting to the law of cause and effect. Simply put, in order to evolve, adjustments and changes are necessary.

Keep an open mind

Regardless of your ethnicity, nationality and social beliefs, there are certain foods that cause you to gain fat. Equally, there are foods that help you release fat. With this said, we encourage you to approach this chapter with an open mind—allowing you to discover and develop methods of eating that not only keep pleasure in your food, but honor your desire to attain and maintain a fit, firm and healthy lifestyle. To the contrary, you may decide to resist and maintain a need to eat the way you were raised and or the way many in your family continue to eat—and that's your choice. However, it is our hope that at this point you come to accept that white flour, deep fried and highly processed foods (to name just a few) contribute to deadly diseases and interfere with your ability to permanently release fat and create health. Accepting this reality can serve as a boundary for establishing an empowering relationship with food.

Diet no more

The major difference between the lifestyle we encourage and that of many diets and various commercial weight-loss programs is that we do not favor restrictions, authorized recipes, deprivation, or "legal and illegal" foods. We help you look at food as either healthy or unhealthy— nothing more, nothing less. Considering certain foods as forbidden is a true indicator that you are tagged with a diet mentality. It is this diet mentality that serves as a major roadblock to releasing fat that doesn't come back.

Imagine never feeling deprived or restricted, yet still able to release fat. Sounds inviting, doesn't it? Believe it or not, it all begins with becoming aware that you have a choice; and it is this ability to choose what you eat and don't eat that causes you to break free from the diet mentality. To help you determine whether or not you have a diet mentality, ask yourself the following questions:

- Do I feel restricted?
- Do I feel deprived?
- Do I feel like I'm making a sacrifice?
- Do I feel bad (i.e., guilt, shame, let down) when I eat foods that are unhealthy?
- Do I ever say things like, "I can't have that (i.e., cake, donut)?"

If you answer "yes" to any of the above questions, you are in fact trapped in a diet mentality. We know it may be difficult to accept, but there is light at the end of the tunnel. You can overcome this roadblock by taking responsibility for the choices you make, and being accountable to your values and self-promise to release fat and create health daily. Please understand that no one is perfect, and there may be situations during the next 365 days where your only food option is an unhealthy one.

However, if and when you make unhealthy choices, notice whether or not you feel guilt or judgment toward yourself. You may say things like, "Why did I eat that?" or "I blew it, I messed up." If so, you probably have a diet mentality. Nonetheless, there are people who eat unhealthy and do not experience inner-turmoil. When this is the case, it's likely that these people are in denial, or refuse to accept the reality that what they choose to eat doesn't honor their well being. This type of attitude and behavior is one of the roadblocks that stop people from releasing fat for the last time.

Establishing a healthy appetite for both the food you eat and the thoughts you think is how you experience lasting success.

Food for thought

Establishing a healthy appetite for both the food you eat and the thoughts you think is how you experience lasting success. If you allow your mind to think you're on a diet, you're doomed. Sooner or later, you are likely to snap and go back to your old eating habits. Before long, your old habits will have you back to the weight of your past.

If you don't think you are on a diet, but you feel deprived and restricted, guess what? You are blinded with a diet mentality; therefore you are on a diet. If you want to move past the diet mentality, take this chapter seriously and implement the eating recommendations until you consciously accept the reality of a lifestyle removed from ever dieting again. You will know that you are past dieting when you no longer feel restricted, and understand that you have a choice in every moment of your life—eating what and whenever you want.

How do you know for sure whether or not you are trapped in a diet mentality? The thoughts you think and the words you use are true indicators. For instance, if you hear yourself saying, "I can't eat that," and "That is not allowed," then you are on a diet. When you begin hearing yourself think and say things like, "I can eat whatever and whenever I want—the choice is mine and I prefer to eat something else," then you are not trapped in a diet mentality. Every chapter in this book offers you suggestions and tools for removing the diet mentality from your thoughts and vocabulary.

Moving into a healthier relationship with food is no easy task, however, after reading this chapter you will be much more equipped to succeed. By allowing us to walk you through a day of eating the Wellness Weight-Loss way—you will discover that choosing to eat healthy can be enjoyable. This is all possible by becoming familiar with portion sizes (for breakfast, lunch, dinner and snacks), eating frequency and timing, tracking, the importance of drinking water, and the power of daily planning. All in all, it is our goal to empower you with a road map to a lifestyle that has no restrictions and does not endorse concepts like "authorized foods" or "cheat days."

If you haven't heard, LIFESTYLE literally means a whole way of living—100 percent of the time.

To cheat or not to cheat

Have you ever heard someone recommend to eat healthy Monday through Friday, but have your way (cheat day or free day) on the weekend? As one of our clients did the math, this would mean a lifestyle where you eat healthy 71.5 percent of the time and eat unhealthy 28.5 percent of the time. Believe it or not, folks, there are weight-loss programs and people who advocate this approach to healthy living. Some programs feel that having one day to eat whatever you want is beneficial psychologically. We say hogwash to such statements. If you haven't heard, LIFESTYLE literally means a whole way of living—100 percent of the time. People ask us all the time whether or not we believe in a free day and we always respond by saying, "Everyday is a free day."

Have you made a decision to release fat? If so, shortly after making this decision, did you feel deprived—craving sweets, chocolate, and high-fat and refined foods? As you were craving these foods that you don't typically eat, did you notice the communication going on in your head? You start telling yourself that this is the last time...you will succeed... you have the willpower and discipline to fulfill your self-promise. But, somehow, for some odd reason you can't seem to understand, you find yourself sitting at the kitchen table eating that very thing you felt deprived of. Sound familiar?

It's hard to imagine going from eating practically anything you want, whenever you want, to never having a donut or fried food again. Even those with somewhat strict eating habits can find themselves having periodic splurges (i.e., ice cream, French fries). So it's wise to remember that whatever its form—donut, pizza, cocktail or fried shrimp—unhealthy foods are nonetheless unhealthy.

As with any food, healthy or unhealthy, its effects on the body largely depend on the amount consumed, with caloric excess causing fat gain. So, you eat reasonably all week, watching your portions only to have your goal disrupted by what many refer to as a "free day" or "cheat day;" the widely accepted method of postponing unhealthy cravings until that one day per week where you engage into conscious, yet reckless consumption. With that said, the choice of a free day or weekly cheat may open the door to sabotaging your weight-loss efforts.

Meet Josephine

Josephine was a keen member of a health club and she insisted on having a free day. Unfortunately, this free day seemed to be implemented when Josephine experienced major cravings. It was obvious that Josephine was always having a free day. For instance, she said her free day was every Saturday, however, one Friday night at a dinner party and as a result of her friend's pressure, Josephine decided to have her free day a day earlier.

Josephine wanted to evolve into a lifestyle that improved her health—resulting in a fit and toned body, but the weekly cheat day proved to be the very thing that held her from making the quantum leap into eating and being healthy 100 percent of the time. This is not to say that a piece of chocolate or an occasional dessert is out of the question, because it's not. Going for a healthy piece of dark chocolate and a dessert that is not made with disease-linked ingredients like trans fatty acids is definitely an option.

Cheat and free days are nothing short of a temporary fix. We encourage you to discover how you can BE healthy 100 percent of the time. So, BEWARE of those who endorse weekly cheats—the same as you would be cautious of someone offering you a snort of cocaine once per week. That one day can be the one step toward sabotaging what is important to you.

Size matters

Between 1977 and 1996, portion sizes for key food groups grew markedly in the United States, not only at fast-food restaurants but also in homes and at conventional restaurants. The authors who provided this data, Samara Joy Nielsen and Barry M. Popkin of the University of North Carolina at Chapel Hill, found that as serving sizes have grown over the past 20 years for all categories—pizza remained the only exception.

The data revealed that over the past 20 years:

- Hamburgers have expanded by 23 percent;
- A plate of Mexican food is 27 percent larger;
- Soft drinks have increased in size by 52 percent;
- Snacks, whether they are potato chips, pretzels or crackers, are 60 percent larger.

The prevalence of adult obesity in the United States has increased from 14.5 percent in 1971 to 30.9 percent in 1999.

Not surprisingly, the prevalence of adult obesity in the United States has increased from 14.5 percent in 1971 to 30.9 percent in 1999. The blame isn't solely on restaurants. It's the responsibility of you—the consumer—to take control of what you put in your mouth. The restaurants are simply providing the consumer with what he or she wants. This "value sizing" marketing philosophy is nothing more than giving you more food for your dollar.

We can overcome the battle of obesity. Your plate doesn't have to be stacked against you. So, the first step in regaining control of your weight is learning what we mean when we say, "Size matters."

The following guidelines can help you estimate portion sizes. Keep in mind that these proposed portions are not intended to restrict how much you eat—but to help you take control of how much you eat.

Breakfast, lunch and dinner

Combine a portion of protein and a portion of carbs at breakfast, lunch and dinner. A portion size is the same as:

- the palm of your hand not to exceed the first knuckle
- a clinched fist or tennis ball
- a deck of cards
- a cassette tape
- a minimum of 20 grams

Protein example: It's lunch and you eat a chicken breast that is no bigger than the palm of your hand (three to six ounces). An example for breakfast would be five egg whites or four egg whites with one whole egg. Dinner could be a salmon fillet that extends from the base of your palm to your first knuckle.

Fibrous carbohydrate example: It's dinner and you eat a sweet potato that is no bigger than your fist or a tennis ball. Another example for breakfast would be a slice of Ezekiel toast. Lunch could be a rounded handful of wild rice.

TIP: When eating breakfast, lunch and dinner, ask yourself two questions: "Where's my protein?" and "Where is my carbohydrate?" We encourage you to eat a protein and a fibrous carbohydrate with each of your three meals. When it comes to vegetables, they're the exception. Even though they are part of your fibrous carbohydrate portion, we recommend you go with one to three fists sizes in addition to or instead of a fibrous carbohydrate (i.e., sweet potato, wild rice, 100 percent whole-wheat bread). *(See Appendix B for more meal ideas)*. Depending on your hunger and the fact that you are not eating a sweet potato, for instance, eat one to three portions of vegetables.

When eating breakfast, lunch and dinner, ask yourself two questions: "Where's my protein?" and "Where is my carbohydrate?" We encourage you to eat a protein and a fibrous carbohydrate with each of your three meals.

Snacks

A portion size for a snack can either be a protein, carbohydrate or a combination. A snack portion is the same size as:

- the palm of your hand not to exceed the first knuckle
- a clinched fist or tennis ball
- a deck of cards
- a cassette tape

Snack examples: You eat breakfast at 7 a.m. and at around 10 a.m. you eat an apple for your snack. You could have easily eaten a pear, cup of strawberries or slice of 100 percent whole wheat bread with all natural peanut butter. It is encouraged that your snack is at least 80 calories and does not exceed 200 calories for women and 300 for men. *(See Appendix B for more snack ideas)*.

More tips that might help:

- Use smaller plates and dishes so your portions won't look lost.

- There is no need to measure your food every time you eat. If you feel it is necessary for you to get an idea of how much your dishes, bowls and glasses will hold, measure once. After that, visualize the portion size. But more importantly, trust your body and portion perception to tell you when it's enough!

Visual Cue	Approx. Size	Foods
Fist or baseball	1 cup	Green salad, yogurt, med. piece of fruit, baked potato
Rounded handful	1/2 cup	Diced fruit, cooked vegetables, pasta, rice
Golf ball or large egg	1/4 cup	Dried fruit, like raisins
Cassette tape	3 ounces	Meat, poultry
Check book	3 ounces	Fish
Thumb	1 tablespoon	All natural peanut or almond butter

Frequency

Have you ever heard that eating five or six meals a day is a great way to lose weight? Although this may sound odd, it's true. Eating three meals plus snacking is a surefire method for shedding the pounds. Even if you consume the same number of calories, you will release more fat if you spread them throughout the day.

Researchers at Tufts University in Boston found that older women (average age 72) who ate mini-meals of 250 and 500 calories burned the same amount of calories per day as 25-year-old women. However, when they consumed 1,000-calorie meals, they burned 60 fewer calories than the younger women. Fact is: in order to keep your metabolism working efficiently, maximize your fat burning potential, increase your energy and experience less hunger and fewer cravings, we encourage you to eat every two to three hours. It has been our experience time and again that when our clients begin their day with breakfast and eat every two to three hours, they are 30 times more successful than those who eat sporadically and skip meals—only to binge later.

Please understand that you are not always going to be hungry. For this reason we encourage you to consider this philosophy: "eat to live, not "live to eat."

Timing is everything

Meal timing is of great importance, not only for digestion, but also for helping you keep your metabolism operating in high gear. As each day wears on, not eating in a timely manner can cause you to become so hungry that you forget about your plan, your goal and the reasons why you want to release fat. When you find yourself hungry, the only thing that matters is satisfying your hunger. When this is the case, vending machines and the donuts sitting in the reception area at work become the solution to your hunger and energy pangs.

Within one hour of waking, unless you are performing cardiovascular exercise, it is very important that you are eating breakfast. Why? Because, when you go to sleep at night, your body goes into a fast, and this fast is broken when you eat breakfast. Matter of fact, this is why we have the word breakfast; it means to break the fast. The clock starts with breakfast—allowing no more than three hours to go by before you eat either a snack or meal. If your timing is off, your body takes over and begins to conserve fuel by burning calories more slowly.

Eating every two to three hours reassures your body that there is no impending famine and that it's okay to "spend" its calories.

You want your body to know that it is getting food on a regular basis; therefore, it will not conserve energy. Eating every two to three hours reassures your body that there is no impending famine and that it's okay to "spend" its calories. This puts you in a position to burn or use the calories you eat rather than storing them. This also helps your body facilitate a healthy fat loss, muscle gain and regulate your blood sugar—avoiding the afternoon lows and drop in energy.

What about late night snacks? We are aware that you have most likely been taught to cease eating at 6 p.m. The good news is that this is a myth. The only thing that matters are what type of foods you are eating. First of all, to stop eating at 6 p.m. and go to bed at 10 p.m. would be a disservice to your metabolism. Remember; eat every two to three hours—even at night if you want to keep your metabolism in high gear. However, it is a good idea to eat your last snack one to two hours prior to going to sleep. It is also helpful to eat low glycemic carbohydrates or protein for your dinner and evening snacks (i.e., vegetables, lean cuts of poultry or fish).

Daily planning

"I am too busy." "I just don't have the time." "I forgot to go grocery shopping." These are common statements expressed by many of our clients. Even though these same clients want to release fat and begin creating health daily, they remain stuck because of their lack of proper planning.

Okay, you have a busy schedule and the fast-paced society we live in makes it difficult to prepare and plan your food for a week, much less a day. Yet, if succeeding is important to you—which we believe it is—daily planning is essential and cannot be overlooked or put on hold.

Planning adds purpose and direction to your ability to succeed. Without a plan, you drift. Without a plan, you will be like a ship at sea with no rudder to guide it to its destination. Consider this analogy: you plan a wedding, you don't just walk into a church and say, "I want to get married."

When you plan, you'll succeed. If you neglect to plan, you will drift and find yourself off course and discouraged. Plan your way to success daily!

Immediately you would be asked, "When and to whom?" Once you sit down with the person who arranges and plans the marriage ceremonies, together along with your fiancé you will enter the process of planning the date, time, etc. Taking the time to plan your wedding thoroughly will make for a great ceremony. We are sure you would do the same thing if you were to plan a vacation or family reunion. Taking the time to plan is not only smart, but also a true predictor that it will be a success. We encourage you to do the same thing with your desire to release fat and create health daily. Take it seriously and keep it a priority, and you will succeed.

When you plan, you'll succeed. If you neglect to plan, you will drift and find yourself off course and discouraged. Plan your way to success daily!

Tracking

Tracking your eating and exercise every day is without a doubt one of the SMARTEST things you can do. All too often people will track in their head, however, writing it down is the most accurate approach, and it helps you maintain accountability to yourself.

In our research and experience with many clients, those who tracked attained greater success than those who didn't. Tracking helps you establish structure and enables you to remain on course. It also gives you a reference to reflect on. Tracking your food will demonstrate to you what worked and provided you optimum results—call it the "blue print" of your success. In our opinion, if you do not to track, you are saying you do not want to be accountable.

One New York study monitored a group of obese patients who complained they couldn't lose weight on 1,200 calories a day. Twelve hundred calories is very low, and unless you are heavily medicated or your thyroid is out of whack, you will lose weight. It may not be primarily fat, however, you will lower your total body weight.

Even though it is common for people to blame their metabolism for not losing weight, under close observation, it was shown that there was nothing metabolically unusual about the patients. Instead, the study found the group was eating, on average, 47 percent more than it claimed and exercising 51 percent less.

Another study at Maastricht University in the Netherlands found that when participants recorded what they ate in a journal, they consumed 26 percent fewer calories. Based on this study, if you are not tracking and you're eating an average of 1,500 calories per day, guess what? You are most likely eating more than 2,000 calories per day. That works out to gaining one pound of fat per week.

When all is said and done, we know the value in tracking and it is up to you to take advantage of this success tool. And when you begin to question why tracking is important, consider the following answers:

- Tracking empowers the accomplishment of your goal.
- Tracking helps you accurately measure your progress.
- Tracking ensures the maximum results for your efforts.
- Tracking positions you to evaluate rather than judge yourself.
- Tracking helps you trouble-shoot and remain on course.
- Tracking provides you with a reference of what works and what doesn't.

A day in the life

Have you ever heard that practice improves performance? In our business we encourage people to focus more on performance enhancement and not on perfect performance. First of all, there is no such thing as perfectionism. And when you focus on perfect performance (eating perfectly), you set yourself up to be let down. If you aim to perform perfectly you will almost always fall short.

When you focus on performance enhancement you learn to evaluate rather than judge. You take time to see the value in your performance and access how you can improve. This is the philosophy we encourage you to take toward daily living. We want you to do everything in your power to perform optimally, however, it is important that you evaluate your day and not judge it.

Consider the following, as it is a typical day of one of our successful clients:

Wake up: 6:15 a.m.
- Cup of coffee with non-fat milk and sugar substitute (Splenda®)

Breakfast: 6:30 a.m.
- One cup of Optimum Power Breakfast cereal with 1 cup of Silk soy milk

Snack: 9:30 a.m.
- One cup of strawberries

Lunch: 12:30 p.m.
- Grilled chicken and black bean salad with olive oil and vinegar dressing

Snack: 3:00 p.m.
- Sliced apple with 1 Tbsp. all natural peanut butter

Dinner: 6:00 p.m.
- Broiled salmon with steamed mixed vegetables

Snack: 8:00 p.m.
- 20 Almonds

Drink up

As you consume our recommended portions of high-quality food, be sure to drink plenty of water. If you are currently drinking a cup, make it a personal quest to increase your water to two cups, then three and so on, until you are drinking a minimum of eight to 12 eight-ounce glasses of water per day.

By replacing one can of soda with a cup of water, you save yourself 54,750 empty calories, or more than 15 pounds, per year. Depending on your daily water intake, your total body weight can vary up to four pounds. For instance, you drink water over the weekend, but neglect to drink much water during the week. Doing this may cause your body to hold on to as much water possible—causing you to weigh more on the scale.

Water is essential. No matter what others say, or what you read about how much is too much or too little, you probably need more water than you're drinking. As we will emphasize in Chapter 19 *(Metabolism Makeover)*, listen to your body and notice the headaches, lack of energy and increased cravings when you are not drinking eight to 12 eight-ounce glasses of water.

Keep your focus on what you want and continue to say "yes" to your desire to experience lasting success.

Maintain focus

To help you maintain focus and keep the taste, convenience and pleasure in your food choices, we have provided you with a sample grocery plan, and meal and snack ideas in Appendix B. As you begin to implement these suggestions, keep in mind our philosophy: Where your focus goes, your energy flows. If you focus on how good your favorite dessert tastes and the feeling you associate with eating it, guess what? You are likely to eat it. However, if you focus on your increased mood and energy, and the joy you feel being fit, you are more likely to eat healthy.

Keep your focus on what you want, and continue to say yes to your desire to experience lasting success. Maintain your focus on the importance of your goal—your self-promise to improve your health and release fat. If you feel that you are an emotional eater, keep in mind that feelings follow thoughts. Get control of the thoughts you think and allow your feelings to be your guide—your compass for your emotional state. By keeping your focus on what is important to you, you will acquire control of your emotional splurges.

When people say it is all in the head, they are correct. Though eating is a physical action, the decision to eat what you eat begins with a thought, then a feeling and finally an action. Focus, focus and focus some more. Keep the focus and you will experience long-term success!

Points to remember:

- Exercise is essential for releasing fat and creating healthy daily; however, what you put in your mouth is of equal importance.
- Regardless of your ethnicity, nationality and social beliefs, there are certain foods that cause you to gain fat.
- Eat a portion of protein and a portion of carbohydrate at breakfast, lunch and dinner.

- Eat frequently, five to six times per day.
- Establishing a healthy appetite for both the foods you eat and the thoughts you think is how you experience lasting success.
- The choice of a free day or weekly cheats may open the door to sabotaging your fat-loss efforts.
- Eat every two to three hours beginning with breakfast.
- Plan and track you food and exercise daily.
- Drink a minimum of eight to 12 cups of water a day.

PART SIX

The Skinny on Fat Loss

19

Metabolism Makeover

"If you learn only methods, you'll be tied to your methods,
but if you learn principles, you can devise your own methods."
—Ralph Waldo Emerson

Do you know someone who survives on Froot Loops and Burger King and still looks great? We all know someone who eats like this, however, most people can't eat these foods and expect to be fit and trim. Unfortunately, even aerobic instructors and personal trainers are not immune. Who hasn't seen at least one aerobic instructor teaching a step class with a noticeable "spare tire?"

We live in a world that complements those who work 10 or more hours, eat one or two meals and down a half-gallon of coffee each day. Arriving home at nine or ten o'clock each night and consuming a bowl of ice cream, a slice of pizza and two beers has become the norm. As a result, this type of lifestyle has proven to be the primary reason more people are discovering an extra 20, 30 or 40 pounds of fat on their bodies. This early-to-rise and late-to-rest work schedule combined with unhealthy eating habits is definitely not the master method for trimming down and leading a healthy lifestyle.

Nevertheless, we encourage you to persevere toward the weight of your youth. As you read this chapter, you are probably going to think that it is too good to be true. After all, your beliefs and habits of thought may be telling you that starving yourself is the only way to shed pounds. The irony of this thought process is that for years, the belief that you have to starve yourself to lose weight is exactly what has prevented many people from getting rid of fat for good. We all know people who've been on diets forever—nibbling on salads and rice cakes to no avail. They may lose a few pounds here and there, but they always seem to gain it back.

We have also witnessed people who are obsessed with working out. They go to the gym everyday, yet their weight and body composition never seems to change.

You can truly eat more, exercise in moderation and slim down—all by increasing your metabolism.

Well, we're here to tell you that it doesn't have to be that way! You can truly eat more, exercise in moderation and slim down—all by increasing your metabolism.

Our goal is to provide you with five surefire methods for making over your metabolism. However, you may choose to continue the pursuit of a quick fix or temporary solution. Why? Well, you may not be convinced that quick, permanent fat loss doesn't exist. After all, we can't expect you to accept what we say as gospel. This is why we encourage you to follow our recommendations for seven days. If you feel it is working for you, go another seven days. A solid effort to makeover your metabolism by implementing these five tips—after 40 days—will turn you into a fat burning machine.

Meet Stacy

If we don't have your attention yet, maybe this story will grab you. When Stacy came to see us she had been on a diet for three years. In her early 20s, standing at 5'7", she weighed in at 175 pounds. She wasn't obese by any means, but at 30 percent body fat, she was headed in an unhealthy direction. The interesting part of this story is that Stacy wasn't an overeater. She ate a few healthy meals per day—mainly salad, vegetables and fish. She worked out six days per week, spending most of her time doing back-to-back aerobic classes and exercising on various pieces of cardio equipment like the treadmill. Stacy was serious, she put in a lot of effort and if she missed a workout, she would go twice the following day to stay on track.

When we first discussed her daily caloric needs and how to rev up her metabolism, Stacy looked worried. Growing up, her mother had struggled with anorexia. She had been taught at a very young age that if you want to be thin, you eat very little, if at all. Together, we were able to identify that the "diet" she had been following over the past several years wasn't getting her the results she wanted; the theory that may have worked for her mother wasn't working for her. Thankfully, Stacy understood that her mother had suffered from a terrible disease and agreed that it was an unhealthy example to follow. Together we made the following agreement: she would follow our eating plan for six weeks. Technically, the first cycle of the Wellness Weight-Loss process is 12 weeks, but we believed that she would get results after six, and would then want to continue. We agreed to help, and she accepted our process whole-heartedly and trusted in our research, education and experience. She even agreed to add resistance training (i.e., weight lifting, strength training) to her exercise routine in place of some cardiovascular training, even though she was afraid of getting big bulky muscles!

During the six weeks, Stacy kept meticulous records. She tracked every calorie, ate five to six meals every day, consumed the recommended amount of water, followed the 21-day induction of choosing healthy alternatives for candy, white and enriched wheat flour, sugar listed first through fourth on any label, breaded or fried foods and alcohol, and she adjusted her exercise program to incorporate our suggestions. Basically, she did everything by the book. At the end of the first three weeks, we measured the results. To her surprise, she lost 12 pounds, dropped two percent body fat, and lost four inches. She couldn't believe it. "But, I didn't do as much cardio and I ate all the time," she exclaimed.

As Stacy continued with the process she learned how important it was to feed her body, and that food wasn't the enemy after all. She began to understand her metabolism and how to exercise more effectively to get the results she wanted. Now, more than three years later, Stacy weighs 135 pounds, and measures in at 14 percent body fat. Stacy remains on top of the world. She now pursues her aspiration of becoming an actress, her weight no longer holding her back from her childhood dream.

Metabolism

Everyone uses the term metabolism. We can't tell you how many times we have heard people tell us that they are overweight because they have a slow metabolism. When we challenge them with the simple question, "What is metabolism?" most people try to make up an explanation, but in the end admit that they don't really know. We have managed to condense the definition of metabolism into the following two sentences: Metabolism refers to the entire network of physical and chemical processes involved in maintaining life. It encompasses all the sequences of chemical reactions that enable us to release and use energy from food, convert one substance to another, and prepare products for excretion and elimination.

Simply put, your body needs water, macronutrients (carbohydrates, fats and proteins) and micronutrients (vitamins and minerals) to function properly. If you neglect to consume these nutrients, you may cause serious harm to your body. For example, a car needs water, electricity, oil and gas to function. If you neglect to provide the car with oil, electricity, water or gas, it will either quit operating or one or more parts will break down, leading to serious problems. Your body is the same. The food you consume directly affects the efficiency of your metabolism. If you have a slow metabolism, it is partly because you overeat and/or diet. Eating more than you need (making yourself tired and sluggish) or dieting (going hungry) are the two primary reasons for slowing your metabolism, which then makes it more difficult to have energy and release fat.

If you find yourself skipping breakfast, getting little sleep, eating a big meal late at night and drinking beer when you get home, guess what? You are not doing your metabolism any good. A slowing metabolism is not solely the result of aging or reduced activities as many people think.

Metabolism makeover

The objective of this chapter is discovering how to improve your natural thermostat for burning fat and increasing your body's metabolic rate. Mastering metabolism will not take up much of your time and it doesn't hurt. Begin with the notion of making your health an important part of your daily life, and believe it or not, integrating proper nutrition and exercise into your busy schedule will prove rewarding. To kick-start your metabolism into high gear, it helps to first assess your daily eating habits, water consumption, nightlife, cardiovascular and resistance training. This assessment and desire to rediscover the fit, firm and fabulous you begins with eating healthy.

Eating healthy

All too often people who want to reduce their body fat begin dieting—eating next to nothing. That's right, dieting is one of the worst things you can do if you want to burn body fat. When you diet, a dramatic and sustained reduction in your metabolic rate takes affect. Your body's ability to burn fat comes to a screeching halt. It also means you are likely to store more body fat as a direct result of eating less. Talk about a plan backfiring!

Eating your way to leanness is nothing short of meal frequency and food quality. Eating five to six times per day keeps your body's metabolic rate high and will help you maintain that all-important muscle tissue. No, this doesn't mean go out and eat pizza on five separate occasions throughout the day. Each of your main meals (breakfast, lunch, and dinner) are to adhere to healthy nutrition basics—low-fat, balanced meals that contain both fibrous carbohydrates and protein, and above all, small portion sizes. Prepare your meals in advance and have a snack between meals.

The keys to this plan are portion sizes and the quality of food you eat. As we explained early on in this book, a portion size is the size of your palm or clenched fist. At breakfast, lunch and dinner we suggest that you consume a portion of protein and a portion of fibrous carbohydrates. If you consider your carbohydrate to be vegetables, fill the rest of your plate with vegetables, but don't exceed three portion sizes. Snacks are typically a carbohydrate, a protein or both, as in low-fat yogurt or almonds.

> *When your body becomes more efficient at processing the food you eat—the faster your metabolism becomes, right? Yes!*

Think about this—instead of stretching your stomach by eating two to three huge meals throughout the day, or consuming all of your daily calories in one sitting, re-program your body by giving it smaller portions of food more often. This tells your body that more food is on it's way very soon; encouraging it to utilize the food you are eating rather than storing it. When your body becomes more efficient at processing the food you eat—the faster your metabolism becomes, right? Yes! Remember the definition of metabolism.

Drink up

Did you know that over 90 percent of the population is considered clinically dehydrated? In healthy, hydrated individuals, 83 percent of their blood is water, 76 percent of their muscles are water and 22 percent of their bone is water. We can live for several weeks without food, but without water, we could die in five days.

Most people will tell you that drinking eight glasses of water is essential to being healthy. Others are aware that you must down an extra glass of water for every cup of dehydrating coffee, and two for alcohol. However, did you know that consuming a responsible amount of water each day keeps your body's metabolic rate in high gear? When the body gets the water it needs to function optimally, you improve endocrine-gland function, more body fat is used as fuel, fluid retention is alleviated and you take stress off your heart, liver, kidneys and joints. Being dehydrated causes your blood to thicken, which slows the circulation of nourishing fluids to your brain, muscles and cells. When this happens your metabolism slows down.

We once had a client share with us the importance of water when getting blood drawn. As the nurse attempted to draw her blood at an annual blood test, the nurse asked, "When was the last time you drank water?" Our client responded with a puzzled look and then said, "I am not sure. Maybe a day or two ago." The nurse recommended she return the following day after getting some water in her body because her blood was too thick—she was having a difficult time getting the blood out! Because blood is composed of 83 percent water, it is imperative that you remain hydrated. If you don't, your blood thickens, making it slow-moving—reducing your metabolism as well.

Drinking ample amounts of water before and after meals and workouts will keep the fat off and your metabolism functioning properly.

Water helps transport nutrients and waste products in and out of cells. Water is an essential nutrient that is involved in every function of the body. Drinking ample amounts of water before and after meals and workouts will keep the fat off and your metabolism functioning properly. How do you know if you're getting enough water? Usually the color of your urine is a good indicator. Pale yellow or clear urine is a symptom of hydration, while dark yellow urine may suggest that it's time to drink more fluids.

One simple method to help you drink all of your water is to fill up a two-quart container first thing in the morning. Carry it around with you wherever you go and make it a goal to finish it by the end of the day. If you are currently drinking fewer than four glasses per day, that may be too big a step for you in the beginning. Make it a priority to add two additional eight-ounce glasses to your current total. Once you have adopted this new habit, add two more and continue this pattern until you are drinking a minimum of eight to 12 eight-ounce glasses of water each and every day.

Nightlife

Sleep! It is a known FACT that your body functions optimally on at least seven to eight hours of sleep each night. Research shows that a chronic lack of rest can slow down your metabolism as much as a sedentary lifestyle. Think about it. There are people who exercise everyday, but get little sleep and therefore are not able to continue progressing with their fat loss efforts.

Sleep is necessary for the adequate production of hormones, including the important growth hormone, which makes us less vulnerable to the diseases of aging. It is at rest that our body is able to build and repair muscle tissue, which is metabolically active. Deep sleep has also been shown to be crucial for the optimal function of our brain.

Sleep deprivation increases levels of cortisol, the stress hormone that increases blood sugar, interferes with memory, retards muscle building, impairs our immune system and promotes abdominal fat. Also, physiological studies involving subjects who were sleeping less than eight hours per night indicated that the subjects were decades older than they actually were! The good news is that once they established a pattern of sleeping nine hours per night, the results improved.

If you don't give yourself sufficient rest to recover from a hard day of physical or mental labor, the need to snooze could trigger a desire for a quick sugar fix. You may also overeat in attempt to boost your energy, and may be too tired to workout. It is clear that if we want to get the most out of exercise and the foods we eat, we must make sleep a top priority. The goal would be to get closer to nine hours of sleep per night, like our hard-working ancestors did back in the early 1900s. Remember, Shakespeare once said that adequate sleep is the chief nourisher of life's feast.

Cardio metabolism

Martial artists, fitness enthusiasts and bodybuilders are constantly trying to figure out the best workout, the most effective cardio program and the quickest way to burn fat. Unfortunately, there are many obstacles in their way. However, when you separate fact from fiction, the key to releasing body fat is burning calories, and you do a whole lot of that during aerobic exercise. Not only do you burn calories during a cardiovascular workout, you continue burning calories once you've finished training. Called excess post exercise oxygen consumption, or EPOC for short, this allows you to burn fat long after you've completed your workout.

Cardiovascular exercise is a major factor in increasing blood flow to working muscles, which in turn boosts your metabolic rate. Combined with healthy eating and added muscle from resistance training, cardio kickboxing and other methods of aerobic (high-intensity) exercise can transform you into a fat-burning machine. If your body has adapted to your cardio workout, it is time to add some variety to your training. By changing the exercises and intensity of your cardio routine, you will "shock" your body into action. When you alter your regular exercise program, your body has no choice but to adapt to the demands placed upon it. In Chapter 20 we explain the finer details of cardio.

Resistance metabolism

Often you'll hear both men and women say that they'll pump some iron after they drop some weight; this is just plain foolish. Resistance exercise facilitates the fat-burning process by preserving the body's most important metabolic regulator—muscle. Skeletal muscle accounts for almost 40 percent of our bodyweight. Most people fail to realize that muscle is much more than something pretty to look at—it's the key to the fat burning process.

---

*The bottom line is:
hit the weight room and introduce your body
to some serious resistance training.*

As you grow older your muscle reduces in size, therefore you burn fewer calories. As you age the elasticity in the muscle weakens and your metabolism slows. By building and/or maintaining muscle you can avoid these concerns. The only way to maintain a fast metabolism, toned body, overall strength, burn fat—and the only way to permanently alter your metabolic rate—is to incorporate resistance training (weight lifting) into your exercise regimen. So, the bottom line is: hit the weight room and introduce your body to some serious resistance training. In Chapter 21 and Appendix C we explain and demonstrate the finer details of resistance training.

Summary

Unfortunately, reducing body fat isn't as simple as denying your body of calories. Your body will not cooperate. If you attempt to reduce your body fat by exercising and eating less, your body will attempt to compensate by metabolizing those calories less efficiently and catabolizing muscle tissue for energy.

Over two years ago, in a landmark study at Rockefeller University in New York, a group of researchers found that if you lose weight, your metabolism slows down and becomes less efficient, therefore, burning fewer calories to do the same work. In short, losing weight in the form of lean muscle tissue is a surefire method for slowing your metabolism.

Similarly, if you gain weight, your metabolism speeds up. If you are going to gain weight, it serves you best if you're adding muscle, simply because added muscle increases your metabolism and burns more calories and fat.

SIDE NOTE: Would you rather add muscle or fat to your body? Obviously, you want to reduce fat and add muscle in its place because one pound of muscle can burn up to 50 calories a day, while fat uses up a measly two to five calories.

Clearly our bodies don't keep us at one weight our entire adult lives. Your body adjusts its metabolic rate depending on age, food intake, lean body mass and amount of physical activity. Adjustments are slow and it seems to be a great deal easier to move up in weight rather than down. With this in mind and knowing how to kick-start your metabolism, make it a model for your lifestyle to look tight wearing white!

Points to remember:

- Metabolism refers to the entire network of physical and chemical processes involved in maintaining life. It encompasses all the sequences of chemical reactions that enable us to release and use energy from foods, convert one substance to another, and prepare products for excretion and elimination.
- Dieting is one of the worst things you can do if you want to burn body fat.
- Eating five to six meals per day keeps your body's metabolic rate high and will help you maintain that all-important muscle tissue.
- In healthy, hydrated individuals, 83 percent of their blood is water, 76 percent of their muscles are water and 22 percent of their bone is water. Most of us could benefit from drinking more water.
- Research shows that a chronic lack of rest can slow down your metabolism as much as a sedentary lifestyle.
- Cardiovascular exercise is a major factor in increasing blood flow to working muscles, which boosts your metabolic rate.
- Resistance exercise facilitates the fat-burning process by preserving the body's most important metabolic regulator—muscle.
- One pound of muscle can burn up to 50 calories a day, while fat uses a measly two to five calories.

20

Cardiovascular Exercise

"A man's health can be judged by which he takes
two at a time—pills or stairs."
—Joan Welsh

Have you ever met someone who loves cardiovascular exercise activities like walking, biking and aerobic classes? Have you ever wondered why they're addicted to such activities? When you meet someone who enjoys the feeling they get from cardio, ask them to explain it, and then ask yourself if you would like to experience the same feeling. Our client, Theresa says, "Cardio is my Prozac—my natural anti-depressant."

Just like clothing fashions, depending on who you talk to, you'll get different responses about cardiovascular exercise (cardio). While many people love the increased energy they get from cardio, others avoid it like the plague. As hard as it is to believe, the thought of enjoying cardio is absurd for many people. "The last thing I want to do is get on some machine for 30 minutes just to say I got my cardio in," announced one of our seminar participants. To our dismay, we have had both sedentary and fitness enthusiasts tell us that cardio is downright dreadful and boring.

Whether you love it or hate it, cardio has its place and we want to explain how you can benefit most from its use. To begin with, "cardio" is short for cardiovascular exercise, and it's crucial for a healthy heart, lungs and vascular system. Secondly, you can't burn fat without performing cardio. Whether it's aerobic (meaning with, or in the presence of, oxygen) or anaerobic (defined as without the presence of oxygen; not requiring oxygen), cardio is how you stimulate the release of fat. Knowing the difference between aerobic and anaerobic may prove valuable as you progress with your exercise. As well, it is to your benefit to be familiar with cardiovascular endurance: summarized as the ability to perform large-muscle movement over a sustained period;

the capacity of the heart-lung system to deliver oxygen for sustained energy production.

Let's take a walk down memory lane (late 1960s to early 1980s) when people used to rush to aerobic classes wearing little wooly tubes around their ankles and calves. Keep in mind that cardio is not typically sought after because of its health benefits, but its ability to burn fat. From the early days of performing cardio-dance-like movements in groups, aerobic classes have continued to grow in popularity, just like the advancement of refining foods. As the American waistline continues to swell in size, so does the growing demand to burn body fat. Some 24.3 million people took aerobic exercise classes in 2001, according to the National Sporting Goods Association, which tracks exercise trends. Then again, we are a far cry from the striped leotard and leg warmers made popular by fitness queen Jane Fonda.

Before the cardio revolution

If you were to go back in time to the early 1900s, you would witness a major movement to refine, process and distribute food to the masses. At the same time you would discover that only a handful of Americans were exercising with intentions of improving cardiovascular health. Today, more people than ever are exercising—not for the sole purpose of improving cardiovascular health, but to burn the excess body fat that that has resulted partly from being sedentary and consuming highly refined, low-fiber foods.

What was believed to be good in the early 1900s has come back to haunt us today. If you want to know why, sit down with practically any weight-loss expert and they will confirm that a major part of the reason Americans have experienced an increase in cardiovascular disease and obesity is due to sedentary lifestyles and current food manufacturing methods that strip foods of their vitamins, minerals and phytochemicals. Highly processed and refined carbs such as soda and many mass-produced breads cause your blood sugar to rise quickly after eating. What goes up fast comes down fast, and you end up feeling tired, lethargic and hungry sooner rather than later. These modern-day foods encourage excess body fat and are linked to lifestyle diseases such as Type 2 diabetes and heart attacks.

To combat the effects of decreased health and increased body fat, people worldwide are turning to cardiovascular exercise. Case in point: In Germany every third child under the age of 12 and every fifth teenager is over fat. In Greece, the land of the highly respected Mediterranean diet, more than 70 percent of the adult men and women are above their ideal body size. Even the Middle East is not exempt as about 60 percent of the women in Egypt are over fat. No longer an American issue, more now than any other time in history, people world-wide are searching out gyms and purchasing exercise equipment. However, this movement was not an overnight occurrence.

"It is easier to maintain good health through proper exercise, diet and emotional balance than it is to regain it once it is lost."

The cardio movement

Since the days of Hippocrates (460 to 377 B.C.) to the days when the Godfather of Physical Fitness Jack LaLanne began popularizing cardio in the late 1930s, to Dr. Kenneth H. Cooper's book, *Aerobics* (1968), and his philosophy of shifting the field of medicine away from disease treatment to disease prevention through aerobic exercise, people have contemplated the role of cardio. A runner at heart, Dr. Cooper made his message clear: "It is easier to maintain good health through proper exercise, diet and emotional balance than it is to regain it once it is lost." However, improved health and running weren't enough to get everyone to take up cardio.

Well, at least not until Jacki Sorensen's *Aerobic Dance* and Judi Sheppard Missett's *Jazzercise* ignited the cardio movement in 1969. And it has progressed steadily since then. Along with the advancement of cardio equipment (i.e., treadmills, eliptical machines), the father of running, Jim Fixx, added to the cardio movement by promoting the idea that exercise can be enjoyable. This philosophy proved true with his bestseller, *"The Complete Book of Running,"* which was published in 1977. Then Jane Fonda and her *"Jane Fonda's Workout"* video captured the aerobic dance style in 1982. And like anything else, people grew bored and yearned for something different, so Gin Miller, who founded the *Step Aerobics* method, came on the scene in 1986 after she injured a knee—an injury she blamed largely on teaching too many classes of high-impact aerobics.

As you can see, cardio methods come and go. Think about it! For awhile there, it seemed like everyone was doing jazzercise or jogging. Then everyone was participating in aerobics classes. A few years ago, kickboxing established itself and Tae-Bo became the rage. And tomorrow, who knows what it'll be?

Cardiovascular exercise trends change for much of the same reasons clothing fashions do: people like a change every now and then, and the fitness industry is always seeking a new trend to supply. But just as the basic suit doesn't go out of style, neither does the basic benefit of cardio and its ability to increase our mood and energy, burn body fat, reverse aging, fight disease and exercise the most important muscle in our body—our heart.

Muscle for muscle, your heart is without question the strongest and most important organ in your body.

Heart healthy

Did you know that the most important muscle in your body is your heart? Muscle for muscle, your heart is without question the strongest and most important organ in your body. In 1614, man scientifically discovered that blood is the carrier of nutrients to every part of the body. This gave further support to the value of the heart muscle and its role as the motor that pumps blood throughout the body.

Like a fuel pump in an automobile, your heart is needed for you to live and perform optimally. Without a fuel pump, your car will not operate. Without a heart, which can pump up to five quarts of blood every minute to every cell in your body—your cells would not get the nutrients or oxygen they need to survive.

If you are not exercising your heart, it will lose its ability to supply your body with nutrients and oxygen. It is your heart, your cardiovascular system that is responsible for the delivery of oxygen-rich blood to all of your tissues. Our cells are completely dependent on oxygen and without it, they die—such as in a stroke or heart attack. Sometimes we forget that every muscle in our body requires exercise to operate more efficiently, including our heart!

Okay, you have a pretty good understanding that cardio is beneficial when it comes to your heart, but what about burning fat? If you thought solving the protein puzzle was confusing, guess what? The debate about which cardio methods are most effective for burning body fat and conditioning the heart can seem quite cluttered. However, to help you determine what is best for you, we have combed through scientific literature, medical journals and client files. In addition, we have interviewed many of our clients who have kept the fat from coming back. The cardio recommendations provided in this book are based on helping you get moving and acquire the results you desire: release body fat and increase cardiovascular health.

Getting started

Now that the decision is made and you are ready to work out, we recommend that you follow your doctor's advice about how much exercise is best for you. Getting the authorization from your doctor to exercise is not only encouraged, but serves as a baseline for where you are to begin. It is important for you to know your fitness level and present health when determining which cardio activity is best for you.

One of the best things you can do if you haven't exercised in a while is to take a first step. After your doctor has given you the okay to get moving, workout a few times and establish a baseline—a point of origin—and then allow time and consistency to condition your body and heart for varied workouts and intensity. The name of the game is to gradually build up to 20 minutes of cardio. Optimally, you will build your cardio up to 30 to 45 minutes four to five times per week. In some cases you may find yourself working up to 60 minutes of cardio six or seven days per week.

But there are cautions. We recommend that you do not begin a vigorous cardio program if you haven't already been active. Then again, what "vigorous" means to us may not mean the same to you. How do you know if you are working too hard or not working hard enough? The answer is intensity.

Intensity

Intensity can be defined as the level of physiological stress on your body during exercise—indicating how hard you are working. The level of intensity depends on your present health, fitness level and reasons for exercising. If you are new to cardio and recently suffered a heart attack, running sprints would not be our recommendation. The fact remains that your present health and fitness level does determine your output—your intensity.

When it comes to cardio, there are several methods of measuring intensity. The one most widely used in the fitness industry is the Target Heart Rate (THR) zone, which involves knowing your heart rate reserve or maximum heart rate. You've probably heard someone say, "If you want to burn fat, you'd better keep your heart rate in the fat-burning zone." The zone they are referring to requires you to take your pulse throughout your exercise session to ensure you're staying within the recommended range (50 to 85 percent of your heart rate reserve or 60 to 90 percent of your maximum heart rate).

However, with the advancement of technology, you can purchase a heart rate monitor and remain aware of your intensity as easily as eyeing your watch. These heart rate monitors are designed to keep you informed about whether or not you are in your THR zone. As well, you can take your heart rate manually at one of two locations; the radial pulse or carotid pulse. Your radial pulse is located on the inside of your wrist just below the base of your thumb, and your carotid pulse is located just below your jaw line on the outer sides of your neck. When taking your pulse however, use your index and middle finger as your thumb has its own pulse and can cause confusion.

Once you have located your pulse, the goal is to figure out how many times your heart beats per minute. To do this, count your pulse for 10 seconds beginning with zero and multiply by six to get your heart rate beats per minute. Use caution when taking your carotid pulse; it is important that you use a gentle touch. Pressing too hard with your fingers could decrease the flow of oxygen to your brain, making you feel dizzy and faint.

Heart rate reserve (HRR) method

To help you calculate your training heart rate zone using the heart rate reserve method (also known as Karvonen method), we have provided a formula below. Although we are providing you with this formula to figure out your heart rate reserve, we will follow up with three additional methods: 1) maximum heart rate, 2) talk test and 3) the rate of perceived exertion. All these methods are designed to help you monitor your intensity and ensure that you are working in your training zone. In short, the HHR is the difference between your maximum heart rate (MaxHR) and resting heart rate.

To increase your cardiovascular fitness and improve your health, train anywhere between 50 and 85 percent of your heart rate reserve. If you're starting out, it's a good idea to begin at the low end of the range and gradually increase.

HRR FORMULA:
1. Subtract your age in years from 220. This is your maximum heart rate.
2. Subtract your resting heart rate. To determine your resting heart rate it is recommended that first thing in the morning for three consecutive days upon waking that you count your pulse for 10 seconds and multiply that number by six. Take the average of the three days to establish your resting heart rate (must be on days that you wake naturally—without an alarm).
3. Multiply your heart rate reserve by the percent of intensity at which you want to train.
4. Add back your resting heart rate.

EXAMPLE:

This is an example for a 50-year-old person with a resting heart rate of 70 beats per minute who wants to train at 40 to 85 percent of his heart rate reserve. First he employs the formula to find the lower end of his range:

1. 220 - 50 = 170
2. 170 - 70 = 100
3. 100 x 40% = 40
4. 40 + 70 = 110 beats per minute

Then he finds his upper limit, 85%

1. 220 - 50 = 170
2. 170 - 70 = 100
3. 100 x 85% = 85
4. 85 + 70 = 155 beats per minute

Once you've determined your heart rate training range (zone), you can use a heart rate monitor to count your heartbeats per minute or manually take your pulse while keeping an eye on a clock or watch. We find it helpful to divide beats per minute by six to get a 10 second heart rate. It is a easier to monitor your pulse for 10 seconds compared to 60 seconds.

Maximum heart rate (MaxHR) method

If you don't know your resting heart rate, and you are not exercising at a super-high intensity level, you can simply calculate your heart rate training zone by subtracting your age from 220 and then multiplying the target heart rate percentage. Consider the following formula for acquiring your target heart rate range (zone):

MaxHR FORMULA:

1. Subtract your age in years from 220. This is your maximum heart rate.
2. Multiply your maximum heart rate by the target heart rate percentage to get heart beats per minute.

EXAMPLE:

This is an example for a 50-year-old person who wants to train at 55 to 90 percent of his MaxHR. We recommend this method when you don't know your resting heart rate. First he employs the formula to find the lower end of his range:

1. 220 - 50 = 170
2. 170 x 55% = 93.5 beats per minute

Then he finds his upper limit, 90%
1. 220 - 70 = 170
2. 170 x 90% = 153 beats per minute

For those of you who prefer not to take a heart rate reading, you can simply exercise at a level that leaves you feeling warm and slightly out of breath, comparable to brisk walking. That would be equivalent to a heart rate range of approximately 55 to 70 percent and would be enough for general fitness conditioning and improve health. This method is commonly referred to as the talk test.

The talk test method

Calculating your heart rate reserve, maximum heart rate, resting heart rate and determining your heart beats per minute can seem more like a cross between a science exam and calculus test. However, there is another method for determining your heart rate training zone—the talk test. It can be summarized with one simple question: Can you talk or are you out of breath? When you are exercising and are still able to talk, you can be fairly sure that you are in an aerobic state (55 to 70 percent of your maximum heart rate).

Being in an aerobic state means oxygen is present and you are indeed burning fat. To monitor and ensure you are in this heart rate training zone, it is important that you can carry on a light conversation while exercising. When you cannot carry on a light conversation, you may be working too hard (without oxygen). If you're not sure if you are working hard enough, pick up the pace.

If you can't engage in a conversation, we recommend you check your level of intensity by singing a verse from "Twinkle, Twinkle, Little Star." If you can't say, "Twinkle, Twinkle, Little Star" in one breath, you are working too hard. At the same time, if you can sing, "Twinkle, Twinkle, Little Star...How I wonder what you are" in one breath, you are not working hard enough.

As you have read, the talk test is good, but may be too vague. If so, consider using our preferred method—the rate of perceived exertion.

The rate of perceived exertion (RPE)

It's one thing to begin cardio, but it is another to know how to gauge your intensity during your workouts. Whether you are walking or using a cardio machine, for best results, knowing what level you are working at does prove beneficial. To save you time, energy and frustration when it comes to monitoring your intensity and getting results, we encourage you to become familiar with the rate of perceived exertion (RPE). This is our preferred method for determining the level of intensity we are working at during exercise.

The RPE method is a self-evaluation that is determined by a simple question: On a scale of 1 to 10, 1 being the lowest and 10 being the highest intensity that you can imagine, how do you feel? We have found that one's RPE and heart rate numbers are often closely related. For example, if your RPE is a 7 out of 10, you are most likely working at 70 percent of your heart rate reserve.

Become familiar with the RPE because we will refer to it when describing cardio routines:

RPE Level	Description
1	Effortless; similar to sitting down and viewing television.
2	Very easy; able to carry on a conversation.
3	Easy; able to talk with a friend and not be out of breath.
4	Moderate effort; you can talk comfortably.
5	Moderate; you can talk but requires some effort.
6	Somewhat difficult; talking requires quite a bit of effort.
7	Difficult; talking is uncomfortable as it requires a significant amount of effort.
8	Very difficult; to talk requires maximum effort.
9-10	Peak effort; to talk is out of the question because you are working at a very high intensity.

Your prescription

Now that you are familiar with how to monitor your intensity, it is time to take action. But before we provide you with a personal prescription for cardio, consider this: most healthcare and exercise specialists agree that 30 minutes of cardio per day is all it takes to have a healthy heart. To the contrary, with Americans getting fatter, the National Academy of Sciences (NAS) issued new dietary guidelines on September 5, 2002 that raised the recommended amount of exercise from 30 to 60 minutes per day. The message from the NAS reflects cold reality—if you want to be lean and fit, it is going to take consistent effort.

We agree that to release fat and improve your health daily, it is necessary to be consistent. However, we recommend that you work up to 45 to 60 minutes of cardio three to five times per week. This is not to say that exercising daily is not recommended, because if you have the time and you enjoy daily exercise, go for it!

The warm up

To maximize the benefits of cardio, warm up for six to 12 minutes as part of your cardio session. Not only will this warm up cause an increase in the temperature of the muscle and connective tissue, thereby reducing the risks of injury, it prepares your cardiovascular system for the upcoming demands—intensity. Also, it allows your cardiovascular system to effectively adjust blood flow from the abdominal area to the active muscles where the need for oxygen is increasing in response to the exercise, while maintaining adequate venous (blood coming back to the heart) return. Some of our clients are tempted to skip the warm-up phase. And we say—stick to the plan! The benefits of warming up can't be stressed enough. If you are simply unable to devote the recommended amount of time for your cardio workout, decrease the period of actual cardio exercise if needed, but don't skip the warm-up phase!

Beginner

If you are currently exercising and have been doing so for a minimum of six weeks—you are no beginner. However, if you are truly a beginner or returning to exercise after a period of inactivity, walking is one of many cardio activities you can start with. In addition to your warm-up, begin with five minutes of cardio a few times per week and gradually work up to 30 minutes over the next three to six weeks. Consider the following when performing cardio in the beginning:

Frequency:	1 to 3 times per week
Duration:	5+ minutes in addition to the warm-up and cool-down
Intensity:	40-50% of heart rate reserve or 55-60% of maximum heart rate
RPE:	4 to 5 rate of perceived exertion (after the warm- up)

Past beginner

Once you have established that you are no longer a beginner, and your body has adapted to the initial demands of exercise, it is time to consider more intense activities like indoor cycling, aerobics, incline walking, hiking, cardio kickboxing, jogging and the use of cardio machines. Consider the following since you have formed the habit of exercising weekly:

Frequency: 3 times per week
Duration: 15-20 minutes in addition to the warm-up and cool-down
Intensity: 50-60% of heart rate reserve or 60-70% of maximum heart rate
RPE: 5 to 6 rate of perceived exertion

Getting fat-specific

You are no longer a beginner, and you have been exercising consistently for six to 12 weeks and you have made some progress. You are now ready for more. It's true that the type of cardio you perform and the approach you take determines the outcome of your efforts.

Have you ever heard that to succeed with fat loss you need to use one particular cardio machine? Or maybe you were told to do high intensity cardio sessions for short and long bouts. Or that that in-door cycling is the best way to burn fat. Moving past the hype and the "he said, she said" jargon, let's take a closer look at the energy systems responsible for optimum fat burning.

There are four energy systems that we utilize during cardio. You have the phosphagen system that is responsible for high intensity, short duration activities that last up to 10 seconds. When this system is activated you are using creatine phosphate and stored Adenosine Triphosphate (ATP) in the muscle. An example of this energy system would be sprinting 50 meters. Second, you have the anaerobic glycolysis energy system that is responsible for cardio activity that lasts from 30 seconds to three minutes. When this system is activated, you are using blood glucose (sugar) and the energy stored in your muscles as fuel. An example of the anaerobic energy system is a half-mile run (800 meters). After the three-minute mark and up to about 20 minutes, the third of the three systems—aerobic glycolysis is at work. When this is the case, you are using glucose in addition to oxygen for fuel. During this aerobic state you are burning a combination of glucose and fatty acids. An example of this energy system is a three-mile run. The fourth energy system is called fatty acid oxidation. This system kicks in after 20 minutes. Its primary source of fuel is fatty acids. An example of this energy system is a marathon.

Now that you have learned a little more about the science behind the energy sources responsible for cardio, let's look at how you can exercise and burn more body fat versus glucose. When performing cardio for more than 20 minutes, you can be assured that approximately 60 percent of the calories being burned are from fat. This energy system is often referred to as fatty acid oxidation where you are using fatty acids (fat) and oxygen as your primary fuel source. This occurs after 20 to 30 minutes of sustained cardio at 60 to 70 percent of your maximum heart rate.

When you perform cardio that is moderate in intensity, but combined with short bursts of high intensity training, you can burn up to 60 percent of your calories from stored carbohydrates (glucose) and approximately 40 percent of your calories from fat. The great thing about this type of training is that you burn more total calories overall.

While it is true that the body burns more overall calories during high intensity interval training (HIIT), it is important to work up to this type of exercising. If you are new to exercise or still in the beginning stages, it is not recommended that you perform HIIT sessions. This is not to say that there aren't major benefits from low intensity activities such as walking. Just as your biceps need to build up strength before they can lift heavy weights, your heart muscle must be conditioned to perform at a higher intensity. As you make progress, your heart will become more efficient at delivering oxygen to the working muscles and it will be able to work at a higher intensity.

> **CAUTION:** Always be safe—your health is first and foremost! If you ever feel faint or dizzy during exercise, discontinue the activity and consult your doctor.

When to exercise

When is the best time to exercise? Is it first thing in the morning or at night prior to bed? Is it before resistance training or after? Along with promoting a healthy heart, cardio combined with healthy nutrition and a resistance (weight training) program is the way to burn the optimal amount of body fat. Influenced by scientific studies, but based on our personal experience and that of many of our clients, we are providing you with the most effective times to perform cardio when the goal is to release body fat. However, we are aware that not everyone is able to perform cardio during the following times:

First Preference—If your lifestyle permits, cardio performed first thing in the morning, on an empty stomach, provides the greatest potential for burning fat.

Second Preference—Performing cardio and resistance (weight) training on separate days has the greatest influence on overall calorie expenditure while also optimizing gains in strength and muscle tissue.

Third Preference—When your lifestyle prohibits you from performing cardio and resistance training on separate days, we recommend you perform cardio after resistance training to promote strength and muscle growth.

Fourth Preference—Performing cardio before resistance training is not recommended, however, it does optimize aerobic performance.

NOTE: Keep in mind—the longer you exercise past 60 minutes, the greater potential for muscle loss.

The plan

Use the Rate of Perceived Exertion (RPE) to monitor your intensity during your cardio workouts. Whether it is first thing in the morning or late in the afternoon, in order to beat the boredom that's commonly associated with cardio, use any cardio machine, or get outside and run or walk; for best results, vary your activities throughout the week.

The exercise routines provided are separated as either an endurance (aerobic) or HIIT workout. For every two endurance workouts during the week, we recommend you perform one HIIT routine. If you decide to do more than what we recommend—take at least one full day off per week.

Endurance workout

With all exercise routines it is encouraged that you warm up for six to 12 minutes at a low intensity. Also, it is important that you allot time to cool down for five to 10 minutes. All too often people will warm up, but skip the cool-down. Take into account that the cool down helps to lower your blood pressure and return blood flow back to your stomach. As well, cooling down helps prevent the sudden pooling of blood in the veins and ensures adequate circulation to the skeletal muscles, heart and brain. It also aids in preventing delayed muscle stiffness and reduces the tendency of post-exercise fainting and dizziness.

1st routine

The goal of this first routine is to boost cardiovascular fitness by working at a low to moderate intensity for more than 20 minutes. To progress with this routine, you simply add 10 minutes every six weeks until you are working out for a total of 60 minutes.

WORKOUT	TIME	RPE *(rate of perceived exertion)*
Warm-up	6 minutes	4-5
Steady intensity	18 minutes	6-7
Cool-down	6 minutes	3-4
TOTAL TIME:	**30 minutes**	

HIIT workout

The goal of the HIIT routine is to boost cardiovascular strength and speed by increasing your ability to train at high intensity, which translates into an elevated metabolism and more total calories burned during and after the workout. To progress with this program, you simply add 30 seconds to the high bursts and subtract 30 seconds from the moderate bursts every four to six weeks until you are performing high bursts for two minutes and moderate bursts for 30 seconds.

2nd Routine

WORKOUT	TIME	RPE *(rate of perceived exertion)*
Warm-up	9 minutes	4-5
Moderate burst	2 minutes	6
High burst	30 seconds	7-8.5
Moderate burst	2 minutes	6
High burst	30 seconds	7-8.5
Moderate burst	2 minutes	6
High burst	30 seconds	7-8.5
Moderate burst	2 minutes	6
High burst	30 seconds	7-8.5
Moderate burst	2 minutes	6
High burst	30 seconds	7-8.5
Moderate burst	2 minutes	6
High burst	30 seconds	7-8.5
Moderate burst	2 minutes	6
High burst	30 seconds	7-8.5
Moderate burst	2 minutes	6
High burst	30 seconds	7-8.5
Cool-down	6 minutes	3-4
TOTAL TIME:	**35 minutes**	

Boredom blues

No matter what city we are in or which fitness center we workout in or present a seminar to, people everywhere consistently share with us their negative association with cardio. The following suggestions are provided to help you counter these blues:

Buddy system. Don't want to be alone? Perform cardio on a machine next to a buddy who is fun to talk to and be around. There may be moments when you are working at high bursts, but during your moderate bursts you can talk lightly and remain inspirational.

Battling boredom. If you are easily bored when performing cardio, split your 30-minute workout in to three sessions—using three different cardio machines, you will not only be more excited about working out, you'll be giving your body the benefits of cross training.

Grooving to the tunes. Studies indicate that people work harder when they're listening to music versus reading a book or magazine. Pre-record your favorite songs and workout to the beat of fast-paced, dance-type music that makes it hard to stand still.

Personal best. Want to make time fly by? Get focused and find a cardio machine or mark out a point when walking that you can establish as your personal best. One day per week, push yourself and break your personal record. It may be walking a mile five seconds faster than the week before or climbing five more floors on the stair master or increasing the incline on the treadmill than the week before.

Television training. While watching television and exercising, boost your intensity every time a commercial comes on. Increase the resistance, add a hill or just go faster. If you are not a fan of television, do the same thing when you hear commercials on the radio.

Setting the mark. Establish a baseline, a minimum amount of intensity you want to perform and stay above that mark. This mark is to be a 7 to 8 on the rate of perceived exertion (RPE). After your warm-up, test yourself and see if you can maintain this level of intensity for 5 minutes. Then challenge yourself weekly to establish the next mark of 10, 15 and 20 minutes—until you reach the 60-minute mark. Then re-evaluate your RPE.

Cardio conclusion

By now you are fully aware of how cardio results in improved heart health and helps in maximizing fat-burning potential. As well, it's a medical fact that cardio reduces risk of heart disease, diabetes, stroke, high blood pressure, and many other conditions, and it also alleviates symptoms of depression and improves well being. All the same, the positives of cardio may not mean you will instantly come to enjoy, like or want to do it. But, then again, you may grow to enjoy the benefits of cardio enough to look forward to it, even if it doesn't rank high on your list of exercise methods. The choice is always yours to make. Remember, "Where your focus goes, your energy flows!"

No matter where you are in your cardiovascular health, you can begin today—making your way to a healthier you, both inside and out.

After reading about why cardio is a healthy choice, you may be thinking to yourself, "I don't have Type 2 diabetes or high cholesterol." Maybe you do or you don't. Regardless, this book is about creating health and releasing fat, and cardio helps you succeed. Also, taking the time to love yourself, care for yourself and give back to yourself is taking care of your body and your health.

We hope that you have grasped a better understanding of why cardio can benefit you, how you can get started, what exercises to perform and when to do it. No matter where you are in your cardiovascular health, you can begin today—making your way to a healthier you, both inside and out.

Points to remember:

- Some 24.3 million people took aerobic exercise classes in 2001, according to the National Sporting Goods Association, which tracks exercise trends. To combat the effect of decreased health and increased body fat, Americans have turned to cardiovascular exercise.
- Muscle for muscle, your heart is without question the strongest and most important organ in your body. If you are not exercising your heart it will digress in its ability to supply your body with nutrients and oxygen.
- Getting the authorization from your doctor to exercise is not only encouraged, but serves as a baseline for where you are to begin.
- Being in an aerobic state means oxygen is present and you are indeed burning fat. To monitor and ensure you are in this heart rate training zone, it is important that you can carry on a light conversation while exercising. When you cannot carry on a

light conversation, you may be working too hard (without oxygen). If you're not sure if you are working hard enough, pick up the pace.

- To save you time, energy and frustration when it comes to monitoring your intensity and getting results, we encourage you to become familiar with the rate of perceived exertion (RPE). This is our preferred method for determining the level of intensity we are working at during exercise.

- We agree that to release fat and improve your health daily, it is necessary to be consistent. We recommend that you work up to 45 to 60 minutes of cardio three to five times per week.

- In order for you to maximize the benefits of cardio and prevent injury, warm up for six to 12 minutes as part of your cardio session.

- Cardiovascular exercise performed first thing in the morning, on an empty stomach, provides the greatest potential for burning fat but may also burn muscle protein.

- All too often people will warm up, but skip the cool-down. Take into account that the cool-down helps to lower your blood pressure and return blood flow back to your heart and other organs like your stomach.

- It's a medical fact that cardio reduces risk of heart disease, diabetes, stroke, high blood pressure, and many other conditions, and it also alleviates symptoms of depression and improves well being.

21

The Role of Resistance Training

"Lack of activity destroys the good condition of every human being,
while movement and methodical physical exercise save it and preserve it."
—Plato

Did you know that you can change your body shape without liposuction and long bouts of cardiovascular exercise? Beyond the health and metabolic benefits, resistance training is simply the most effective method for changing your body composition. If you think that cardiovascular exercise (cardio) is enough—think again! Cardio alone is not enough if you want to alter the shape of your body. The fact is, if you are shaped like a pear and you only perform cardio, you will remain shaped like a pear—just smaller. Resistance training is how you dramatically change the contour of your body.

Resistance training is not only useful for building lean muscle tissue, which is a key factor for burning fat, it also strengthens and thickens bones (important for dramatically slowing down osteoporosis), helps relieve symptoms of arthritis, builds strength, increases tolerance for activities of daily living (functional fitness), and reverses a number of age related problems such as fatigue, poor balance and difficulty in walking. Studies also show that resistance training improves glucose tolerance and insulin sensitivity in people who have diabetes or are at risk of developing Type 2 diabetes.

Resistance training

What is resistance training? Often referred to as strength training or weight lifting, resistance training involves any physical training that uses weights—dumbbells, barbells and weight-lifting machines, to name a few—to perform isometric, isokinetic or isotonic exercises to strengthen and develop muscles. An isometric exercise involves muscle contractions that do not change the muscle length. For instance, ask the average ten-year-old to show you his muscles and he will more than likely lift his arm up, make a fist, and pull it towards his ear—squeezing the biceps muscle. He might even say, "Here, feel this," as he motions you to feel his bicep while he holds this isometric contraction.

In addition to improving the look and tone of your body, resistance training decreases the natural progression of muscle loss.

The isokinetic method of resistance training refers to exercises that vary the force throughout the range of motion. A great example of this is the use of rubberized tubing. The tension you feel when using these resistance bands changes as you work through the exercise. The further you pull the tubing away from the center, the greater the resistance. It almost feels like the tubing may snap as you pull and stretch it while performing the exercise.

Last of all, you have isotonic or dynamic constant resistance, which refers to exercises that have a constant load (force) throughout the range of motion. This is not limited to lifting barbells or dumbbells, but includes working your muscles against your own body weight (i.e., push-up, squat) and with a variety of plate-loaded machines and cables that are attached to pulleys and a stack of weight plates.

Regardless of which method you choose, over time and with repeated activity, your muscle fibers get stronger and thicker. Subsequently, you are able to work against a greater force (lift heavier weights).

In addition to improving the look and tone of your body, resistance training decreases the natural progression of muscle loss. Medical research has shown that resistance training is responsible for the following benefits:

- Strengthens the muscular system
- Strengthens the skeletal system
- Improves bone density (decreases the risk of osteoporosis)
- Increases metabolism
- Increases fat-burning potential
- Improves posture
- Improves coordination and balance
- Improves mood
- Increases blood circulation

- Slows atrophy (loss) of the muscles
- Aids in hypertension control
- Aids in cholesterol control
- Aids in prevention of Type 2 diabetes
- Aids in the prevention of heart disease and certain cancers

The benefits of resistance training are becoming more and more apparent and documented by medical professionals. According to the Sporting Goods Manufacturers Association (SGMA), resistance training has recently taken a front seat next to aerobic exercise in popularity, with an estimated 40 million people performing resistance training. Particularly for women, resistance training has grown in popularity. The SGMA reports that the number of women who train with free weights increased 134 percent between 1990 and 1999, from 8.3 million to 19.4 million. Regardless of age or gender, the benefits of resistance training are rapidly becoming an essential fitness and health component of many people's lifestyles.

Bringing clarity to resistance training

What comes to mind when you think of resistance training? Unfortunately, most people (specifically women) think of bodybuilding and the fear of gaining a massive amount of muscle, and even looking like a steroid-enhanced freak. This concern couldn't be further from the truth. First of all, women don't have enough testosterone to create big, bulky muscles. Further, many female bodybuilders put more than just resistance training into looking MASSIVE. In short, it is not uncommon for female bodybuilders to eat excessive amounts of calories, lift weights twice a day and supplement their body with various forms of steroids.

Resistance training is not only for bodybuilders, but also for anyone wanting to improve health and keep the released fat from coming back. Again...resistance training is for anyone.

To recap and provide you with more examples of resistance training, please note that it can be done anywhere—with or without weights. You can perform resistance training with your own body as experienced with exercises like squats, crunches (sit-ups) and when executing chin- and push-ups, just to name a few. You can even use household products when resistance training. However, to greatly benefit from this type of activity it helps to understand that the greater the demand (heavier the force), the more your muscles expand (breakdown and become stronger).

Weight-bearing exercise

We would like to bring clarity to the term "weight-bearing exercise," since it is often recommended by physicians and mentioned in the same breath as resistance training.

Like muscle, bone is alive and responds to both resistance training and weight-bearing exercise by becoming stronger and stimulating tissue growth. At this point, you may be asking yourself, "What's the difference between resistance training and weight-bearing exercise?" Simply put, "weight-bearing" means that your muscles and skeleton supports your own body weight. For instance, a weight-bearing exercise can include such activities as walking, hiking, jogging, playing tennis and dancing. On the other hand, exercises such as swimming and bicycling are not weight bearing, but are nevertheless helpful because of their positive effects on fitness.

If you are standing still, you are supporting your own body weight, therefore this activity would be weight bearing. Lying down on your stomach is not weight bearing. However once you begin to push yourself up, you are partially supporting your body weight and then engaged in a weight-bearing activity. Dancing on your feet is a weight-bearing activity, whereas dancing while seated is not.

Examples of weight-bearing activities:
> Basketball
> Cardio Kickboxing
> Yoga
> Tennis
> Gardening
> Golf
> Walking, Jogging and Running
> Dancing
> Push-ups
> Squats
> Lunges

Weight-bearing activities that involve the support of your body weight with your legs may prove beneficial in preventing falls that lead to fractures of the head of the femur (thigh bone that attaches at the hip). The more often our feet are in contact with the ground, the denser these bones become.

Living proof

Although the concept of resistance training is becoming clearer, you may remain sedentary or action-less because you can't imagine yourself grunting and growling your way to improved health. This perception of resistance training may cause you to take up weight-bearing exercises instead. You may think to yourself, "Weight-bearing exercises are all I need to build muscle. My goal is not to enter a bodybuilding competition." This may be true in essence, however; weight-bearing exercises may not be enough to bring about the results you desire. Every weight-bearing step you take sends pulses of electrical energy up and down the lengths of your bones, however, these pulsating currents of bio-electricity may not offer you a great enough demand (force) for your muscles to expand (breakdown and become stronger).

Resistance training improves quality of life, now and in your golden years.

Case in point: in a landmark study published in 1990, a group of nine 90+ year-old nursing home residents in the Boston area saw their leg strength improve by 174 percent and their walking speed increase by 48 percent, after just eight weeks of resistance training. The researchers who conducted this study and many others believe resistance training can actually reverse aging, with the oldest and weakest showing the greatest improvement. In the aforementioned study, keep in mind that the participants didn't dance, golf or play basketball. They performed resistance training (i.e. lifted weights).

Another study conducted by the United States Department of Agriculture (USDA) Human Nutrition Research Center on Aging discovered that resistance training is key in slowing the aging process. They discovered after a year-long study of women aged 50 to 70 that strength, balance and physical activity decline significantly. Such losses lead to falls—the great risk for fractures in the elderly. On the flip side, it is possible for anyone at any age to reverse and prevent such declines.

In this year-long study, 20 of the 39 volunteers strengthened muscles on pneumatic equipment for just 40 minutes twice a week. The resistance was set at 80 percent of maximum load (resistance) each could handle at a given session. Meanwhile, a control group of 19 of the 39 women continued their normal lifestyle. At the end of the year, the trained group had gained one percent more bone density in the hip and spine compared to a 2.5 percent loss in the control group. The trained muscles had strength increases from about 35 to 76 percent above the control group. Balance improved 14 percent. And spontaneous physical activity—excluding the resistance training sessions—increased by an average 27 percent, whereas it decreased in the control group by about the same amount.

What do these studies confirm? Resistance training improves quality of life now and during your golden years.

Use it or lose it

Have you ever heard the saying, "Use it or lose it?" This statement is very true when it comes to your lean muscle tissue. For instance, if you neglect intense physical activity all together, you may lose as much as 40 percent of your lean muscle tissue by the age of 80. Such shrinkage and loss of muscle makes you weaker, slows down your metabolism and negatively effects your body composition. It's been reported by various medical, health and fitness-related organizations that you can lose up to a half pound of muscle every year after age 25. For this reason alone, it is in your best interest to be consistent with your resistance training.

One pound of muscle can burn up to 50 calories a day, while fat can burn only two to five calories per day.

Consider this: one pound of muscle can burn up to 50 calories a day, while fat can burn only two to five calories per day. When less energy is needed for daily metabolic function, calories that were used by muscle are now stored as fat. The gradual loss of muscle tissue in sedentary adults leads to a five percent reduction in the metabolic rate every decade of life—making you more frail and prone to falls and other health related issues in later years.

It is unrealistic to blame your difficulties with managing your weight solely on age, genetics or chronic over-eating. It's also the result of an inadequate amount of muscle tissue in your body. As shocking as it may be to first learn of this unspoken phenomenon, you can build muscle at any age—regardless of gender.

In our opinion, the process of losing muscle is more insidious and crippling than osteoporosis, however, many people are unaware of this phenomenon until they experience difficulty walking up stairs or getting up from the sofa. Matter of fact, you probably didn't know that the gradual erosion of muscle is the major reason elderly North Americans are forced to move into nursing homes. As we stated earlier—by performing resistance training you become stronger, build muscle and therefore, slow down or help prevent age-related problems such as fatigue, poor balance and difficulty in walking.

"Why does this happen?" "Why am I just now learning about this?" and "What can I do to prevent or stop this from happening?" are questions many of our clients ask us once they learn the value of lean muscle tissue. No one is exempt from age-related muscle loss. However, before you confront your doctor and question why you're not informed, it wasn't until a few years ago that medical experts put a name to this phenomenon: sarcopenia, derived from the Greek words for vanishing flesh. In the mid-1990s, several labs across the country launched the first major studies of the subject.

Today, a new understanding of age-related muscle loss is beginning to emerge, along with some hopeful indications. Far from being as unavoidable as gray hair and wrinkles, sarcopenia can be reversed or slowed significantly by resistance training.

Muscle matters

When you have more muscle on your body, you burn more calories than someone who doesn't, even when you're both sitting still. This is because muscle requires more oxygen and more calories to sustain itself than body fat. Even while we sleep our skeletal muscles are responsible for more than 25 percent of our calorie use.

When you adhere to a low-calorie, reckless nutrition plan, your body disrupts your fat-burning potential by catabolizing (breaking down) lean muscle tissue, therefore, slowing your metabolism. Equally, if dieting doesn't decompose your muscle, more than likely the culprit responsible for your muscle loss will be decreased activity or a sedentary lifestyle.

Consider this example: A 140-pound woman who is 28 percent body fat (39 pounds of fat and 101 pounds of lean body mass) loses four pounds of fat and gains four pounds of muscle. She still weighs 140 pounds, but now 25 percent body fat (35 pounds are fat and 105 pounds are lean body mass). Every pound of muscle gained through resistance training increases your metabolic rate by up to 50 calories a day. Therefore, by gaining four pounds of lean muscle tissue, like the 140-pound woman, you may burn up to 200 extra calories per day, even at rest.

Muscle loss equates to a slower metabolism

People constantly share with us how their metabolism slows as they age. What they don't realize is how much muscle they lose largely determines how many calories they burn. So, as you lose this muscle, you slow your metabolism. Consequently, the more muscle you have, the faster your metabolic rate.

As we explained in Chapter 19, metabolism refers to the entire network of physical and chemical processes involved in maintaining life. It encompasses all the sequences of chemical reactions that enable us to release and use energy from food, convert one substance to another, and prepare products for excretion and elimination. With this said, muscle requires a significant amount and constant supply of energy to exist. Muscle cells have the ability to increase their workload faster and to a greater extent than any other cell in the body. There is a constant exchange of nutrients and waste products at the cellular level of the muscles. As a result, the more muscle you have—the more activity and chemical processes involved—the higher your metabolism.

Anna and her metabolic muscle disaster

Meet Anna, a 165-pound woman standing 5'5" with a body-fat percentage of 34 (56 pounds of fat and 109 pounds of lean body mass). Ready to get back to her high school weight of 10 years ago, Anna decided after meeting with us that she wanted quick results. The thought of losing one to two pounds a week was too slow. So, Anna decided to go with a high protein/low carbohydrate diet. She did inform us that after she dropped a few pounds she would return and learn how to eat healthy.

Six months later, Anna returned and weighed in at 130 pounds with a body-fat percentage of 32.3 percent (42 pounds of fat and 88 pounds of lean body mass). Anna couldn't understand why after losing 35 pounds, her body-fat percentage had only dropped 1.5 percent. As we explained the importance of lean muscle tissue, Anna remained puzzled (in denial), yet convinced that her approach was working for her. She didn't seem a bit concerned with the fact that of her 35-pound weight loss, 60 percent of it (21 out of the 35 pounds) was lean body mass—mostly in the form of muscle tissue.

Set on maintaining her new body weight of 130 pounds, Anna went on and continued to train aerobically five times per week. But, as the holidays crept up on her, in no time Anna was quickly adding on the pounds, and before you could say, "I told you so," she was back up and over 165—now weighing 170 pounds.

Exercising more and moving into deep depression, Anna decided to give us another opportunity. Without judgment, we sat down with Anna, conducted a body composition analysis for which we learned she had a body-fat percentage of 37 percent (63 pounds of fat and 107 pounds of lean body mass). Immediately, Anna bowed her head in tears. She was ready for change—she wanted something different. Frustrated and still not convinced that resistance training would help her release the fat and, more importantly keep it off, Anna pulled herself together and appeared to be more motivated than ever. Nonetheless, she didn't enroll into the Wellness Weight-Loss process. Anna had lost the weight before and she said she would get down to 130 and promised us that she would then take up resistance training.

In Anna's own words she said, "I will do the cardio first. Get my weight down and then build some muscle." This statement rang loud and clear to us that Anna wasn't hearing a word we were saying. We wished her well, provided a few recommendations and she left our office.

Two years went by and Anna experimented with a half dozen or so diets, and finally she returned to our office ready for a lifestyle change. It was great to see Anna again. A lot had changed in her life and she truly was ready for a lifestyle change. We conducted a body composition analysis and learned that her total body weight was 179 pounds with a body-fat percentage of 41.9 percent (75 pounds of fat and 104 pounds of lean body mass). When we first met Anna she had 109 pounds of lean body mass—now down five pounds, which equates to a slowed metabolism of up to 250 calories per day. This muscle loss and change in body composition took place in less than three years. Imagine what happens to those who gain weight, lose weight and continue this cycle for 10, 20, 30 years or more.

Anna eventually learned the importance of lean muscle tissue. We educated her on sarcopenia and its effects over time. Today Anna continues her cardio workouts, eats healthy all the time and lifts weights twice a week. Anna is a great example of someone who resisted the truth. Fortunately, Anna is aware now—she knows the deal—and is a true advocate of resistance training. Prior to completing this book, we met with Anna and conducted a body composition analysis and learned that she had settled in to a lean 23 percent body fat. Anna hasn't been this fit since high school. If you were to ask her, she would say she is more fit today than any other time in her life.

Low-calorie dieting is often another culprit responsible for causing your body to go into a famine state— slowing the metabolism even more.

The next step

Along with losing muscle as we age, low-calorie dieting is often another culprit responsible for causing your body to go into a famine state— slowing the metabolism even more. However, just as you can build strength and add muscle to your human frame at any age, the same remains true for increasing your metabolism through resistance training and a healthy nutrition plan.

Where do you start? Do you hire a personal trainer? Can you simply purchase a resistance-training book and get started? Before you rush out and spend hundreds of dollars purchasing equipment, employing a personal trainer and enrolling into a health club, first become familiar with the basics.

With a wide array of philosophies and methods being preached and promoted on how to best perform resistance training, there are five basic facts we want you to become familiar with:

Proper Warm-Up—After you have approval from your physician to engage in resistance training, prior to performing the exercises, it is to your benefit to perform a cardiovascular warm-up as we explained in Chapter 20 *(Cardiovascular Exercise)* for six to 12 minutes, followed by a series of stretches (see Appendix D).

Muscle Building Basics—To build muscle and improve strength it is best to perform eight to 12 repetitions. Building muscle is also known as hypertrophy. Because hypertrophy involves the tearing and rebuilding of muscle tissue, adequate rest between this type of workout is imperative.

Strength Building Basics—To build maximum strength it is best to perform one to three reps for a specific muscle group. Simply put, to build strength you benefit most from lifting heavy enough weight (resistance) that you cannot—without the help of a friend—perform more than three reps. You may have heard the term one rep max (1RM), which means the amount of weight that you can lift only one time. Obviously, this type of training is for competitive athletes who train specifically for strength and would not want to be included in any beginner program.

Muscle Endurance Basics—Endurance training basically means the ability of a muscle to contract repeatedly against a moderate resistance. To train for muscle endurance it is best to perform more than 12 reps using a light to moderate weight. We recommend you do not exceed 20 reps at a time because it can cause unnecessary wear and tear on the joints and connective tissue. Just look at the causes of conditions like tennis elbow or carpal tunnel syndrome. Simply put, if you can perform more than 20 repetitions—increase the weight.

Work Large to Small—To get the most out of your exercise sessions, work large muscles (compound exercises) first and then finish with the smaller muscles (isolation exercises). Because many smaller muscles assist in large muscle group exercises working them first would position you to lack the strength and intensity needed to train the big muscle groups effectively. For example: imagine exhausting your triceps muscles and then performing three sets of push-ups. You would probably fall on your face and wouldn't get the full benefit of the push-ups.

Have the gym membership, now what?

There is definitely a learning curve involved when beginning to use weights or perform resistance training. It takes time to understand the proper performance of technique. In the beginning—for the first three to four weeks—the results will be neuromuscular in nature. This means that you are recruiting previously inactive nerves in the muscle (motor units). However, as you establish a baseline or foundation, you will improve in coordination and become more confident. In no time you will begin to feel your muscles working as you perform the exercises. Frankly put, you will start to feel the burn in your muscles as you increase the intensity of your workout.

Whether you decide to use a health club, employ a personal trainer, purchase resistance equipment or participate in group classes, there are a few guidelines you want to keep in mind as you begin and continue progressing with your resistance training.

The F.R.R.I.T. principle

- **Frequency.** The duration and number of times per week you exercise is what we mean by frequency. One of the most common questions we are asked is, "How often and for how long should I exercise?" We recommend you adhere to the American College of Sports Medicine's (ACSM) suggestions: cardiovascular exercise 20 to 60 minutes, three to five days a week, and resistance or strength training two to three days a week for 30 minutes. When the NAS issued their guidelines they were referring to 60 minutes of total exercise per day.

- **Reps and sets.** A repetition (rep) is one complete action of an exercise. A set is defined as the number of successive reps performed without rest. If you are new to resistance training, we recommend you perform one set of eight to 10 exercises for 10 to 15 reps during your first week; two sets your second week and by the fourth week, increase to three sets. This will allow your muscles and nervous system to gradually adapt to the demands that you are placing on them and prepare your body for a slightly heavier load of eight reps by the sixth week. There will definitely be a trial and error period in the beginning to properly assess your weights and perform the proper technique—be patient. Once you have been consistent with resistance training for six weeks, we encourage you to perform a total of four sets. Your first set of 15 reps with a lighter weight will be considered your warm up. The three remaining sets will be as follows: second set, 12 reps; your third set, 10 reps; and your fourth set, eight reps. The goal is to increase the resistance (weight) with each set as you decrease the number of reps.

Week One One set 10-15 reps	**Week Two** Two sets 10-15 reps	**Week Three** Two sets 10-15 reps	**Week Four** Three sets 10-15 reps	**Week Six** Four sets 15-12-10-8 reps

Note: If your body-fat percentage is over 32 percent for women and 25 percent for men, or if you have high blood pressure, continue with muscle endurance training of three sets of 15 reps until your body-fat percentage is under the above numbers and your blood pressure is under control.

- **Rest.** It is highly recommended that you rest 30 to 60 seconds between sets for the same muscle group (i.e. back, legs, shoulders, chest, biceps, triceps). However, an active rest is the exception: resting one muscle group while working another as in a circuit or what is coined "superset." For example, you may choose to save time by completing an exercise set for chest (i.e., push-up), followed by an immediate set for back without rest. At some point, you will want to take a break to allow your muscles to recover so you may continue to lift the same or greater amount of weight. Too little rest between exercises will not give you enough time to replenish the energy needed within the muscle to complete each set with intensity. It is also recommended that you rest 48 hours after working a muscle group. For instance, if you train your whole body on Monday, wait a minimum of 48 hours before performing resistance exercises again. Note: cardio and muscular endurance training can be performed daily as long as your muscles aren't too sore.

- **Intensity.** Intensity can be defined as performing each rep through a full range of motion—completing each set to muscle fatigue or failure. If you are new to resistance training, we want you to work with enough resistance (weight) that you can perform the exercise for 10 to 15 reps for the first six weeks. To ensure you are working with enough resistance, it is important that the weight is heavy enough that you cannot perform 16 reps without the help of a friend or training partner. By the sixth week we encourage you to perform no more than 12 reps in a set—unless it is a warm-up set of 15 reps. Following the warm-up set, if you can perform 13 reps— the resistance (weight) is too easy for you. Remember, the goal is to completely fatigue the muscle without sacrificing proper form and technique. Safety and injury prevention are always a priority. The bottom line: If you can perform more than 15 reps, the weight is too light. Conversely, if you cannot perform at least eight reps, the weight is too heavy.

- **Timing (rhythm).** The rhythm of a repetition has a major impact on injury prevention and strength development. Using momentum and lifting with speed places a great deal of stress on the muscles and the connective tissue (tendons and ligaments), especially at the beginning of the movement. In order to reduce the risk of injury and increase the effectiveness of each repetition, we recommend that you take two seconds during the lifting phase (the concentric motion) and three to four seconds to lower the weight—during the eccentric phase of the exercise. It is always a good idea to take a pause at the peak of the contraction and contract (squeeze) the muscle. It is also of value to exhale when the muscle is exerting the greatest force and inhale during the eccentric phase. Example: when performing a squat, as you decent toward the ground (the eccentric phase), count to three or four and inhale. As you ascend (the concentric phase), count to two and exhale.

Muscle burns fat

Okay, you accept the fact that muscle is important and you will get around to adding resistance training to your weekly routine. However, you have this belief that it is best to first get your body fat down and then begin resistance training with hopes of toning up. If you have these thoughts taking up space in your mind, consider this important fact: it is muscle that burns fat when performing cardiovascular exercise. Therefore, if you aren't doing what is necessary to preserve and build your muscle, you are going to lose your muscle, lowering your fat-burning potential.

When you perform cardiovascular excercise, fat is released into your blood stream and carried to your muscle to be burned.

Now that you are aware that muscle is a fundamental component of your metabolism, it is vital that you keep as much of this muscle as possible when you are releasing fat. The most effective method for keeping muscle is performing resistance training. As well, the most effective method for burning fat is performing cardiovascular exercise, as we explained in Chapter 20.

When you perform cardiovascular exercise, fat is released into your blood stream and carried to your muscle to be burned. When the muscle doesn't burn the fat, the excess makes its way to your liver where it is metabolized and then re-entered into your blood, and more often than not stored in what we refer to as trouble areas (fat depots).

When you perform resistance training, it is a fact that you elevate your metabolism during the hours following your workout—that is, you burn more calories over the next 48 hours. However, you are not burning fat when performing resistance training. Why? Because oxygen is not present in your muscles when performing this type of exercise, and it is the presence of oxygen that makes it possible for your muscles to burn fat. (If necessary, review the energy systems in Chapter 20).

To get the most out of your resistance training, we encourage you to eat a balanced meal or at least a snack within one hour after your workout.

So, to get the most out of your resistance training, we encourage you to eat a balanced meal or at least a snack within one hour after your workout. The time following your resistance training is referred to as the anabolic window—the window of opportunity for you to replenish the energy supply in your muscles that is needed to actually re-build the tissue. Prior to your resistance training, we recommend eating a snack such as a slice of toast with natural peanut butter, an apple, protein shake, yogurt or something light—giving yourself a minimum of one hour for digestion prior to training.

When you are performing resistance training with intensity, you are actually creating micro-tears in the muscle. As a result, you are likely to be sore for a few days. Muscle tears along with high acid concentrations and muscle metabolic wastes (lactic acid) are responsible for soreness. It is during the rest and recovery phase that the muscles are using the macronutrients you consume to repair and building in strength. This is why it is so important to eat enough food and get rest 48 hours in between intense resistance workouts.

Time for KFC

The KFC we are referring to is not Kentucky Fried Chicken. The "K" in this acronym stands for knowing what you want. The "F" is a reminder to find out what you're getting. It is one thing to begin resistance training, however it is something different to be aware of the progress you are making. A great example of finding out what you're getting is to monitor your body composition. It is important that you are aware of whether or not you are building, maintaining or losing muscle and fat. The "C" is for changing what you do until you get what you want. Simply put: if you're not progressing—change what you're doing. For a detailed resistance and stretching program, refer to Appendix C.

Points to remember:

- Resistance training is the way you dramatically change the shape of your body.
- The number of women who train with free weights increased 134 percent between 1990 and 1999, from 8.3 million to 19.4 million.
- Women don't have enough testosterone to create big, bulky muscles.
- Like muscle, bone is alive and responds to both resistance training and weight-bearing exercise by becoming stronger and stimulating tissue growth.
- Weight-bearing exercise is an activity where your muscles and skeleton supports your own body weight.
- In a landmark study published in 1990, a group of nine 90+ year old nursing home residents in the Boston area saw their leg strength improve by 174 percent, and their walking speed increase by 48 percent after just eight weeks of resistance training.
- If you neglect intense physical activity all together, you may lose as much as 40 percent of your lean muscle tissue by the age of 80.
- One pound of muscle can burn up to 50 calories a day, while fat can burn only two to five calories per day.
- It is reported that you can lose up to a half pound of muscle every year after age 25.
- When you adhere to a low-calorie, reckless nutrition plan, your body disrupts your fat-burning potential by catabolizing (breaking down) lean muscle tissue, therefore, slowing your metabolism.
- Muscle cells have the ability to increase their workload faster and to a greater extent than any other cell in the body.
- Muscle burns fat.
- Refer to the Appendix C for the resistance program and stretching illustrations.

Wellness Weight-Loss

It's a lifestyle ..not a diet!

PART SEVEN

Resolve to Evolve

22

Knowing and Doing

"Within the self, there is a central force of character that unifies thought and actions. When you are not in accordance with your goals, you may feel indecision, conflict, or malaise; when you are, a sense of self-confidence and well being will surround you"
—I Tao Te Ching no.45

"I know what to eat." "I know what I need to do." "I know what I should be doing." Do any of these statements sound familiar? Of the thousands of people we have worked with, the statement that rings true with most of them begins with: "I know…" When it comes to following through with what's in their best interest, however, it seems to be a task easier said than done.

Doing what you know has to be the ultimate cliché when it comes to actions speaking louder than words. Think about it: If all you had to do was know, then being fit, firm and healthy would come easy. Helping our clients bridge the gap between knowing and doing is one of the things we do best.

Despite everything people say about knowing what to do, most of them continue to remain stuck—action-less. Understanding that this is the case, we remain compassionate because we know that following through with what you know is not an easy task. On one hand, we believe in Earl Nightingale's affirmation that you become what you think about most. However, on the other hand, we know that just thinking about what you want or feel that you need is simply not enough. That's why we look forward to sharing with you two essentials that will help you be the person you want by successfully bridging the gap between knowing and doing.

Your foundation

Before we introduce two essentials of bridging the gap between knowing and doing, it is important that you become aware of the distinction between what needs and wants are—and what they're not. Here's an easy question: "Do you want to lose weight or feel you need to lose weight?" "Do you want to eat healthy or feel you need to eat healthy?" Regardless of how you answer, please keep in mind that "wanting" and "needing" are two different things, and our goal is to help you put into perspective the concept of wants versus needs. Read and reflect on the following definitions before you proceed:

People, for the most part, base the bulk of their daily actions on maintaining what it is they want, rather than what they truly need.

NEEDS: Living essentials: air, water, shelter, food and defecation. You can't sustain life without these basic needs being met.

WANTS: Things that are above and beyond life's essentials, including money-oriented comforts, as well as services and products that many people associate with an increased quality of life.

People, for the most part, base the bulk of their daily actions on maintaining what they want, rather than what they truly need. Many people would rush to disagree with this statement, claiming that their decisions are based on a combination of both wants and needs. When such an objection arises, we always ask, "Can you share with me one thing that you do out of need?" After a few moments of thought, most people redefine their need as a want.

Consider this: You don't work because you need to work. You work because you want to have electricity, shelter, etc. You don't eat healthy because you need to lose weight and feel good. You eat healthy because you want to lose weight and feel good. Based on our experience with many clients, if you feel you need to lose weight, you will probably put off taking action. Whereas, once you want to lose weight, you have made a decision and that means you're ready to take action.

We know many of you are thinking, "I do need to work." Well, whether you want to believe it or not—you don't. No one is holding a gun to your head, forcing you to work. It is your choice. You could easily choose to be homeless, live with your parents or go on welfare. We agree that going to work is being responsible, however, it is still a choice.

Get excited

People don't get excited about **NEEDING** to do anything (i.e., dishes, cleaning, exercising). People get excited when they **WANT** something (i.e., release fat, take a vacation, purchase a new car). Think about it! If your doctor says to you, "You need to lose weight." How does that make you feel? Is it motivating to need something?

Vocabulary

All too often people believe they take action based on needs, however, in reality it is actually their wants that serve as the motivation for those actions. We are experts in the psychology of weight loss and human actions. One of the key determinants in whether or not you succeed is discovered in the words you use. Knowing that words are an expression of your thoughts, we pay close attention to your vocabulary.

For instance, do you ever say the following:

"I need to do something about my weight."
"I need to eat healthier."

Using the word "need" tells us that you are putting off making a decision. The word "need" is similar to the word "try" and the phase "I think" as they clarity the fact that procrastination is present.

Instead of saying the aforementioned, say the following:

"I want to do something about my weight."
"I want to eat healthier."

Taking the "need" out of your vocabulary and replacing it with "want" is a surefire method of helping you become decisive. We have learned after working with many people that those who are able to define their wants most clearly, are more likely to do what is necessary to succeed, ultimately bridging the gap between knowing what to do and doing what they know.

Eat to live or live to eat

Ask yourself, "Do I eat to live or live to eat?" Though eating is definitely a need, it is obvious that you eat because you want to live. You don't eat because you need to live.

Regardless of how you have thought and expressed yourself up to this point, you are more likely to take action when you want something, rather than when you "need" it. People often verbalize the need to lose weight, eat healthy and exercise, but they rarely act on it. Quite often people may say, "I need to lose weight," but continue to procrastinate. On the flip side, when people say, "I want to lose weight," they are one step away from taking action. Why? Taking action is usually prompted by knowing what you want, not what you need.

Momentum

As you begin to use the word "want" in place of "need," you will notice a new sense of momentum. Wanting is powerful and we encourage you to "want" your way to a diet-free and healthier lifestyle. Nonetheless, make it part of your mission to acquire professional and credible assistance as you empower yourself and your "wants."

First essential

Now that you want to release fat, you are in a better position to bridge the gap between knowing and doing. To jump start this process, we would like you to become familiar with the first of two essentials: self-suggestion. We precede "suggestion" with the reflexive "self" because we are talking about you and only you. If you didn't already know, suggestions are very powerful sources of persuasion. When positive in nature, suggestions act as the driving forces behind why we continue to strive for what we desire most.

What exactly are suggestions? Suggestions are thoughts that are known to be the communication link between the conscious and subconscious mind. Hypnotherapy is based primarily on planting suggestions. For instance, if a licensed hypnotist were to offer you a suggestion that you would be willing to accept, with repetition, you might begin to act on what he or she has suggested. Point blank, hypnotherapy is all about self-suggestion or, shall we say self-hypnotherapy.

More on hypnotherapy

Hypnotherapy is based primarily on stimulating the subconscious mind through the delivery and acceptance of suggestions. Simply put, hypnotherapy is a means of preparing your subconscious mind to take orders for which it will then act upon later. It is important for you to know that even with hypnotherapy, it helps to receive suggestions (orders) over and over again through repetition before they are interpreted by your subconscious mind.

We are not recommending that you rush out and schedule a session with a hypnotist. Instead what we are suggesting is that you take advantage of this first essential and begin reinforcing your goals via empowering statements and self-suggestions; you are the administrator of your own thoughts. Though you will continually receive suggestions from friends, relatives, books and television programs, it is you who ultimately decides which suggestions become "self-suggestions."

In Chapter 9 *(Friend or Foe?)* we shared with you how the questions you ask yourself determine how you think; the same is true here. Instead of asking yourself, "Why can't I lose weight?" replace that question with, "How can I release fat and enjoy the process?" Become your own best friend; ask yourself positive questions, and be weary of outside influences that may conflict with the direction you're headed.

Though you will continually receive suggestions from friends, relatives, books and television programs, it is you who ultimately decides which suggestions become "self-suggestions."

Misguidance

In today's world we are overloaded with information. It's everywhere. We have the Internet, libraries, magazines, trade papers, direct mail and thousands of books claiming to have the solution to weight loss. These are definitely booming times for businesses offering weight loss products and services. The reason for this is simple—supply and demand.

Americans are spending a significant amount of money each year on gym memberships, home exercise equipment and weight-loss products and services. The economic cost of obesity in the United States alone is over $100 billion. These numbers have attracted the attention of many weight-loss specialists, physicians, fitness trainers, acupuncturists and even chiropractors. It seems more and more that everyone knows not only how to lose weight, but how to help you lose weight.

Unfortunately, advice on how to best lose weight is now coming from so many different sources, that it all too often causes more confusion than clarity. Everyone knows what to do, how to do it and why their approach is the best. As a result of all the confusion, it is likely that you will find yourself misguided by the acceptance of outside suggestions. Consider this situation: you meet someone who lost weight on a high protein/low carbohydrate diet and his or her experience now becomes a suggestion to you. The next thing you know, you are taking steps in a different direction—making their experience your own self-suggestion.

Stick to your guns as you move forward with the Wellness Weight-Loss process. In order to do this it helps to heighten your protection filter and not allow outside sources to detour you from what is true in essence; increased activity and/or fewer calories consumed will cause a caloric deficit and therefore a reduction in fat.

With the Wellness Weight-Loss process you are reversing the causes of excess body fat by creating healthy daily habits. Wellness Weight-Loss is a lifestyle approach, with no gimmicks, no shortcuts, and no fads. The suggestion that you are reinforcing with the Wellness Weight-Loss process is a lifestyle that not only increases your energy, but also enhances the aesthetics of your body and improves your overall well being.

Whatever the suggestion, be it healthy or unhealthy, it is likely to begin growing roots. Remember, it is a well-known fact that you are likely to believe whatever you repeat to yourself—whether or not that statement is true or false. If you repeat a lie over and over, you will eventually accept that lie as truth. Be weary of outside suggestions. Again, always filter information before accepting it as part of your beliefs (habits of thought).

Self-suggestion is a powerful tool, however, it is important that it is used carefully and with resolve. When used consistently, you are likely to throw off any outside influences that otherwise would disrupt your potential. We encourage you to reinforce your suggestions daily and compare this process to that of a seed. Be patient—the harvest is coming!

Self-suggestion formula:

First: Find a quiet place where you will not be disturbed and repeat out loud your written goal of how much body fat you're going to release, the target date for its achievement, and a description of what actions you're going to take in order for your goal to become a reality. If you have not established your goal, refer back to and re-read Chapters 11 and 13.

For example: Suppose you intend to release 25 pounds by the first of June (12 weeks), and you intend to exercise a minimum of three days per week, drink a minimum of eight glasses of water daily and follow the Wellness Weight-Loss process. Your written statement of purpose will be similar to the following:

"On June 1, 2004, I will weigh a maximum of 170 pounds. I will achieve this goal by adhering to the Wellness Weight-Loss process which means eating healthy, exercising regularly and planning daily."

Second: Repeat this statement first thing in the morning and last thing at night until you reach your goal.

Third: Place a written copy of your statement where it can be seen first thing in the morning and last thing at night; read it out loud prior to sleep, and immediately after waking until it has been learned.

Remember, as you follow these instructions, you are applying the first essential of self-suggestion. What this means is that you are providing your subconscious mind with daily suggestions to act upon. These daily suggestions will help you follow through with what you know.

The fact is, the larger the gap between knowing and doing, the lower the level of your self-esteem.

Second essential

What's the big deal about not doing the things you know? What's so horrible about avoiding exercise like the plague when you know it improves your overall health? When you know which foods are healthy, but you eat unhealthily, how does that affect you? The fact is, the larger the gap between knowing and doing, the lower your level of self-esteem.

Self-esteem, in our opinion, is the most overlooked essential in terms of getting control of your weight and health. How you value yourself is the by-product of how much inner-worth and importance you experience every moment of your life. The term self-esteem has become a cliché, but the essence of the word relates to how a person regards him or her self. How much unconditional love and acceptance you give yourself determines the strength of your self-esteem. Sincerely, how much you like yourself is what determines your level of self-esteem.

Before we continue, please note that we are talking about how you value yourself, and no one else. We are not referring to spouses, parents, boss, siblings or children; we are referring to you. In order for you to better understand your self-esteem and the role it plays in bridging the gap between knowing and doing, it is important for you to first realize it is an inside job. You do for yourself or it doesn't get done.

Your current degree of self-esteem is where it is because of your total life's experiences. Your self-esteem is not based on one or two things that happened in your past, it is a culmination of your entire life. However, regardless of past experiences, decisions you've made and actions you have taken, it's what you do beginning today and each and everyday that will determine in which direction your self-esteem will move.

There is no shelf life on self-esteem; each day we either build or sabotage it—there is no gray area. It is either black or white and you are in charge of what it will be. If you want to build your self-esteem it helps to remain in the present and accept all previous experiences. It is important to realize and accept that you cannot change the past—what others have done to you, what you have done to someone else or what you have done to yourself. The past is history and the only person you can change is you.

Self-esteem starts with honoring all of the promises you make to yourself.

Self-esteem begins with...

What does it take for you to gain inner-worth and importance? How do you begin to earn value and significance? Self-esteem starts with honoring all of the promises you make to yourself. In order to do this, it is important that you take the time to nurture and care for yourself. It's time to make you a priority. As you begin investing in yourself you will discover it isn't an easy task. This can be attributed to the fact that we live in a hurry-up-and-go world that recognizes and rewards what you do for others more than what you do for yourself.

How is it that caring for yourself carries with it a penalty? Why is it that many women and men think it's selfish to take care of themselves? What makes being selfish so bad? Please understand that when we use the word selfish we are referring to the opposite of someone who is self-centered or self-absorbed.

We define being selfish as giving to yourself so that you are better able to give to others. Being selfish is not mistreating others or thinking you are the almighty. When the late Mother Theresa was asked why she dedicated her life to helping the poor in Calcutta, she said, "It brought me joy." Does the joy she received from helping others make her selfish? Mother Theresa is a great example of someone who valued self-love, for that is what helped her to be "others-oriented".

Imagine the following scenario: you are flying on an airplane with your five- and nine-year-old boys. The flight attendant gives you specific instructions as to what to do if the oxygen masks drop down from the enclosed area above your seat: "You have seven to eight seconds to mask yourself and then help your children put their masks on."

Depending on altitude, if you don't get your mask on quickly you may slip into unconsciousness and therefore not be able to help your children. However, if you neglect to care for yourself first, you are also placing your children in harm's way. It might seem difficult in a panic situation to imagine doing for yourself first, but if you don't, you will be doing a disservice to your children. In a scenario like this, not caring for yourself first may prove disastrous for your loved ones.

Now, consider this possibility: the oxygen masks drop down from overhead and you decide to place the mask on your five-year-old and then turn to help your nine-year-old. Once you get your older son's mask on however, you discover your five year old has taken his mask off. Why? Because small children always do what their parents do, and since your mask isn't on, your son is thinking, "Why should I keep my mask on?" On the flip side, when you put your mask on first, then turn to the five-year-old to put his mask on and then turn to your older son, guess what: he already has his mask on.

Looking out for your children is putting your mask on first. Taking care of yourself is how you make the biggest impact on those closest to you. When you take care of yourself, you give the best of who you are to those you love the most. It is taking responsibility for yourself that empowers you to become others-oriented.

If you are a parent or not, please nurture yourself. Love yourself and be kind to yourself and you will notice more and more each day that you can give more love to those closest to you. If you do not take time out for yourself and continue doing only for others, you are going to find yourself living a big chunk of your life trying to out perform, produce and pretend to the entire world that you are okay. When this is the case you will return home after a crazy day of doing for everyone else but yourself—burned out. If you are feeling burned out, ask yourself, "Do I have my mask in place and am I taking care of myself first?" When you take care of yourself and put yourself first, you will begin to follow through on what you know.

As you have read, we could easily write an entire book on self-esteem and its relationship with weight management. However, because of time and space restraints, we encourage you to consider our audio program and workbook: *Esteem Your 'Self' for a Diet-Free Life!* In the end, when all is said and done, a higher level of self-esteem will require a permanent investment into the five dimensions of wellness: spiritual (living in harmony), physical (physical/physiological well-being), intellectual (open to learn), emotional (coping skills), and social (support systems).

We strongly encourage you to reflect upon these five dimensions. Taking time to reflect and ensure that adequate attention is being given to each dimension will prove to be a great foundation for building your self-esteem. Remember, self-esteem is how you value yourself and it is enhanced by taking the time to care, nurture and love you. Make time for yourself and you will be better able to love those closest to you.

Points to remember:

- Doing what you know has to be the ultimate cliché when it comes to actions speaking louder than words.
- When you want to release fat, your scope of options is broadened and you're more likely to succeed.
- Positive suggestions act as the driving force as to why you continue to strive for what you desire most.
- Increased activity and/or fewer calories consumed will cause a caloric deficit and therefore a reduction in weight.
- Motivation is important in not only getting started, but also following through, remaining on course and getting back on track when and if you fall off.
- The larger the gap between knowing and doing, the lower your level of self-esteem.
- How you esteem yourself is the by-product of how much inner-worth and importance you experience every moment of your life.
- When you put your mask on first (take care of yourself) you will be better able to help others.

23

Conquering Procrastination

"If we did all of the things we were capable of,
we would literally astound ourselves."
—Thomas A. Edison

Have you ever procrastinated? After all you have learned and having read 22 chapters, will you procrastinate? People share with us all the time that they have put off their fat loss goals for far too long. Why do you think people procrastinate when it comes to fat loss? More importantly, why do you find yourself procrastinating?

Technically, procrastination means avoiding a specific task or job that is to be accomplished.

All the same, this technical explanation doesn't begin to capture the many emotions triggered by the word. For most of us, especially when it comes to releasing fat, the word "procrastination" reminds us of past experiences when we have felt guilty, lazy, inadequate, anxious or stupid—or some combination of these. It also implies a value judgment: if you procrastinate, you are bad, and as such, you lack worth as a person. Procrastination is about not getting things done on time and the torture you put yourself through to complete them. It's about promises made to change, but not being able to keep them for reasons you don't u nderstand, don't accept, or don't know what to do about. Examples of procrastination include the following:

- The electric bill that doesn't get paid on time
- The frustration of being behind...again
- The late charges for movie rentals that cost more than the video to rent
- The promise to never put things off...again
- The waiting for the last minute to complete a project and then stressing about it the night before

- The phone calls that don't get returned
- The wall you come up against when you attempt to lose weight...again

---

Procrastination makes no task easy...when it comes to doing the things you already know, it helps that procrastination is overcome by conviction.

It's all these things and more. Procrastination makes no task easy. Most people assume the reason they procrastinate is because they lack willpower and discipline. The reality is that people who procrastinate demonstrate quite a bit of will power and discipline in many other areas of their life. However, when faced with following through on certain goals or self-promises such as releasing fat, they get stuck and often experience emotions of helplessness, powerlessness, being overwhelmed, being out of control, and feeling sad or resentful.

Understanding and overcoming procrastination is a tall order, however, it can be conquered. There are no ifs, ands or buts about it. We have interviewed and coached countless people who have successfully won the battle of the bulge. Through this we've learned that all of them came to a point in their life where they made a decision to alter their lifestyle. Alternatively, those who lack skills in decision-making are more likely to fall victim to the confinements of procrastination.

When it comes to doing the things you already know, it helps that procrastination is overcome by conviction. If not, you may remain immobilized when it comes to your weight. Like obesity, procrastination is a silent killer and is best dealt with seriously. It will continue to creep in and cause you to remain stuck—action-less. Therefore, it is to your benefit that you solve your procrastination issues.

Take a closer look at whether the cause of your immobilization is poor time management; if so, it is necessary for you to learn and develop time management skills. For instance, eating every three hours is fundamental in releasing fat and keeping it off.

Getting started

If you are skillful in managing your time, but find yourself not utilizing these skills, you may require additional attention. However, in the meantime, contemplate the following reasons for not taking the first step toward a leaner and healthier you:

- LACK OF RELEVANCE. If something is neither relevant nor meaningful to you personally, it may be difficult to get motivated even in the beginning. One solution is to discover meaning in why you want to release fat and alter your lifestyle.

- ACCEPTANCE OF ANOTHER'S GOALS. If everyone but you is insisting that you need to lose weight and it is not something you want to do, it is very likely that you will be reluctant to spend the necessary time to see a weight-loss goal through to conclusion. There is no point starting unless you really want to do it yourself.

- PERFECTIONISM. If you believe your weight-loss goal is unreachable, it may discourage you from following through with your self-promise. Perfectionism is proven to stop many people from attempting fat loss for the sole reason they want to be perfect. Remember, perfection is unattainable. It does not exist.

- EVALUATION ANXIETY. Since others' responses to your lifestyle change are not under your direct control, overvaluing these responses can create the kind of anxiety that will interfere with you following through and accomplishing your goal. For instance, someone may say, "You are no fun anymore—I like the old you better."

- AMBIGUITY. If you are uncertain of what is expected of you, it may be difficult to get started. This is why we welcome all inquiries, concerns and questions regarding the Wellness Weight-Loss process. We are merely an e-mail away from answering your questions.

- FEAR OF THE UNKNOWN. Beginning a fat-releasing program and not having any idea of how well you are going to do can be frightening. Many people put off starting a fat-loss program because of the uncertainty. The Wellness Weight-Loss process is safe and we are here to support you. We encourage you to recognize the fact that fear of the unknown is conquered by enthusiasm of the present. Fear of the future is a waste of energy because it does not exist.

- INABILITY TO HANDLE THE TASK. We have learned that many people avoid lifestyle changes because they lack the skills or ability to remain on track. For this reason we encourage you to ask us questions. You are not alone, and we are here to help you broaden your resources.

Underlying cause

Procrastination takes on many faces. However, once you acknowledge the underlying causes of your procrastination, you can move toward removing this roadblock to success. Consider the following questions:

1. Do you act as if being over fat will go away if you avoid thinking about it? Let's face it, being over fat is not likely to disappear, no matter how much you ignore it.
2. Do you underestimate the planning involved in altering your eating habits? Do you tell yourself that a lifestyle of eating healthy doesn't involve much planning? In reality it is likely to require a minimum of one hour per week.
3. Have you misled yourself into believing that a mediocre performance or lesser standards are acceptable? For example, you may feel that you have succeeded in all other aspects of your life, including career, relationships and finances, to name just a few. However, the only area that you have not conquered is your weight. Have you accepted lower standards for your physical appearance and health? If this is the case, you may be avoiding the decision to alter your lifestyle so much that you are unable to support your fat loss efforts. This form of avoidance can prevent you from consciously making choices about long-term management of your weight.
4. Do you kid yourself by substituting one worthy activity for another? Suppose you do laundry instead of exercise. Valuing clean clothes is excellent, but if that value takes priority over the time you have allotted for exercise, you are procrastinating.
5. Do you believe that repeated delays are harmless? An example is putting off eating after a workout so you can check your e-mail. If you still haven't eaten after five-minutes on the Internet, you may stay in cyberspace for the most part of the evening, inevitably compromising your fat loss efforts.
6. Do you dramatize a commitment to healthy eating rather than actually doing it? An example is buying healthy foods (i.e., vegetables, fruit) and rarely eating them.
7. What about planning rather than doing? Are you an over-planner? An example is spending such an enormous amount of time planning that you never take action.
8. Do you persevere on only one portion of your desire to release fat? An example is performing resistance training (i.e. lifting weights, strength train) but not dealing with the necessities of

cardiovascular (aerobic) exercise. Resistance and cardiovascular exercise are both equally important in the fat-loss process.

9. Do you become paralyzed in deciding between alternative choices? An example involves spending so much time deciding between joining two health clubs that you have difficulty actually getting underway with your exercise program.

Following through

Now that you have brought clarity to some of the most common examples of how you may procrastinate, it is time for some effective planning. Fortunately, most of the work has been done for you regarding nutrition and exercise. The Wellness Weight-Loss process is your plan and will prove its weight in gold.

Your biggest obstacle may come if you think you don't need assistance or some method of consistent reinforcement. Until your lifestyle is such that you have made it a habit to exercise regularly and eat healthy (all the time), take advantage of our support system. We have many methods of coaching in place (i.e., office visits, Internet coaching). Consider the following steps for ensuring your follow through:

- Take baby steps. Releasing fat may seem overwhelming at times— smaller steps may seem more manageable. For example, instead of expecting to release five pounds of fat per week, we suggest you let go of one to two pounds per week.

- Distribute the baby steps reasonably within a given time frame. "Reasonably" is the key word; allot sufficient time for each step. Do not fool yourself by believing you can do more than is humanly possible. This is why we recommend 12-week increments, combined with setting and achieving short-term goals along the way.

- Realize that it is natural to want variety in your food choices as you move toward a healthier lifestyle. For this reason we believe it helps to intersperse rewards, relaxation and gratification for the efforts put forth. However, a reward does not mean all you can eat pizza; instead, purchase a new blouse or go for a weekend get-a-way for instance. This will help you feel less resentful of the efforts you're making.

- Assess dilemmas when they arise and resolve them quickly. Remember, becoming skilled at making decisions is synonymous with conquering procrastination. Keep track of daily progress and how each day fits together with the next to form the whole picture. Reassess time commitments as necessary.

- When you come to the 24 action steps in Chapter 24, take your time and complete each task before moving to the next one. There is no hurry. The one step at a time process is how you are going to carry your momentum over to the next day, then the next and for the rest of your life.

We've shared with you the basics of what procrastination means and why people procrastinate. We've also provided some methods of conquering procrastination. Of course, there is still much more that could be said about why people procrastinate when it comes to releasing fat and creating health.

Going directly to the cause and reversing it is fundamental in conquering procrastination.

It takes a lot of work to conquer procrastination, and we'd be insincere if we said it's easy. It takes the ability to establish priorities, manage time, to set goals and to break them down into manageable pieces—if conquering procrastination is the ultimate objective. Before you can do these things however, be aware of the reasons why you have been unable to follow through in the first place.

Going directly to the cause and reversing it is fundamental in conquering procrastination. For instance, if you experience a situation where you are hungry and all you have available is a vending machine, what do you do? When you go to the cause, it's obvious that a lack of planning put you in this situation. Therefore, to avoid situations like this in the future, decide right now that you want to improve your ability to plan ahead. That would be a way to reverse the cause in this scenario.

To help our clients remain empowered and equipped with food, we have established the Wellness Kit. We invite you to learn more about our Wellness Kit and how it can benefit you by visiting our online store at **www.wellnessweightloss.net.**

Make the decision

Procrastination is basically your perception of how you see things. Surprisingly, it is quite typical for most of us to perceive taking action as more painful than doing nothing. You may be thinking that when it comes to fat loss, the reward of releasing fat after all these years is much more pleasurable than remaining fat. Though this may be true, what you consider more real at the time—the moment—is the realization that taking action to release fat means experiencing some discomfort.

When releasing fat increases your energy, self-esteem and health, why is it that so many people remain over fat? With all the great things that result from releasing fat, you would think there would be a line of people eagerly wanting to get started. Unfortunately, what separates those who do from those who don't is making a decision.

Every positive change in your life begins with a clear decision that you are either going to do something or stop doing something. For the most part, people are over fat because they have not yet decided to commit to releasing the fat. Making the decision is very powerful, and once made, watch out because the power behind deciding to release fat is a true predictor of success!

The only component necessary after making the decision to release fat and create health is consistent reinforcement. Whether it is a friend, support group or a Wellness Weight-Loss coach, having someone to check in with and reinforce your commitment is the surest method for continued progress. At least until you are no longer trapped in a diet mentality and your new lifestyle becomes a habit.

Points to remember:

- Procrastination refers to avoiding a specific task or job that is to be accomplished. It's about things not getting done on time and the torture you go through to complete them.
- Procrastination is about promises you make to yourself to change, but not being able to keep them for reasons you don't understand, don't accept or don't know what to do about.
- The antidote to procrastination is decisiveness.
- For the most part, people are over fat because they have not yet decided to release fat.

24

Bottom Line

"If we could give every individual the right amount of
nourishment and exercise, not too little and not too much,
we would have found the safest way to health."
—Hippocrates

Nine out of ten women feel they are overweight, and nearly as many men want to get rid of excess body fat. Many of these women and men are willing to do just about anything to look and feel better. We have met people who've attempted to use massage, liposuction, lotions and creams, and even extreme methods of exercise to get the fat off their body. And let's not forget those who take diet supplements, like pills, potions and miracle liquids hoping they'll do the trick.

What is the answer? What really works? The bottom line: focus, regular exercise, healthy food and habits of thought (beliefs). Exercise is important. According to the National Weight Control Registry, the nation's most successful fat-droppers work off about 2,800 calories a week. However, it is the "two-armed table pushback" that is the most determining factor in the fight against fat.

The fact remains that when it comes to releasing fat, what you eat and don't eat will either help or hurt you. Here's one example: walking or running a mile burns roughly 100 calories. A pound of fat is 3,500 calories. That's 35 miles per pound, or almost a marathon and a 10-miler combined.

To exercise, but neglect a habit of healthy nutrition is like running a race without running shoes. We have witnessed this first hand in one of our offices located inside a health club. Day in and day out, we observe hundreds of people exercising daily, sometimes twice per day, making very little—if any—progress aesthetically. Most people we have met in health clubs see very little change when it comes to fat loss.

What is blocking these people? Why aren't they succeeding and getting in the best physical shape of their life? As we have said time and again, you can be fit, but still fat. You can exercise like there is no tomorrow, but unless you are practicing healthy eating habits, your progress may be short-lived. If you think nutrition doesn't play a roll, consider this: in our first year of working within a health club, we observed three aesthetically healthy club members having heart attacks.

People who learn to eat healthy, yet neglect to exercise, may see results on the scale, but most of the weight they lose is lean muscle tissue.

On the other side of the equation, people who learn to eat healthy, yet neglect to exercise, may see results on the scale, but most of the weight they lose is lean muscle tissue. Therefore, they're actually slowing down their metabolism. Healthy eating by itself is not the "be all, end all" to releasing fat that doesn't come back. Ironically, those who eat healthy are quick to blame their lack of exercise as the reason they're not more fit and firm. On the flip side, those who exercise regularly point the finger at their eating habits.

The benefit of implementing both healthy eating and regular exercise along with mental focus provides you with a race that keeps you on course to the finish line. Once you accept this, it's only a matter of time before you are where you want to be.

Gearing up

As your Wellness Weight-Loss coaches, we are focused on helping you create health and release fat that doesn't come back. To do this, we want you to understand how you can take action and remain on course.

The solution sounds simple, and it really is: Where your focus goes, your energy flows! This clear-cut principle works, and has for all time. If you can't seem to get moving or have fallen off course, check your level of focus, as it is often overlooked and under-estimated.

Becky's butterscotch pie

When we first met Becky, she shared with us how much she loved butterscotch pie. Made with practically all sugar, this southern pie is nothing short of a fat pill. During the early stages of the Wellness Weight-Loss process, Becky found herself eating this pie when visiting her mother. When Becky returned from vacation and we conducted a body composition analysis, she had gained nearly five pounds of fat. Becky was so frustrated that she thought about giving up. Satisfied with blaming her emotions for sabotaging her progress, it was tough motivating Becky to get back on course. Nonetheless, she regrouped and decided to continue her pursuit to create health and release fat.

Considering the state Becky was in, we quickly coached her on the principle: Where your focus goes, your energy flows! Prior to visiting her mother's house, Becky promised herself that she would continue eating healthy and that her goal was more important than a slice of pie. Although Becky was aware that the pie was unhealthy and fattening, it didn't take long before she was sitting at the table reasoning and justifying how a little pie was not going to interfere with her long-term success. In her mind, she focused on the fact that she had been doing well and it was time for a reward. Sound familiar?

What happened to Becky happens to many people. There is no doubt that she was focused on eating healthy when she arrived at her mother's house. However, once she walked into her mother's kitchen, her focus shifted from her weight-loss goal and the reasons why she promised herself to continue eating healthy, to how good the pie smelled and how she remembered it tasting. As Becky's focus grew stronger toward the benefits and pleasure of the pie, she no longer thought about her weight-loss goals until after the pie was eaten.

Seven months later, Becky was gearing up for another visit to her mother's house. This time was going to be different however, because Becky had altered her association with pie. Instead of focusing on how the pie would taste and how good it smelled, Becky looked past the immediate gratification of eating the pie. Becky's focus had shifted and the thought of eating the pie meant destruction of her desire to evolve with her lifestyle. You see, Becky kept her focus on her weight-loss goal and how great it felt to choose her way to success. Eating the pie in Becky's mind meant slowing down her progress and putting what was truly important to her on hold. The focus Becky maintained while at her mother's house was a defining experience in her life. Although she chose not to eat the pie, Becky did thank her mother with grace and love.

Becky has learned a great deal about focus, and she knows that if she wants her energy to flow in a certain direction, focus is essential. Learning to focus takes practice and that means keeping what you desire most in your thoughts—conscious and subconscious. Like Becky, we encourage you to practice being focused, and it will become a core component of your habits of thought.

Your reality is your own

Have you ever had someone gossip about how they know someone who can eat whatever he or she wants and not gain a pound? If you haven't, there are many people on this earth who are perceived for some reason as being able to eat practically anything and not gain weight. Before you draw conclusions about why they can get away with such actions and you can't, consider the reality that you have no idea whether or not they are suffering from bulimia or some other diet-related illness. We have had visibly thin clients share with us that they suffered from bulimia for nearly 30 years and kept it a secret. No one knew, not even their spouses. You have no idea what people are going through in their mind and body. You do not know whether or not they are healthy on the inside, suffering from some illness or have a parasite feasting in their body. What's important, however, is what's real for you.

Are you aware that by the time you were seven years of age, your body had acquired somewhere between 30 to over 250 billion fat cells that will be with you until the day you die? These fat cells are not going anywhere and depending on your number, other genetics, activity, eating habits and hormones, you are more or less likely to store body fat. It may not seem fair, but it is a reality and it is up to you to either accept or resist it.

Acceptance goes like this: What's real for someone else may not be real for you. So, in order for you to make your reality your own, consider the following:

- Stop comparing yourself to others.
- Take ownership of your life and be accountable to yourself.
- Be your own best friend and learn to evaluate your behavior and not judge it.
- Take control of your destiny by doing for you what no one else can do.

A matter of balance

Focus! Take control! Just do it! These statements sound good, but the action they imply is easier said than done. To bring the role of balance into perspective, take a few minutes and ponder the following questions: Do you find yourself doing more for others than you do for yourself? Do you feel fulfilled with your life? Now imagine this scenario: You return home from work after a long day tired and mentally exhausted. Your goal is to exercise after work, but you decide to go home and rest instead. You feel beat up. After you arrive home you hear this voice in your head saying, "You should exercise—what about your weight-loss goal?" To shut the voice up you think to yourself, "Why not?" and the next thing you realize—you're nurturing yourself with some tasty treats (i.e., cookies, ice cream, wine). Following your emotional feast the voice returns and it is louder than ever. You become more frustrated and depressed about how you behaved.

No longer your own best friend, you begin to judge yourself and say things like, "I have no willpower" and "What's wrong with me?" Then, you look over at the sink and notice the stack of dirty dishes. These dishes remind you of the dirty clothes that are sitting on the washer and the dinner your family expects. The thought of eating dinner becomes even more bothersome because your family doesn't want to eat what you are cooking. Can you just hear their response? "I don't want that diet food. I want regular food." Soon, you notice your mind is overwhelmed with a stream of things to do, and you conclude that you will not get everything done. As this becomes the daily routine for many women, peace of mind is placed on your personal wish list and seems out of grasp for now.

Feeling overwhelmed and out of balance is not beyond resolving.

The good news: feeling overwhelmed and out of balance is not beyond resolving. The antidote is applied by building your self-esteem, conquering procrastination, feeling like you are making progress and coming into balance with your life. Sounds good so far, but how do you accomplish this? The answer isn't simple. It's not solely about downscaling either, but first learning to accept what's not in your control. This is no easy solution, but it works! Remember; the only person you can control is you—the only person you can change is you. When you find yourself frustrated, annoyed, angry and overwhelmed, ask yourself, "What am I attempting to control?" This question will help you come face to face with what you are attempting to control. Once answered, ask yourself, "Is this something I can change, or is it out of my control?" If you can change it, then take action. If you can't, you will be faced with a decision: You can either resist by continuing your efforts to control what is out of your control, or you can begin moving into acceptance.

The bottom line

The principle of acceptance says that you do not have to like, enjoy or want something (i.e., food, exercise), yet it is what it is. If a person isn't successful at lasting fat loss, you can be assured that he or she resisted some truth or reality at one point or another. Maybe it was the decision to go on eating unhealthy food that blocked their progress. Maybe they remained stuck because they decided not to take responsibility and become accountable for their choices. But somewhere along the line, they refused to accept the truth and/or take action.

The bottom line is to continue focusing on what you want, not on what you don't want. This includes accepting the reality that you create health and experience lasting fat loss by: regular exercise, healthy eating, daily planning of meals and snacks, tracking, scheduling time for grocery shopping and maintaining focus and a desire to evolve as a person. Regardless of where you've been—what matters is where you're going.

Keep your focus on long-term success,
and you will be able to maintain your gains.

Going forward

To help you continue making progress, we encourage you to come back to this book, read the chapters that capture your interest and re-read the entire book every three or six months. Each time you read this book, you will learn something new. Remember the saying, "You will only hear what you are ready to learn?" Each time you re-read a chapter you will become aware of concepts you didn't notice before. You will also begin noticing that you have made significant progress since the first day you discovered this book. Additionally, visit our web site, **www.wellnessweightloss.net**, and keep current with food and exercise methods. Revisit the 24 action steps provided below. These action steps provide you with a step-by-step approach to getting started, moving forward and the building foundation to evolve for the rest of your life.

Begin with the first action step—complete it and move on to the next one. Continue this process until you have completed all 24 action steps. We wrote this book to help you evolve with your lifestyle, and each action step is symbolic of one hour in a day. It is our message that you evolve with your life 24 hours a day, 365 days a year.

Keep your focus on long-term success, and you will be able to maintain your gains. This is your life to live and enjoy as you create health daily and mature with increased energy, vitality and the wisdom to do for you what no one else can.

Even though it is a fact that you cannot turn back the clock and start your life over—it is also a fact that beginning today—you can move forward and create a new future. Make life a journey that you enjoy, because when it is all said and done, there is no finish line.

ACTION STEP #1: Conduct a body composition analysis (BCA). Refer to Appendix A or visit our web site to learn more about how to conduct a BCA (measure your body-fat percentage). Make sure your BCA includes measurements and total body weight. This first action step is essential in your journey to release fat that doesn't come back. Remember, no longer are you concerned with your total body weight, but with your percentage of body fat and measurements.

ACTION STEP #2: Re-read and complete the exercises in Chapter 13 (Goal Getting) where you learn to set clear, specific, measurable, realistic and written goals. Decide what you want and why you want it.

ACTION STEP #3: Use the power of self-suggestion as explained in Chapter 22 (Knowing and Doing). Read and review daily to keep you focused, motivated and on track.

ACTION STEP #4: Become a label detective and choose products that are not highly processed and refined. To help you succeed we recommend you LOOK FOR SUGAR! On the labels of highly processed and refined foods, sugar will be listed in the first four ingredients. Look for sugar in all its hidden identities. Dextrose, corn syrup, maltodextrin, fructose, lactose, sucrose, maltose, malt syrup, honey, brown rice syrup, molasses, modified food starch and corn starch are, in fact, sugar.

ACTION STEP #5: Plan a grocery list for the next seven days and go shopping. Remember, "Failure to plan is planning to fail."

ACTION STEP #6: Track (write down) what you eat and the time you eat it until you are at your desired body-fat percentage for a minimum of three months. We strongly encourage you to eat every two to three hours. Take a look at Chapter 18 where we emphasize the importance of tracking.

ACTION STEP #7: Practice portion control with your meals and snacks as explained throughout this book, specifically in Chapter 18.

ACTION STEP #8: Increase the amount of water you drink to a minimum of eight to 12 eight-ounce glasses per day. The easiest way to ensure that you are drinking enough water is to track it daily.

ACTION STEP #9: Schedule an appointment to visit your family physician for medical clearance prior to beginning to exercise.

ACTION STEP #10: Make a plan to perform cardiovascular exercise a minimum of three days per week for 20 to 30 minutes each time. Make an appointment to exercise and stick to it. There are 168 hours in a week, and once you work up to three hours per week, this works out to less than three percent of your time. Refer to Chapter 20 for a refresher on cardiovascular exercise.

ACTION STEP #11: Take 10 to 15 minutes at the end of each week and reflect on the progress you have made. Taking time to reflect and ponder on the things you have learned, the people you have met, and the choices you have made is a surefire way to remain empowered and assured that you are evolving.

ACTION STEP #12: When it comes to eating carbohydrates (carbs) we encourage you to choose fibrous carbs of color. For example, instead of a white potato, eat a yam or sweet potato. Instead of white rice, eat brown or wild rice. Instead of white bread, eat 100 percent whole wheat, stone ground or whole grain sprouted bread. Other fibrous carbs include green leafy vegetables, whole grains and colorful fruits like apples, pears, peaches, kiwi, cantaloupe and berries.

ACTION STEP #13: Grill, broil, poach, stir-fry or bake your meat, poultry or fish instead of deep-frying. As well, we encourage you to cook with healthy oils (i.e., olive, grape seed, flax seed) as expressed in Chapter 15.

ACTION STEP #14: Word power and phrases: If you haven't already empowered your vocabulary both in the words you speak and the thoughts you think, it is time to replace self-defeating words, phrases and thoughts such as "I have to," "try," and "I can't." Plan to read Chapters 1, 3 and 9 within the next 10 days.

ACTION STEP #15: Take a look at the amount of saturated fat you are eating each day. We recommend you establish a boundary not to exceed 10 grams of saturated fat if you eat under 2,000 calories per day. If you are consuming more than 2,000 calories we recommend you eat less than 20 grams of saturated fat per day. For health reasons we encourage you to choose products that are trans-fat free (look at the ingredients for the words hydrogenated, partially hydrogenated and fractionated oils).

ACTION STEP #16: For continued progress, choose foods and pastries that are not made with white flours, including unbleached, wheat, enriched, semolina and durum. Instead, when it comes to bread and pasta, choose products made with stone-ground whole-wheat, corn, buckwheat and 100 percent whole-wheat flour. Our bread of choice,

Ezekiel, is available in practically any grocery store. Manufactured by Food for Life (www.foodforlife.com); visit them online for a list of other products. If you have a wheat allergy, consider kumut or spelt flour. Also available are non-wheat flours like soy and lentil.

ACTION STEP #17: Perform resistance training a minimum of twice per week. Review Chapter 21 and Appendix C for specific details.

ACTION STEP #18: It is time for a progress evaluation. From this day forth, plan to conduct a body composition analysis once a month—or at the most, twice a month—to ensure you are moving in the direction you desire. We consider routine body composition analysis the same as screening for breast and prostate cancer.

ACTION STEP #19: Eat a portion of protein (i.e., tofu, chicken, fish) and extra vegetables for dinner. This means replacing the potato, yam, bread, etc., you may have been eating with vegetables. In addition, it is to your benefit to eat fruit during the day and snack on protein and/or vegetables in the evening. Doing this will help you continue releasing fat.

ACTION STEP #20: Evaluate your daily consumption of fiber. For seven days write down how much fiber you are eating. You can do this by using the food values chart in Appendix B, visiting our web site for ideas and taking action by eating a minimum of five fruits and vegetables per day (i.e., a cup of raspberries yields over eight grams of fiber). Reminder, we encourage you to eat 25 to 40 grams of fiber per day. It is also a great time to review Chapter 17.

ACTION STEP #21: Alcohol yields seven calories per gram and this sugar-consumed drink is nothing short of empty calories. Cut down or cut out the alcohol to continue making progress. If you are drinking three days a week, cut down to twice per week. After a few weeks, cut back to once per week. If you are drinking hard alcohol like vodka, rum, etc., we encourage you to shift to red wine. From a health standpoint, we recommend no more than two four-ounce glasses of wine in a day.

ACTION STEP #22: Track the number of hours you sleep for the next seven days. After seven days of implementing this action step and increasing hours of sleep, we have had many clients break plateaus. Plan to sleep a minimum of seven hours (preferably eight or nine) each and every night so that you maximize your fat burning potential.

ACTION STEP #23: Go fishing! Unless you are a vegan, vegetarian or simply despise or are allergic to fish, begin eating fish like salmon once or twice per week. More often than not, when people share with us that they do not like fish, what they are really saying is they don't like how the fish is cooked. You are at the point in this process where being creative and experimenting with various methods like broiling, stir-fry, and marinades can make the biggest difference in taste. Visit our web site for ideas as you implement fish into your diet.

ACTION STEP #24: Experiment with one new healthy recipe every 14 days. Remember, courage to risk is synonymous with higher self-esteem.

Appendix A
Body Composition Analysis

You've read **Fat That Doesn't Come Back** and you are ready to learn more about conducting a body composition analysis (BCA). By conducting a BCA you are able to divide your body into two parts: lean body mass and fat mass. Your lean body mass is composed of muscle, water, bones, connective tissue, internal organs and blood (everything but fat), and your fat mass is just that—the amount of fat you have on your body. Determining how much of your total body weight is fat mass will result in your percentage of body fat. Simply put, this percentage indicates the amount of your total body weight that is composed of fat.

Learning how to measure and monitor your body-fat percentage lets you know whether you are building and maintaining muscle and/or releasing body fat. Now, as we stated in Chapter 1 and regardless of age, for men who aspire to achieve optimum health, we recommend a body- fat percentage of no more than 15. With regard to women, we recommend no more than 22 percent. However, if you are taking hormone replacements, beta-blockers, birth control pills, selective serotonin re-uptake inhibitors (i.e., Prozac, Zoloft) or any other medication that may affect your hormonal balance, you may add an additional five percent to our recommendation and still be considered healthy (men no more than 20 and women, 27 percent).

Getting started

Even though you may step on the scale as often as brushing your teeth, by now you are aware that the scale by itself is a poor indicator of your body composition. However, we hope you haven't tossed it in the trash. Many BCA methods require your body weight as part of the equation to determine your percentage of body fat.

At the present, there are a wide variety of methods used to measure body fat. Four of the most popular are hydrostatic (underwater) weighing, skin fold testing (calipers), bioelectrical impedance (i.e. Tanita scale) and near-infrared interactance (i.e. Futrex 5000). Regardless of the method you use to measure your percentage of body fat, we encourage you to pick one and stick with it. Why? Because there is already a degree of error with the various methods, and jumping from one BCA to another may not indicate your true progress or regress. Utilizing the same test method positions you to accurately measure and track your gains and losses.

> *Regardless of the method you choose to measure your percentage of body fat, we encourage you to pick one and stick with it.*

Once you have chosen your testing method, conduct a BCA every two to four weeks. Again, it is imperative that you track your progress by writing down the date and outcome of your BCA. We also recommend that when you conduct a BCA, it's done around the same time of the day while wearing tight fitting clothes. As we said earlier, by sticking with the same method under the same or very similar circumstances, the degree of error is reduced.

Outside BCA

Before we walk you through the process of conducting a BCA in the privacy of your home, you may decide to venture out and have a BCA conducted at a health club, commercial weight-loss clinic, college or medical office. Regardless of the method you choose, it is important that keep track of your progress and repeat the test every two to four weeks until you are at your desired body composition. By doing this you will no longer be guessing what you are losing—you will be 100 percent aware of your results.

After you achieve your desired body composition, we encourage you to continue to conduct a BCA every three to six months. We also recommend that you consider the following tips when seeking a BCA:

- Choose a qualified technician with ample experience.
- Have follow-up evaluations performed by the same person.
- Don't concern yourself with decimals, fractions and error ranges. Remember; what's important is that you are reducing body fat over time.
- Medical and fitness experts tend to differ on what is recommended as healthy body fat ranges. However, make it your goal to reach optimum health and attain the body fat percentage we mentioned above and in Chapter 1.

In-house BCA

After venturing out, visiting our web site and learning more about the various methods of conducting a BCA, you may decide that being submerged in water or having a stranger pinch your fat is out of the question. For this reason and simple convenience, we have provided you with an in-house method that even the godfather of fitness and health, Jack LaLanne, says cannot be debated: body measurements and a mirror.

In order for you to conduct an in-house BCA you are going to need a few things: a cloth measuring tape, highly accurate digital scale and a camera of some sort. And it doesn't hurt to enlist a "pound pal" to help you obtain accurate measurements in addition to providing you with ongoing support.

The question of accuracy

We first learned of this in-house method by one of our clients and we have tested a wide array of people—comparing our in-house results with bioelectrical impedance, near-infrared interactance and hydrostatic (underwater) weighing methods. The results have been consistent. Using the hydrostatic weighing method, which is considered the "gold standard" when conducting a BCA as our base, the in-house method is often within two percent accuracy. In comparison to the other methods, our in-house method gets the gold star.

The only negative is the more fit a person is, the more likely the in-house method will measure him or her around three percent higher. The opposite happens with people who are "skinny fat" as they tend to measure up to five percent lower than the underwater testing. So, if you are an extreme athlete or someone who exercises 10 or more hours per week—performing both resistance training and cardiovascular exercise—the error rate can be up to three percent. To put this into perspective, if you are tested with the hydrostatic weighing method and your body-fat percentage is six percent, the in-house method may measure you at nine percent. The opposite end of the spectrum is for those who are sedentary, unfit, but appear thin (skinny fat)—the hydrostatic weighing method may measure them at 30 percent and our in-house method may say 25 percent.

The man behind the method

After using the in-house BCA formula and coming to appreciate and respect its accuracy, we went on a mission to learn of its origin. The man who wrote the best-selling book, *Fit or Fat,* Covert Bailey is the source behind this amazing BCA method. Not surprisingly, Covert Bailey has always been a pioneer in the fitness and health community and it gives us great pleasure to acknowledge him and his work to help people transition from fatness to fitness. So, when you are done reading this book, go to your local book store and read up on this living legend. Take our word for it, Covert Bailey knows his stuff!

Measuring basics

First things first. You need a cloth measuring tape. Secondly, a journal to record your results, and last but not least, have fun and take your time. As you practice and improve on these skills, the process will get easier. To achieve accurate measurements, we recommend that your wear tight fitting clothing with bare arms and legs.

Okay, the prerequisites are out of the way. Now for the operating instructions: when measuring limbs such as your thigh and arm, measure your dominant side. Simply put, if you are right-handed, measure your right thigh and vice versa if you are left-handed. When taking and tracking measurements, be precise and consistent with where you measure. To help matters, we have provided measuring instructions.

Right Calf: It is important that you distribute your body weight evenly on both feet. Your point of measure will be somewhere between the ankle and the knee at the widest point of your calf muscle. It is also best to tighten the tape measure so it is firm but not squeezing the skin.

Right Thigh: Keeping your feet at hip width and your body weight evenly distributed in the middle. It is important to measure the upper part of your thigh (between the hip bone and knee cap) at its widest part. It is also best to tighten the tape measure so it is firm but not squeezing the skin.

Hips: Stand with your feet at hip width and keep your body weight evenly distributed in the middle. Wrap the tape measure around your hips and with the use of a mirror, place the tape measure at the peak of your buttock. Take a close look to ensure the tape measure is at an even height all the way around your hip area. Tighten the tape measure so it is firm but not squeezing the skin.

Waist (MEN): Stand tall with your feet at hip width and your body weight evenly distributed in the middle. It won't benefit you to suck everything in; instead just relax and breathe regularly as though no one is watching. Wrap the tape measure around your waist and place the tape measure one inch below your belly button or at the peak of the belly (which ever is widest). Take a close look to ensure the tape measure is at an even height all the way around your waist. Tighten the tape measure so it is firm but not squeezing the skin.

Waist (WOMEN): Stand tall with your feet at hips width and your body weight evenly distributed in the middle. It won't benefit you to suck everything in; instead just relax and breathe regularly as though no one is watching. Wrap the tape measure around your waist and place the tape measure one inch above your belly button. Take a close look to ensure the tape measure is at an even height all the way around your waist. Tighten the tape measure so it is firm but not squeezing the skin. Look straight ahead into a mirror when reading the measurement. Looking down can actually expand your waistline, giving you and inaccurate reading.

Chest (MEN): Stand tall with your feet at hips width and your body weight evenly distributed in the middle. Wrap the tape measure around your chest and place the tape measure at the peak of your chest (typically across your nipples). Take a close look to ensure the tape measure is at an even height all the way around your chest. Tighten the tape measure so it is firm but not squeezing the skin.

Chest (WOMEN): Stand tall with your feet at hips width and your body weight evenly distributed in the middle. Wrap the tape measure around your chest and place the tape measure at the peak of your chest. Take a close look to ensure the tape measure is at an even height all the way around your chest. Tighten the tape measure so it is firm but not squeezing the skin.

Forearm (MEN): Make a fist with your dominant hand so that your forearm is contracted and measure at the widest part between the wrist and the elbow. Tighten the tape measure so it is firm but not squeezing the skin.

Wrist: Place the tape measure just above the bony protuberance at the base of your baby finger (toward the hand). Tighten the tape measure so it is firm but not squeezing the skin.

Bicep: Place the tape measure between the shoulder and elbow of your dominant arm; centered on your bicep with your arm extended out to the side with your palm facing the ceiling. Tighten the tape measure so it is firm but not squeezing the skin.

The measuring formula

Okay, now that you have conducted and recorded all of the necessary measurements, let's plug them into the Covert body fat analysis equation. Then, once we have your body-fat percentage, we will be one step closer to discovering how much of your body weight is fat and how much lean body mass you have on your frame.

Women 30 years or younger—calculating body fat percentage
If you are a woman who is 30 years or younger, it is necessary that you use the measurements of your hips, thigh, calf and wrist. After you have these measurements, you will calculate the following formula:

hips + (.80 x thigh) – (2 x calf) – wrist = percentage of body fat

Consider the following measurements for example:
hips = 40"; thigh = 21"; calf = 14 _", wrist = 6"

The calculation using the above scenario (example) is as follows:
40 + (.80 x 21 = 16.8) – (2 x 14.5 = 29) – 6 = 21.8 percent body fat

Women at least 31 years of age—calculating body fat percentage
If you are a woman who is at least 31 years of age, it is necessary that you use the measurements of your hips, thigh, calf and wrist. After you have these measurements, you will calculate the following formula:

hips + thigh – (2 x calf) – wrist = percentage of body fat

Consider the following measurements for example:
hips = 39 1/2"; thigh = 19"; calf = 12 1/2"; wrist = 6"

The calculation using the above scenario (example) is as follows:
39.5 + 19 – (2 x 12.5 = 25) – 6 = 27.5 percent of body fat

Men 30 years or younger—calculating body fat of percentage
If you are a man who is 30 years or younger, it is necessary that you use the measurements of your waist, hips, forearm and wrist. After you have these measurements, you will calculate the following formula:

waist = (1/2 hips) – (3 x forearm) – wrist = percentage of body fat

Consider the following measurements for example:
waist = 30 1/4"; hips = 36"; forearm = 10.5"; wrist = 6 1/4"

The calculation using the above scenario (example) is as follows:
30.25 + (.5 x 36 = 18) – (3 x 10.5 = 31.5) – 6.25 = 10.5 percent of body fat

Men at least 31 years of age—calculating body fat percentage
If you are a man who is at least 31 years of age, it is necessary that you that you use the measurements of your waist, hips, forearm and wrist. After you have these measurements, you will calculate the following formula:

waist + (1/2 hips) – (2.7 x forearm) – wrist = percentage of body fat

Consider the following measurements for example:

waist = 37"; hips = 41"; forearm = 11"; wrist = 6 1/2"

The calculation using the above scenario (example) is as follows:

37 + (.5 x 41 = 20.5) – (2.7 x 11 = 29.7) – 6.5 = 21.3 percent of body fat

Calculating your BCA

Once you know your percentage of body fat, step onto the scale in order to learn your total body weight; then, you can determine your lean body mass and fat mass. To calculate your fat mass you simply multiply your total body weight by your body fat percentage. You then subtract your fat mass from your total body weight to get your lean body mass.

Consider the following example: Let's say you weigh 200 pounds and your body-fat percentage is 15, you simply multiply 200 pounds by .15 (percent of body fat) to get your fat mass, which in this scenario is 30 pounds. To learn your lean body mass you subtract your fat mass (30 pounds) from your total body weight of 200 and your lean body mass is 170 pounds.

200 pounds of total body weight x .15 = 30 pounds of fat
200 pounds – 30 pounds of fat = 170 pounds of lean body mass

Example #2: If your body-fat percentage is 28 and your total body weight is 160 pounds: multiply 160 by .28 to get your fat mass, which in this example is 45 pounds. You then subtract your fat mass (45 pounds) from your total body weight (160 pounds) to get your lean body mass, which in this example is 115 pounds.

160 pounds of total body weight x .28 = 45 pounds of fat
160 pounds – 45 pounds of fat = 115 pounds of lean body mass

Conclusion

Hopefully you can see how important this equation is when it comes to measuring your future progress. By conducting a BCA on a regular basis you can determine if you are losing body fat or lean body mass!

If you have any questions regarding the various methods of conducting a BCA, please visit us on the Internet at:

www.WellnessWeightloss.net.

On our web site we explain the finer details of the various methods of conducting a BCA in addition to related links. As well, if you have specific questions, send us an e-mail. We are here to help you.

Appendix B
Meal and Snack Suggestions

Do you consider yourself a planner? If not, now is a great opportunity to make weekly and daily planning part of your lifestyle. Why? When it comes to food—the absolute healthiest way to release fat that doesn't come back is to plan—prepare healthy meals in advance. This may not seem easy at first; however, it is a principle that has been proven time and time again.

To ensure your success, it helps to prepare snacks and meals ahead of time. For instance, you can freeze a bunch of meals on Sunday, take leftovers to work or get up early and pre-cook your meals for each day. If you do not plan your meals, you may find yourself feeling hungry, snacking at vending machines and visiting fast food restaurants. Not planning means you either go without or pick up something quick—making it difficult to eat your way to a fit and healthy body.

Frequency

Keep in mind that we are not talking about planning one meal. We are talking about planning and eating five, six and sometimes even seven or eight times each day. Eating several times each day speeds up your metabolism, whereas eating one large meal or even three for that matter can slow your metabolism. As odd as it may seem at first, frequent eating of small portions is a surefire principle for revving up your metabolism and helping you release fat.

To help you grasp this concept, we want you to think of frequent eating as fuel—equal to the gasoline you put in your car. Your metabolism is the engine and it needs gasoline to operate. In this analogy, your car runs out of gasoline every three hours and in order to avoid going on empty, it is necessary that you fuel it in a timely manner.

You can only go three hours on a tank full of gasoline; therefore, the longer you go without eating, the slower your metabolism becomes.

The absolutely worst thing you can do is skip meals—not refill your tank!!! So, if you don't want to run out of gasoline—planning is crucial. Equally, if you want to be successful with releasing fat that doesn't come back, eating every two to three hours takes planning.

Quality food

As you become skilled at eating in a timely manner, it's also important that you eat quality foods. Eating a fried donut and candy bar every two to three hours is not what we mean by quality food.

Back to the car analogy: imagine what would happen if you pumped diesel fuel into your car. As you begin to drive away from the service station you can't help but notice the black smoke coming out of the tail pipe. The next thing you notice, the car isn't running smoothly and it stops. You get towed to a service station and into the garage where the mechanic asks, "What are you burning for fuel?" You reply by saying, "Diesel."

The mechanic giggles and recommends that you pump gasoline in to your car. You do this and your car works great. The black smoke disappears and the engine operates smoothly. You think to yourself, "That mechanic is so smart. He is awesome!"

Having the mechanic inform you that proper fuel will help you get more out of your vehicle is equal to our recommending proper nutrition for your body. Eating food that is too oily and high in unhealthy fats and highly refined carbohydrates is a prime example of doing more harm to your body than good. Unhealthy foods stick to you and clog you up the same as diesel fuel damages a car that operates on gasoline.

As we are forever evolving with our eating habits, our bodies continue to remain lean and healthy. Our clients experience the same thing that has happened to us. By simply eating quality foods on a frequent basis, you can expect to find yourself waking up to a lean and healthy body everyday. So, don't be surprised when your blood pressure goes down, Type 2 diabetes is reversed and you no longer need the cholesterol and hypertension pills your doctor said you would take for the remainder of your life.

Example of a weekly grocery list

We have provided you with an example of a weekly grocery list. This list is broken down not only to help give you an idea of how to put one together, but to reinforce what is considered a protein and carbohydrate. (Some products may contain both protein and carbs so we categorized foods according to the dominant macronutrient.)

PROTEIN GROUP

Omega (DHA Omega-3) or **egg substitute** (we suggest 100% Egg White sold in cartons near the cottage cheese)

Skinless chicken breasts (bone or filet)

Ground turkey or chicken breast (instead of ground beef)

Turkey breast

Canned tuna in water (in moderation)

Canned salmon in water

Fresh fish (i.e., halibut, cod, salmon, flounder, tuna, snapper, tilapia)

Very lean cuts of meat

Low-fat or non-fat cottage cheese

Other low fat dairy products like skim milk

Original soy milk (Silk or Sun brands taste great)

Protein powder of your choosing (look for hidden sugars in their secret identities!)

Turkey bacon or **veggie bacon**

Veggie products: patties, deli meats, tofu, cheese, sausages (Morning Star Farms, Boca, California, Lightlife and Yves brands taste the best)

Legumes (lentils)

CARBOHYDRATE GROUP

Cereal: Old Fashion Oatmeal (not the instant kind), Kashi Go Lean, Optimum Power Breakfast, Optimum Slim or Flax Plus

Bread: Ezekiel (regular or Sesame) or 100% Stone ground or sprouted 100% whole-wheat breads

Tortillas: Ezekiel or La Tortilla Factory Low-Carb

Crackers: Ak-mak, TLC, Light Ry Krisp, or Wasa

Rice: Brown or wild (wild is the healthiest)

Yogurt: soy or dairy low-fat or nonfat (sweetened with fruit juice)

Fruit: grapefruit, tomatoes, apples, oranges, peaches, nectarines, pears, watermelon, strawberries, blueberries, blackberries, cherries, papaya, mangos, cantaloupe, honeydew, mangos, unsweetened applesauce and bananas

Vegetables: red leaf, green leaf, or romaine lettuce, spinach, collard greens, broccoli, cauliflower, zucchini, squash, turnip, cucumbers, asparagus, green and/or red peppers, green beans, peas, yams, sweet potatoes, mushrooms, onion, egg plant, lemons and limes

Pasta: whole grain or buckwheat pasta

Tomato sauce: Classico Tomato and Basil, or Bartelli brands (no sugar added)

Beans: garbanzo, pinto, black, kidney, navy, and lima

Flour: Bake with soy, 100% stone ground whole wheat, bran, and oat or rye flour instead of white. Also, you can always substitute vanilla protein powder for some of the flour.

SPICES, CONDIMENTS, DRESSINGS AND MARINADES

Spices and herbs: Mrs. Dash, McCormick's or Ralph's salt free varieties, pepper, garlic, fresh herbs of choice.

Condiments: salsa, mustard, soyanaise or veganaise, natural peanut, almond or soy butter, 100% fruit jam (sweetened with fruit juice) and Smart Balance butter.

Dressings: Annie's Naturals and Newman's Own brands or make your own with lemon juice, apple cider vinegar, olive oil and spices of choice.

Marinades: Braggs Liquid Amino's—great for marinades or as a soy sauce substitute, Golden Dip Lemon and Herb, Annie's Naturals or the Ginger Peoples brands.

All meals (breakfast, lunch and dinner ideas) contain a balance (portion) of carbs and protein. As well, the snack examples are either a carb, protein or combination of the two.

VEGETARIAN NOTE: Substitute any of the meat, poultry or fish entrees with grilled, baked or sautéed tofu, or any other soy products of choice.

Breakfast ideas

Breakfast #1
Eat a cup of fresh or frozen washed and drained blueberries drain with a cup of low-fat or non-fat cottage cheese.

Breakfast #2
Drink a smoothie by blending ice, a cup of skim milk or soymilk with one level scoop of protein powder and one cup of fruit (i.e. banana, berries).

Breakfast #3
Eat a cup of Optimum Power Breakfast cereal with a cup of soy or non-fat milk.

Breakfast #4 (Oatmeal)
Cook a half-cup of old fashion oats (not instant) with half a banana and a half-teaspoon of cinnamon. Once the oats are cooked, mix in one level scoop of vanilla protein powder.

Breakfast #5

Beat eight ounces of an egg substitute or seven egg whites in a bowl. Spray a frying pan with non-stick spray like Pam and then scramble the eggs. Spice it up with any variety of Mrs. Dash spices. Toast one slice of Ezekiel bread and put a half-tablespoon of natural peanut or almond butter on the top.

Breakfast #6

In a rush? Toast two slices of Ezekiel bread and top them with one tablespoon of natural peanut butter.

Breakfast #7

In a blender combine one ripe banana, quarter cup of old fashion oats (oatmeal), half a level scoop of vanilla protein powder, half-teaspoon cinnamon, half carton egg substitute or four egg whites, then blend until mixed. Use this mixture to make Power Pancakes by pouring 4 inch by 4 inch cakes into a non-stick frying pan. Eating five of these pancakes topped with unsweetened applesauce or low-calories (diabetic) sugar free syrup makes for a well-balanced breakfast.

Breakfast #8

Create an egg white omelet by mixing a half carton of egg substitute (i.e.100% Egg Whites or Egg Beaters), or five egg whites with 1/4 medium diced bell pepper, one medium diced tomato and cook on skillet with non-stick cooking spray. You can also add one slice of Veggie Slices "Pepper Jack" cheese, Mrs. Dash spices and/or top with salsa. (Onions and mushrooms are optional).

NOTE: Begin your day with at least one eight-ounce cup of water. If you drink coffee, we recommend you choose not to add processed sugars and creamers such as Coffee-Mate, Half and Half or any flavored non-dairy creamers. Most creamers (both dry and liquid) have unhealthy trans fatty acids (look for the words hydrogenation, partially hydrogenated or fractionated oils). You are far better off adding regular non-fat or soy milk to your coffee.

Keep in mind, that a six-ounce cup of coffee with one teaspoon of granulated sugar and one tablespoon of Half and Half yields 40 calories. If you want to add sweetener, WE RECOMMEND using Stevia, a naturally sweet Brazilian herb found in health food stores or the sugar substitute Splenda®.

Lastly, a cup of coffee without sugar or cream will only give you four calories!

Snack ideas

For optimum results in releasing fat and remaining lean, we recommend that you choose to snack on small portions of food in between meals. We suggest snacking on carbohydrates that are low in sugar and high in fiber or lean quality protein sources that are low in saturated fat. An example of an evening snack would be a high fiber piece of fruit like one cup of berries, an apple or a pear or a small portion of nuts such as 20 almonds or walnuts. You could also choose a protein source like low-fat cottage cheese, four to five scrambled egg whites or a few hard-boiled eggs (minus the yolk if you have high cholesterol), a protein shake, and a two-ounce can of tuna, chicken or salmon (in water) topped with fresh salsa.

The following are a variety of day time snacks: an apple, pear, orange, mango, one cup cubed cantaloupe or honeydew melon, one cup strawberries, one cup blueberries, half-cup of grapes, one cup unsweetened apple sauce, three cups of air popped popcorn, one-third cup trail mix, sliced apple with one tablespoon natural peanut butter, half-cup low-fat cottage cheese with diced strawberries, two celery sticks (about seven inches long) with one tablespoon natural peanut butter, one slice of Ezekiel toast with one tablespoon 100 percent fruit jam, eight-ounce low-fat fruit yogurt (sweetened with fruit juice), a protein shake, one cup sugar/fat free Jell-o, three ounces fresh roasted nitrate-free deli turkey (breast meat), a sliced tomato, half-cup kidney, black or pinto beans, a medium baked yam or sweet potato with cinnamon or one cup of raw vegetables.

When you are ready for more snack ideas, consider our homemade fruit bar (see wellnessweightloss.net for recipe). Supplement bars are also an option for people on the go; however, check the ingredients to ensure the bars are free of unhealthy trans fatty acids (hydrogenated and fractionated oils).

Lunch ideas

Lunch #1
Mix half a six-ounce can of salmon, tuna or chicken (drained in water) with two tablespoons of low-fat cottage cheese (it tastes better than it sounds) or mustard. Serve on two slices of Ezekiel bread. Feel free to put tomato and lettuce on the sandwich. Serve with a salad or vegetable of choice such as a sliced cucumber, half-cup baby carrots, broccoli or cauliflower.

Lunch #2
Grill, bake or broil four ounces of skinless chicken breast. (Use a marinade of your choice). Serve with one medium sweet potato topped with two

tablespoons of salsa and/or a touch of Mrs. Dash spices and a side of fresh steamed vegetables.

Lunch #3
Prepare a tuna salad by mixing half a six-ounce can of tuna (drained in water) with two cups romaine lettuce, one sliced tomato, half diced bell pepper, half-cup drained and rinsed black or garbanzo beans. Top with the juice of two lemon wedges or two tablespoons of vinaigrette dressing.

Lunch #4
Grill or pan fry your veggie burger of choice and make a sandwich on a sprouted or 100% stone ground whole grain bun with mustard, sliced tomato, and lettuce.

Lunch #5
Bake or grill four ounces of skinless chicken breast and sandwich it with a sprouted or 100% stone ground whole grain bun with tomato, lettuce and mustard.

NOTE: If you use condiments to add flavor to your food, keep in mind that one tablespoon of mayonnaise can add as much as 100 calories to your meal; one tablespoon of ketchup adds 15 calories, while mustard contains ZERO calories and carbohydrates.

Lunch #6
Create a simple, yet tasty lunch by baking, grilling or broiling four ounces of skinless chicken breast, slice and put in one Ezekiel 10-inch or two six-inch La Tortilla Factory Low-Carb tortillas. Add half-cup black or pinto beans that have been drained, rinsed and heated. Top with a slice of soy cheese and fresh salsa (veggies are a great addition; steer clear of such fat trappers as sour cream and guacamole).

Lunch #7
Thinly slice four ounces of grilled chicken or turkey. Sauté some bell peppers and onions using a non-stick spray, and create chicken or turkey fajitas. Serve with one 10-inch Ezekiel or two six-inch La Tortilla Factory Low-Carb tortillas flavored with fresh salsa. If a tortilla isn't a tortilla unless it comes with cheese, we recommend Veggie Slices "Pepper Jack" cheese—no saturated fat in this kind!

Did you know that a cheeseburger, fries and soft drink may contain over 1500 calories? That is a whole day's worth of food for most people who are interested in releasing fat. Which would you rather do, eat all day and release body fat or eat once a day and gain fat?

Dinner ideas

Dinner #1

Grill, broil or bake a four-ounce skinless chicken breast, (use a marinade of your choice), and serve with two cups of fresh salad topped with one to two tablespoons of Annie's Natural dressing.

Dinner #2

Bake four ounces of a flatfish (sole or flounder) of your choice and serve with half-cup of cooked wild rice and eight to 10 spears of steamed asparagus

Dinner #3

Broil or grill four ounces skinless chicken breast, (use a marinade of your choice), and serve with one to two cups sautéed sliced bell pepper, onion, and tomato wedges in one tablespoon of grape seed oil with fresh garlic and spices.

Dinner #4

Make some spaghetti marinara with ground turkey breast. Take a quarter package of dry spaghetti, boil, then combine with four ounces pan fried ground turkey breast and sautéed bell pepper add half to one cup of Classico Tomato and Basil sauce. Enjoy!

Dinner # 5

Grill or broil four-ounce salmon with lemon herb marinade. Serve with half-cup baked yam and a half-cup cooked spinach.

Dinner #6

Grill or broil four ounces of halibut and serve with half-cup of cooked wild rice and one cup of steamed broccoli.

NOTE: Feel free to substitute fish entrees with a fish of your choice such as sea bass, halibut trout or tilapia. Cold water fish is usually high in protein and contains healthy fat. A word of caution: shark, swordfish, tilefish, and tuna fillets have higher mercury content than any other types of fish. It has been recommended that pregnant women and children avoid these species of fish all together.

Dinner # 7

Make a stir fry by dicing up four ounces of tofu or chicken breast. Cook, then combine with sautéed and diced zucchini squash (about three inches long), half bell pepper, two-ounce onions, fresh garlic or ginger, one-tablespoon olive oil and two to three tablespoons of Bragg Liquid Aminos or any Annie's Naturals marinade.

SUGGESTION: You can replace any of our suggested vegetables with a different vegetable if you so desire. Also, if you haven't exercised yet, wait at least 60 minutes after your meal before you hit the gym or start those crunches. If you just got back from the gym, we recommend that you eat within 30 minutes after your workout in order to replenish your body with nutrients, stimulate muscle growth and to keep your metabolism elevated. If you haven't worked out and are eating dinner late, we recommend that you skip the starchy carbs like the rice, pasta and sweet potatoes, and instead double your portion of vegetables.

Healthy alternatives

With an emphasis on releasing fat through creating health and evolving with your lifestyle, we felt it would be beneficial to give you an idea of how you can evolve with your food choices. Simply put, if you are currently eating white bread, we recommend you give whole-wheat bread a try. After making the transition from white to whole wheat, a next baby step would be to go from whole wheat to Ezekiel or stone ground bread for instance.

INSTEAD OF THIS:	TRY THIS:
White bread	Stone ground wheat bread
Whole wheat bread	Ezekiel or sprouted grain bread
Cream of Wheat	Old-fashioned oatmeal
Cheerios	Optimum Power Breakfast
White rice	Brown or wild rice
White potato	Sweet potato or yam
Microwave popcorn	Air popped popcorn
Margarine/butter	Smart Balance
Cream sauce	Tomato based sauce
Cream soup	Clear soup
Ranch dressing	Italian dressing
Corn oil	Olive or grape seed oil
2% milk	1% or skim milk
Feta cheese	Ricotta cheese
Cheddar cheese	Soy cheese
Soda	Carbonated water
Cheeseburger	Boca burger with soy cheese
Hamburger	Grilled chicken burger
Fried French fries	Baked French fries
Fried chicken	BBQ or broiled chicken
Pork bacon	Turkey or soy bacon
Packaged deli meat	Fresh deli meat

INSTEAD OF THIS:	TRY THIS:
Iceberg lettuce	Green leaf or romaine lettuce
Chocolate bar	Carb Control bar by EAS
Chips	Kettle Chips
Doritos	Blue Corn or Bean Tortilla chips
Candy	Diabetic candy or dried fruit
Ice cream	Soy ice cream
Dessert	Yogurt with fresh fruit

Food values chart—nutrition approximation analysis

FRUITS AND VEGETABLES

Food Item	Portion Size	Calories	Carbs	Protein	Fat	Fiber
Apple	1 large	125	32 g	>1 g	0.8 g	5.7 g
Applesauce unsweetened	1 cup	105	27.5 g	0.4 g	0.1 g	2.9 g
Apricots	3 small	50	12 g	2 g	0.4 g	2.5 g
Artichoke	1 med. cooked	60	13 g	4 g	0.2 g	6.5 g
Asparagus	1 cup cooked	43	8 g	5 g	0.6 g	2.9 g
Avocado	1/2 med.	153	6 g	2 g	15 g	4.2 g
Banana	1 med.	109	28 g	1 g	0.6 g	2.8 g
Bell Pepper	1 large	44	11 g	2 g	0.3 g	3.0 g
Blackberries	1 cup	75	18 g	1 g	0.6 g	7.6 g
Blueberries	1 cup	81	21 g	1 g	0.6 g	3.9 g
Broccoli	1 cup cooked	44	8 g	5 g	0.6 g	4.7 g
Cantaloupe	1 cup	62	15 g	2 g	0.5 g	1.4 g
Carrots	1 cup cooked	70	16 g	2 g	0.3 g	5.2 g
Cauliflower	1 cup cooked	29	5 g	2 g	0.6 g	3.3 g
Celery	1 cup chopped	20	4 g	1 g	0.2 g	2.0 g
Cherries	1 cup	104	24 g	2 g	1.4 g	3.3 g
Collard Greens	1 cup cooked	40	9 g	4 g	0.7 g	5.3 g
Corn	1 cup	177	41 g	5 g	2.1 g	4.6 g
Cranberries	1 cup	47	12 g	>1 g	0.2 g	4.0 g
Cucumber	1 cup sliced	14	3 g	>1 g	0.2 g	0.8 g
Dates	2 oz.	156	42 g	1 g	0.3 g	4.3 g
Figs	2 med.	74	19 g	1 g	0.3 g	3.3 g
Grapefruit	1/2 med.	39	10 g	1 g	0.1 g	1.3 g
Grapes	1 cup	114	29 g	1 g	0.9 g	1.6 g
Honeydew	1 cup	62	16 g	1 g	0.2 g	1.1 g
Kiwifruit	2 med.	93	23 g	2 g	0.7 g	5.0 g

Food Item	Portion	Calories	Carbs	Protein	Fat	Fiber
Lemon Juice	1/2 cup	15	5 g	0 g	0 g	0.2 g
Lime Juice	1/2 cup	17	6 g	0 g	0.1 g	0.3 g
Mango	1 med.	135	35 g	1 g	0.6 g	3.7 g
Mushrooms	1 oz.	84	21 g	3 g	0.3 g	3.2 g
Nectarine	1 med.	67	16 g	1 g	0.6 g	2.2 g
Orange	1 med.	64	16 g	1 g	0.1 g	3.4 g
Papaya	1 cup cubed	55	14 g	1 g	0.2 g	2.5 g
Peach	1 med.	42	11 g	1 g	0.1 g	2.0 g
Pear	1 med.	98	25 g	1 g	0.7 g	4.0 g
Peas	1 cup cooked	134	25 g	9 g	0.4 g	8.8 g
Potato	4 oz. baked	133	31 g	3 g	0.1 g	2.9 g
Prunes	1/4 cup	102	27 g	1 g	0.2 g	3.0 g
Raisins	1/4 cup	107	29 g	1 g	0.2 g	2.5 g
Raspberries	1 cup	60	14 g	1 g	0.7 g	8.4 g
Romaine Lettuce	2 cups raw	16	3 g	2 g	0.2 g	1.9 g
Spinach	2 cups raw	13	2 g	2 g	0.2 g	1.6 g
Squash	1 cup cooked	36	8 g	2 g	0.6 g	2.5 g
Strawberries	1 cup	46	11 g	1 g	0.6 g	3.5 g
Sweet Potato	1 med.	143	34 g	3 g	0.1 g	3.7 g
Tomato	1 med.	48	11 g	2 g	0.8 g	2.5 g
Watermelon	1 cup	49	11 g	1 g	0.7 g	0.8 g

GRAINS, BEANS AND LEGUMES

Food Item	Portion Size	Calories	Carbs	Protein	Fat	Sat Fat	Fiber
Ak-mak Crackers	5 crackers	116	19 g	4.6 g	2.3 g	0.5 g	3.5 g
Barley Pearls	1 cup cooked	193	44 g	4 g	0.7 g	0.2 g	6 g
Black Beans	1/2 cup cooked	110	19 g	7 g	1.0 g	0 g	7 g
Brown Rice	1 cup cooked	216	45 g	5 g	1.8 g	0.4 g	3.5 g
Buckwheat Flour	1/2 cup dry	200	42 g	7.5 g	1.8 g	0.5 g	6 g
Buckwheat Pasta	1 cup cooked	113	24 g	6 g	0.1 g	0 g	1.3 g
Durum Semolina Pasta	1 cup cooked	197	40 g	7 g	0.9 g	0.1 g	2.4 g
Edamame Beans	1/2 cup cooked	127	10 g	11 g	5.8 g	0.7 g	3.8 g
Ezekiel Bread	1 slice	80	14 g	4 g	0.5 g	0 g	3 g

GRAINS, BEANS AND LEGUMES (cont.)

Food Item	Portion Size	Calories	Carbs	Protein	Fat	Sat Fat	Fiber
Flax Plus Cereal	1 cup	133	29.3 g	5.3 g	2.0 g	0 g	4 g
Garbanzo Beans	1/2 cup cooked	135	23 g	7 g	2.1 g	0.2 g	6.2 g
Go Lean Cereal	1 cup	160	37.3 g	10.7 g	1.3 g	0 g	13.3 g
Kidney Beans	1/2 cup cooked	120	21 g	7 g	0.5 g	0 g	6 g
Lentils	1/2 cup cooked	115	20 g	9 g	0.4 g	0.1 g	7.8 g
Light Ry Krisp Crackers	2 crackers	45	10 g	2 g	0 g	0 g	2 g
Millet - Pearls	1 cup cooked	191	38 g	5.3 g	1.6 g	0.3 g	2.1 g
Oatmeal	1/2 cup dry	150	27 g	5 g	3 g	0.5 g	4 g
Oat Flour	1 cup	360	60 g	15 g	6 g	0 g	12 g
Optimum Power Cereal	1 cup	190	40 g	8 g	2.5 g	0 g	10 g
Optimum Slim Cereal	1 cup	200	42 g	10 g	1 g	0 g	12 g
Pinto Beans	1/2 cup cooked	117	22 g	7 g	0.4 g	0.1 g	7.4 g
Popcorn air popped	1 cup	31	6.2 g	1 g	0.3 g	0 g	1.2 g
Soy Flour	1/2 cup	122	9 g	11 g	5.8 g	0.8 g	2.7 g
Tortilla - *Ezekiel*	1 - 10 inch	150	24 g	6 g	3.5 g	0.5 g	5 g
Tortilla – low carb							
"La Tortilla Factory"	1 small	60	12 g	5 g	2 g	0 g	9 g
Wasa Fiber Rye Crackers	2 crackers	60	14 g	2 g	1 g	0 g	2 g
Wheat Bran	2 Tbsp.	16	5 g	1 g	0.3 g	0.1 g	3.1 g
Wheat Germ	2 Tbsp.	52	7 g	3 g	1.4 g	0.2 g	1.9 g
Whole Wheat Flour	1/2 cup	134	29 g	5 g	0.7 g	0.1 g	4.8 g
Whole Wheat Pasta	1 cup cooked	174	37 g	8 g	0.8 g	0.1 g	3.9 g
Wild Rice	1 cup cooked	164	34 g	6 g	0.3 g	0 g	1.5 g

MEAT, POULTRY, FISH, DAIRY, SOY PROTEIN

Food Item	Portion Size	Calories	Carbs	Protein	Fat	Sat Fat	Fiber
Beef - filet mingon	3 oz. cooked	188	0 g	24 g	2 g	1 g	0 g
Beef – sirloin	3 oz. cooked	183	0 g	25 g	8.5 g	3.5 g	0 g
Buffalo	3 oz. cooked	120	0 g	24 g	2.0 g	1 g	0 g
Cheese - goat	1 oz.	82	0 g	6 g	6.5 g	4.5 g	0 g
Cheese - part skim mozzarella	1 oz.	79	0.9 g	7.8 g	4.9 g	3.1 g	0 g
Cheese - part skim ricotta	1/4 cup	96	2.5 g	6.7 g	6.4 g	4.1 g	0 g
Chicken - breast	3 oz. cooked	140	0 g	26 g	3 g	1 g	0 g
Chicken - canned	3 oz.	119	0 g	21.6 g	3 g	0.8 g	0 g
Chicken - thigh	3 oz. cooked	178	0 g	22 g	9.3 g	2.6 g	0 g
Cottage cheese nonfat	1 cup	140	10 g	26 g	0 g	0 g	0 g
Cottage cheese – 2%	1/2 cup	100	5 g	14 g	2.5 g	1.5 g	0 g
Egg Beaters	1/2 cup	60	2 g	12 g	0 g	0 g	0 g
Egg whites	1/2 cup	61	0 g	12.8 g	0 g	0 g	0 g
Egg – regular	1 whole	75	1 g	6 g	5 g	2 g	0 g
Egg - omega 3 (DHA)	1 whole	70	>1 g	6 g	4.5 g	1.5 g	0 g
Fish - cod	3 oz. cooked	93	0 g	20.2 g	0.8 g	0.1 g	0 g
Fish – halibut	3 oz. cooked	119	0 g	23 g	2.5 g	0.4 g	0 g
Fish - salmon, Atlantic	3 oz. cooked	164	0 g	24.2 g	6.6 g	1.4 g	0 g
Fish – salmon canned	3 oz. drained	89	0 g	15.5 g	2.2 g	1.1 g	0 g
Fish - sea bass	3 oz. cooked	112	0 g	21.2 g	2.3 g	0.6 g	0 g
Fish – snapper	3 oz. cooked	109	0 g	21 g	1 g	0 g	0 g
Fish – sole	3 oz. cooked	100	0 g	21 g	1 g	0 g	0 g
Fish – trout	3 oz. cooked	144	0 g	21 g	6.1 g	1.8 g	0 g
Fish - tuna fillet	3 oz. cooked	130	0.3 g	23.3 g	3.4 g	0.7 g	0 g
Fish - tuna solid white canned in water	3 oz. drained	135	0 g	21 g	4.5 g	0.5 g	0 g
Milk – nonfat	1 cup	86	12 g	9 g	0.4 g	0.3 g	0 g
Milk – 1 %	1 cup	102	12 g	8 g	2.6 g	1.6 g	0 g

MEAT, POULTRY, FISH, DAIRY, SOY PROTEIN (cont.)

Food Item	Portion Size	Calories	Carbs	Protein	Fat	Sat Fat	Fiber
Shrimp	3 oz. cooked	84	0 g	18 g	0.9 g	0.3 g	0 g
Soy bacon, *Morning Star Farms*	2 slices	60	2 g	2 g	4.5 g	0.5 g	> 1 g
Soy burger - *Boca*	1 patty	80	8 g	13 g	0 g	0 g	4 g
Soy burger *Morning Star Farms*	1 patty	100	6 g	13 g	2 g	0 g	3 g
Soy cheese – *Pepper Jack Veggie Slices*	1 slice	40	0.6 g	4 g	2 g	0 g	0 g
Soy – ground round *Lightlife Brand*	2 oz.	70	5 g	12 g	0 g	0 g	3 g
Soy milk *Silk*	1 cup	100	8 g	7g	4 g	0 g	0 g
Soy – tofu firm	3 oz.	42	3.6 g	13.5 g	7.5 g	0.9 g	2.1 g
Turkey bacon	1 thick slice	54	0.4 g	4 g	3.9 g	1.2 g	0 g
Turkey breast	3 oz. roasted	120	0 g	28 g	1 g	1 g	0 g
Turkey breast, ground	3 oz. cooked	120	0 g	26 g	1.5 g	0.5 g	0 g
Yogurt - *Continental*	12 oz.	190	38 g	12 g	0 g	0 g	0 g

NUTS, SEEDS, OILS AND FAT SOURCES

Food Item	Portion Size	Calories	Carbs	Protein	Fat	Sat Fat	Fiber
Almonds	1 oz.	167	6 g	6 g	15 g	1.4 g	3.1 g
Almond butter	1 Tbsp.	101	3.4 g	2.4 g	9.5 g	0.9 g	0.6 g
Almond oil	1 Tbsp.	120	0 g	0 g	13.6 g	1.1 g	0 g
Avocado	1/2 med.	153	6 g	2 g	15 g	2.2 g	4.2 g
Brazil nuts	1 oz.	186	4 g	4 g	19 g	4.6 g	1.5 g
Chestnuts	6 roasted	124	27 g	2 g	1.1 g	0.2 g	2.6 g
Canola Oil	1 Tbsp.	120	0 g	0 g	13.6 g	1.1 g	0 g
Grape seed oil	1 Tbsp.	120	0 g	0 g	14 g	0 g	0 g
Flaxseeds	1 Tbsp.	47	4 g	2 g	4.1 g	0.4 g	3.3 g
Flaxseed oil	1 Tbsp.	120	0 g	0 g	13.6 g	1.2 g	0 g
Olives	6 big ones	74	5 g	1 g	6.3 g	0.8 g	2.3 g

NUTS, SEEDS, OILS AND FAT SOURCES (cont.)

Food Item	Portion Size	Calories	Carbs	Protein	Fat	Sat Fat	Fiber
Olive oil	1 Tbsp.	119	0 g	0 g	14 g	1.8 g	0 g
Peanuts	1 oz.	166	6 g	7 g	14 g	2.0 g	2.3 g
Peanut butter	1 Tbsp.	95	4 g	3 g	8.2 g	1.7 g	0.9 g
Safflower oil	1 Tbsp.	120	0 g	0 g	13.6 g	1.2 g	0 g
Smart Balance	1 Tbsp.	80	0 g	0 g	9 g	2.5 g	0 g
Soyanaise	1 Tbsp.	30	1 g	0 g	3 g	0 g	0 g
Soybean oil	1 Tbsp	120	0 g	0 g	13.6 g	1.1 g	0 g
Soy nuts	1 oz.	130	9 g	10 g	6 g	0 g	2 g
Sunflower seeds	1 oz.	165	5.5 g	6.6 g	14.1 g	1.5 g	2 g
Walnuts	1 oz.	182	5 g	4 g	18 g	1.6 g	1.4 g
Walnut oil	1 Tbsp.	120	0 g	0 g	13.6 g	1.2 g	0 g

Conclusion

We invite you to visit us on the Internet and take advantage of our weekly recipes. In the meantime, focus on keeping the taste by using healthy marinades, fresh garlic, ginger and herbs. The idea that healthy food is bland and boring is far from the truth. Once you cleanse your pallet and open your eyes, you will see a variety of healthy yet great tasting foods!

Points to remember:

- Plan your grocery shopping, meals and snacks daily.
- When you go grocery shopping, spend most of your time on the outside of the store and dash into the middle isles for items like bread, cereals, whole grain pasta, tomato sauce, beans, spices, olive oil, canned chicken or fish, toiletries, and cleaning supplies.
- Take a multi-vitamin daily.
- Eat every two to three hours.
- Eat your last meal/snack no more than three hours before bed.
- Eat a portion of protein and carbohydrate with breakfast, lunch and dinner.
- A snack can be either a portion of protein, carbohydrate or a combination as in trail mix for instance.
- Eat five to eight servings or fresh fruit and vegetables per day. Frozen varieties are healthier than canned ones.
- Choose to grill, bake, broil or poach your lean meats, poultry or fish.
- Experiment with healthier options to your favorite food choices. When you keep your eyes open to new possibilities—you will surely find them!

Appendix C
Exercise Program Guide

First of all, let us begin this appendix by saying that it is impossible to design a generic program that works for everyone. When we design an exercise program, we customize it for our clients after we get to know them and by asking a lot of questions. In short, we sit down with each client, one-on-one and conduct a body composition analysis after we discuss their exercise history, personal goals, current and previous injuries and health concerns. There just isn't one generic program that will suit everyone's personal needs.

We have outlined some basic exercise guidelines and principles that can be applied to a wide variety of individuals. The two programs provided will however, increase your strength, boost your metabolism, burn calories, increase your energy, improve the efficiency of your heart and lungs, make daily physical activities seem easier, tone your muscles, stimulate the increase in bone density, increase the release of mood enhancing endorphins, improve your over all health and help you release fat.

All of the exercises are safe and effective. We have carefully selected exercises that will provide the greatest benefit to you with minimal risk. What this means is that we have omitted any exercises that may put your joints at risk for injury. For example, bench dips are a great exercise for the triceps muscles (the back of the arm). However, there is a high probability of developing several damaging shoulder ailments such as impingement syndrome (ouch!) or rotator cuff tears. Instead of ignoring these risk factors, we chose triceps exercises like the lying triceps extension (skull crusher) and kickback. These exercises offer excellent toning benefits for this muscle group, without any risk to the shoulder joint.

Below we have provided you with two exercise programs. If you work out in a health club with a variety of machines you may choose to substitute some of the resistance exercises for machines. The important part is to have a plan. We witness many people everyday who wander around the gym going from machine to machine and performing the exercises that they "feel like" doing at the time. This can lead to muscle imbalances, weakness and plateaus. Similar to having a grocery list before you go shopping—it is to your benefit to have a workout plan before you start to exercise!

Basic exercise guidelines:

- Consult a physician prior to beginning any exercise program.
- If you ever feel faint or dizzy during exercise, stop and consult your physician.
- Always perform a low-moderate intensity cardiovascular warm up for six to 12 minutes prior to any type of exercise.
- There a two main types of cardiovascular training methods, a) shorter duration higher intensity type sessions i.e. 30 minutes of interval training or b) longer duration moderate intensity type training i.e. walking for 45 to 60 minutes. If you are a beginner, stick with low to moderate intensity cardio sessions of 15 to 20 minutes and slowly work up to a longer duration.
- For a combination of metabolic, strength and toning benefits, perform three to four sets of eight to 12 repetitions per resistance exercise. (Beginners start with one set and build up to three to four sets).
- Always stretch your muscles after your body is warmed up—either before you begin your resistance exercises, or as a cool down after your resistance or cardio session.
- Variety is the key to your success—change your program every 30 days by increasing your weights, the number of repetitions or increasing your duration or intensity of your cardio sessions. Keep your body and mind stimulated by doing something different every four weeks.
- Some soreness may occur during the next two days after performing the resistance exercises. If you are still sore on the day you are supposed to perform weights, do cardio instead and go back to the weights the next day. Soreness that lasts more than two days requires more rest and recovery.

NOTE: Please review Chapters 20 and 21 for more specific exercise details.

Level I program:

This program is designed for individuals that are new to exercise or resistance training, may have been inactive for at least three months, or may not have the time or the energy to workout with weights more than twice per week. It is a very effective program that will yield results. You may choose to stick with this program or advance to the Level II program after six to 12 weeks. Bear in mind that variety is the key to success. If you decide to stay with this program, be sure to change some of the exercises, increase the weight (load), or increase the duration and/or the intensity of the cardio sessions every four to six weeks.

Here is what your week may look like:

Monday
- 6-12 minute cardio warm up
- 30 minutes of weights (total body circuit), 1-4 sets, 8-12 reps
- 10-15 minutes of stretching

Tuesday
- Cardio low to moderate intensity of 20 to 45 minutes (depending on your level and ability)

Wednesday
- Cardio low to moderate intensity of 20 to 45 minutes (depending on your level and ability)

Thursday
- 6-12 minute cardio warm up
- 30 minutes of weights (total body circuit) 1-4 sets, 8-12 reps
- 10-15 minutes of stretching

Friday
- Cardio low to moderate intensity of 20 to 45 minutes (depending on your level and ability)

Saturday
- Cardio low to moderate intensity of 20 to 45 minutes (depending on your level and ability)

Sunday - OFF

Monday	Tuesday	Wednesday	Thursday	Friday	Saturday	Sunday
Weights	Cardio	Cardio	Weights	Cardio	Cardio	Rest
Total Body	20 to 45	20 to 45	Total Body	20 to 45	20 to 45	
1-4 sets	minutes	minutes	1-4 sets	minutes	minutes	
8-12 reps			8-12 reps			

TOTAL BODY CIRCUIT
Twice per week. Example: Monday and Thursday

- 6-12 minute Cardio Warm-Up (i.e., brisk walk, jog, variety of cardio equipment, dancing, or the warm up segment of a workout tape).
- Squat—choose from the variations (photos 1A to 3B)
- Overhead Shoulder Press (photos 15A and 15B)
- One Arm Row (photos 7A to 7B)
- Push Up—choose from the variation (photos 10A to 12B)
- Biceps Curls (photos 19A and 19B)
- Lying Triceps Extension (photos 17A and 17B)
- Crunch (photos 22A and 22B)
- Alternate Arm/Leg Lift (photos 21A and 21B)
- Cool-Down—stretching

Level II program

This program is designed for individuals at a higher fitness level with more experience exercising. We recommend that you start with the Level I program if you are unable to perform 45 minutes of continuous cardiovascular activity at a moderate intensity. The Level II program consists of cardiovascular interval training—short high intensity burst followed by moderate intensity recovery periods. Also, we have split the resistance routine into two separate workouts—referred to as a two-day split.

A two-day split allows you to perform more exercises per muscle group. This is considered more intense because you hit the muscle from different angles, recruiting more muscle fibers. This can create additional tears in the muscle, which requires longer rest periods in-between workout sessions—resulting in greater strength and muscle growth. Although you could do this with a total body workout as in the Level I program, adding additional sets would make the workout long. The longer the workout, the more likely you are to lack intensity during those last few exercises. By performing a two-day split we have less muscle to focus on, therefore, we can execute more sets per muscle group. Make sense?

Also, you will want to alternate Day 1 and Day 2. One week you perform two day ones and the next week you perform two day twos. For example: During week one you may perform "Day 1" on Monday, "Day 2" on Wednesday and perform "Day 1" again on Friday. During week two you may perform "Day 2" on Monday, "Day 1" on Wednesday and "Day 2" on Friday. Repeat this cycle.

Here is what your week will look like:

Monday
- 6-12 minute cardio warm up
- Day One (Chest, back and shoulders), 3-4 sets, 8-12 reps
- 10-15 minutes of stretching

Tuesday
- Cardio: moderate intensity with high intensity intervals for 30 to 45 minutes

Wednesday
- 6-12 minute cardio warm up
- Day Two (Legs and arms), 3-4 sets, 8-12 reps
- 10-15 minutes of stretching

Thursday
- Cardio: moderate intensity with high intensity intervals for 30 to 45 minutes

Friday
- 6-12 minute cardio warm up
- Day One (Chest, back and shoulders), 3-4 sets, 8-12 reps
- 10-15 minutes of stretching

Saturday
- Cardio: moderate intensity for 30 to 60 minutes

Sunday – OFF

Note: If you want to add additional cardio sessions on your resistance training days, for best results we encourage you to perform your cardio in the morning and weights in the afternoon or at night (depending on your schedule).

Monday	Tuesday	Wednesday	Thursday	Friday	Saturday	Sunday
Weights	Cardio	Weights	Cardio	Weights	Cardio	Rest
Day 1	30 to 45	Day 2	30 to 45	Day 1	30 to 60	
3-4 sets	minutes	3-4 sets	minutes	3-4 sets	minutes	
8-12 reps		8-12 reps		8-12 reps		

Day 1: Chest, Back and Shoulders

6-12 minute Cardio Warm-Up

Overhead Shoulder Press (photos 15A and 15B)

Two Arm Prone Row (photos 8A and 8B)

Incline DB Chest Press (photos 14A and 14B)

One Arm Row (photos 7A and 7B)

Chest Press or Push Up (photos 11A and 11B, 12A and 12B, 13A and 13B)

Reverse Fly (photos 9A and 9B)

Side Lateral Raise (photos 16A and 16B)

Crunch (photos 22A and 22B)

Reverse Crunch (photos 23A and 23B)

Cool-Down – stretching

Day 2: Legs and Arms

6-12 minute Cardio Warm-Up

Squat – bench or free squat (photos 2A and 2B or 3A and 3B)

Standing Calf Raise (photos 6A and 6B)

Lunge – full range of motion (photos 4C to 5B)

Standing Biceps Curl (photos 19 and 19B)

Triceps Kickback (photos 18A and 18B)

Seated Concentration Curl (photos 20A and 20B)

French Press (Lying Triceps Extension) (photos 17A and 17B)

Bicycle (photos 24A and 24B)

Alternate Arm/Leg Lift (photos 21A and 21B)

Cool-Down – stretching

Exercises

Legs:

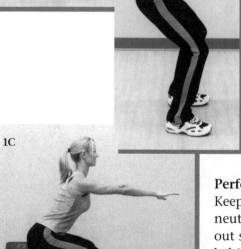

SQUAT

Starting Position:
Start with your feet hip width apart, chest lifted and shoulders pressed down. Look forward to keep your head neutral. Maintain the natural curve of the lower back while pulling your bellybutton into your spine. Keep your hips pressed back and your weight centered over your heels and mid-foot.

Active Phase:
Lower your body toward the floor like you are going to sit in a chair —keeping your knees behind your toes. To start, descend to 45 degrees and eventually work your way to a 90-degree angle where your thighs are parallel to the floor. Exhale as you ascend (push up), keeping your knees slightly bent at the top. Feel free to use a bench for safety and form development *(see photo 1C).*

Performance Tip:
Keep your neck and spine neutral and stick your but-tocks out so that your knees remain behind your toes. Look straight ahead into a mirror to monitor your technique.

BENCH SQUAT W/DUMBBELLS

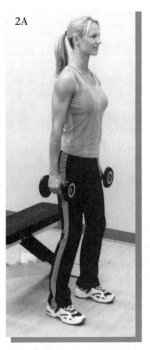

2A

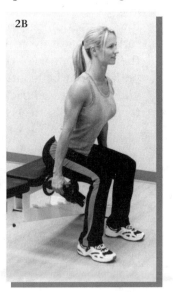

2B

Starting Position/Active Phase:
Perform a squat using the same description as 1A through 1C. Using a bench for support and safety, complete a full range of motion squat while holding a dumbbell in each hand (palms facing in) to increase intensity. Gently touch the bench without resting your total body weight.

Performance Tip: Stand far enough away from the bench so that you can stick your buttocks out as you descend. This will keep the stress off your knees.

FREE SQUAT W/DUMBBELLS
Starting Position/ Active Phase:

Perform all phases of this exercise as described in 1A through 1C. Remember to keep your chest lifted and knees behind your toes. As well, by holding a dumbbell in each hand you increase the intensity.

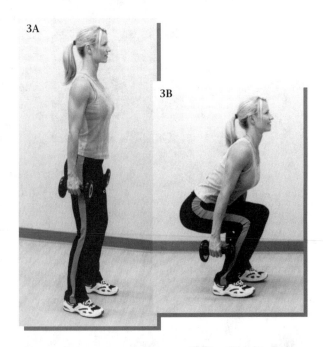

3A

3B

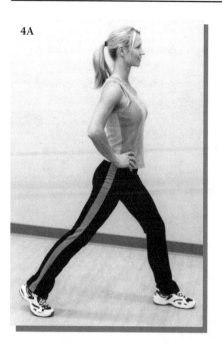

4A

LUNGE

Starting Position:
Standing with your feet hip-width apart, toes pointing straight ahead, take one giant step forward. Elevate your back heel to transfer your weight to the front heel and mid-foot (the back leg is for balance and support).

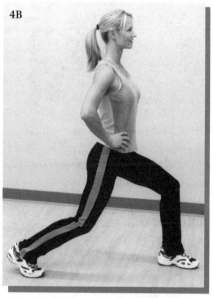

4B

Active Phase:
Maintaining proper posture, bend both legs as you lower the back knee toward the floor. Lower to 45 degrees *(see photo 4B)*, then advance to a 90-degree angle as in photo 4C. Exhale as you ascend to the starting position—keeping your knees slightly bent at the top. When you have completed a full set, repeat on the opposite side. For additional balance, you may hold on to a chair or place one hand on the wall.

Performance Tip:
Stop before your back knee touches the floor. If your front knee passes your toe, take a longer stride forward.

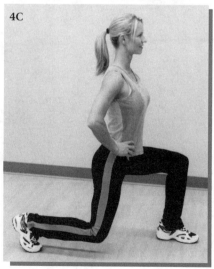

4C

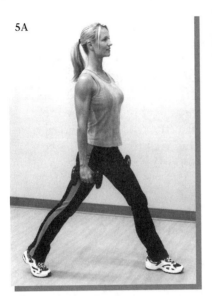

5A

FULL LUNGE W/DUMBBELLS

Starting Position/Active Phase:
Perform a lunge using the same description as with photographs 4A through 4C.

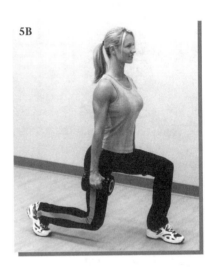

5B

Complete a full range of motion lunge, holding a dumbbell in each hand (palms facing in) for increased intensity.

STANDING CALF RAISE

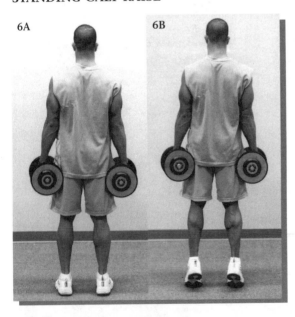

6A   6B

Starting Position:
Stand with your feet hip-width apart, abs tight and hold a dumbbell in each hand with your palms facing inward.

Active Phase:
Keeping your knees straight, exhale as you elevate your heels off the floor as high as you can. At the top of themotion, pause for one second, then, slowly descend to the starting position.

Performance Tip: Keep your abs engaged by pulling your bellybutton in toward your spine for balance. If you are still unstable, hold one dumbbell instead and use the free hand to hold onto a chair or the wall for improved balance.

Back:

ONE ARM ROW

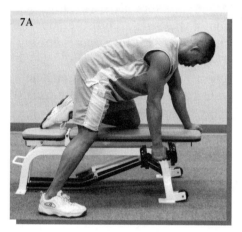

Starting position:
Create a tripod for support by placing your left hand and knee on a bench and your right foot on the floor with your knee slightly bent. Holding a dumbbell in your right hand, start with your arm extended toward the floor. Keep your back flat and parallel with the bench. Keep your arm close to your body and your neck in a neutral position by looking at the bench.

Active Phase:
Exhale as you pull your elbow up toward the ceiling, lifting the dumbbell until it is just about on the same level with your chest. Slowly return the dumbbell to the starting position. When you have completed a full set, follow the same instructions for you're your left arm.

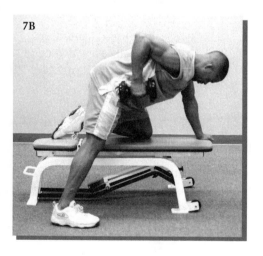

Performance Tip:
When you reach the top of the motion, be sure that your arm is at a 90-degree angle. This will keep the load on your back (lats) muscles and less on your biceps.

TWO ARM PRONE ROW

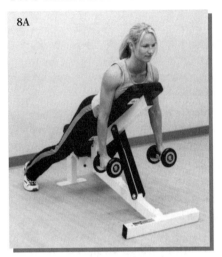

Starting Position: Elevate your bench to a 45-degree angle. Holding a dumbbell in each hand, slowly lower your body to a prone or face down position. Align your shoulders with the top of the bench, and sink your shoulder blades into your spine. This will elevate your chest slightly off the bench and engage your back muscles. Let your arms hang toward the floor—palms facing inward.

Active Phase: Exhale as you pull the dumbbells up close to your lower rib area—keeping your elbows in tight to your body. Bring your shoulder blades together at the top of the movement and contract (squeeze) your mid-back (trapezius and rhomboids). Slowly lower the dumbbells to the starting position.

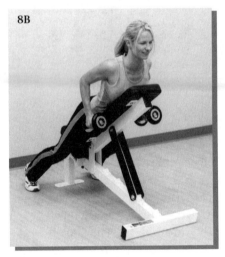

Performance Tip:
Keep your shoulder blades sunk into your spine and chest slightly elevated. This will prevent any rounding of the shoulders that can cause unnecessary stress to your rotator-cuff muscles.

REVERSE FLY

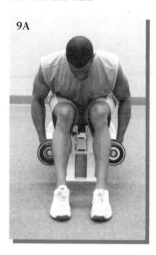

9A

Starting Position:
Sit on the end of a bench with your knees in line with your feet. Keeping your back straight, lean forward at the hips to a 45-degree angle. With your elbows slightly bent, hold a dumbbell in each hand underneath your thighs.

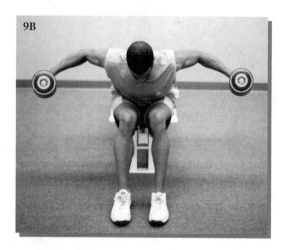

9B

Active Phase:
Keeping your elbows slightly bent and your palms facing in, retract your shoulder blades until your elbows are level with your trunk (torso). You will want to feel your shoulder blades moving toward the center of your spine. Pause for one second at the top, then, slowly lower your arms back to the starting position.

Performance Tip:
Keep your trunk (torso) motionless and lift your arms slowly—with control. Exhale on the way up as you retract your shoulder blades.

Chest:

WALL PUSH UP

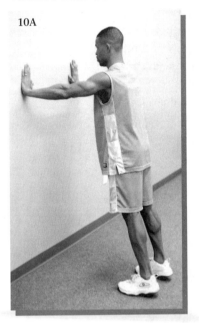

10A

Starting Position:
Place your hands on the wall slightly below shoulder height and wider than shoulder width. Elevate your heels off the floor to transfer some of your body weight to your arms. Keep your elbows slightly bent and pull your bellybutton into your spine.

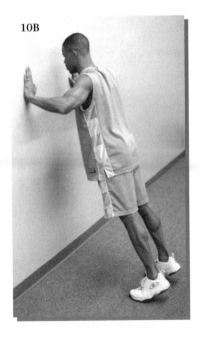

10B

Active Phase:
Slowly lower your body to the wall until your arms are at a 90-degree angle or until your elbows are in line with your shoulders. Exhale as you slowly push your body away from the wall and back to the starting position.

Performance Tip: Sink your scapula (shoulder blades) into your spine to maintain proper posture. Eliminate stress on the joints by keeping your elbows slightly bent at the top and by dropping your elbows just below your shoulders.

FLOOR PUSH UP (SHORT)

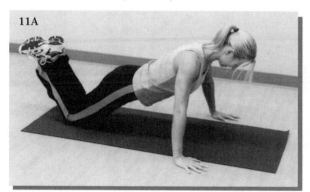

Starting Position: Place your hands on the floor slightly below shoulder height and just wider than shoulder-width apart. Drop your hips so they are level with your trunk and bend your knees so your bodyweight is distributed between your hands and knees.

Active Phase: Slowly lower your body to the floor—stopping when your elbows are level with your trunk (90-degree angle). Exhale as you push up to the starting position. Keep your elbows slightly bent at the top.

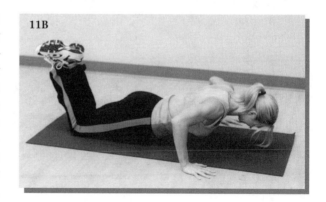

Performance Tip:
Maintain proper body alignment by pulling your bellybutton into your spine, contracting your gluteus maximus (buttocks) and sinking your shoulder blades into your spine.

FLOOR PUSH UP (LONG)

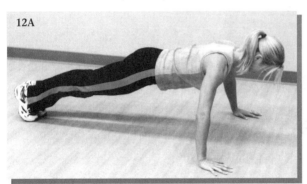

Starting Position: Perform using the same technique as described with photographs 11A and 11B. The only exception is to straighten your legs and keep your weight distributed between your hands and toes.

Performance Tip: Maintain proper body alignment by pulling your belly-button into your spine, contracting your gluteus max-imus (buttocks) and sinking your shoulder blades into your spine.

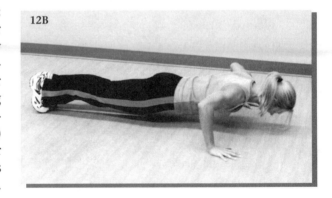

CHEST PRESS

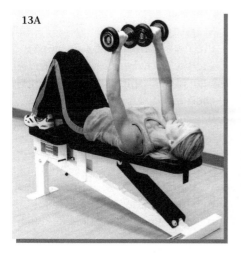

13A

Starting Position: Holding a dumbbell in each hand, lie on your back with your feet on the bench to keep your lower back flat. With your elbows in tight to your body and palms facing in, push the dumbbells up above your sternum—in the center your chest. Rotate your palms so they are facing your knees.

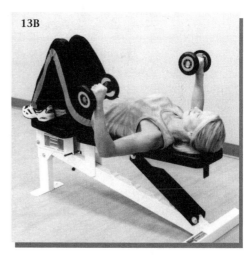

13B

Active Phase: Slowly lower the weight until your elbows are at right angles or level with your trunk. Keep your wrists straight and in line with your elbows. Exhale as you push the weight up to the starting position. Keeping your elbows slightly bent at the top.

Performance Tip:
Be sure to stop when your elbows are level with your trunk. Dipping your elbows past your body can cause unnecessary stress to the shoulder joint.

INCLINE CHEST PRESS

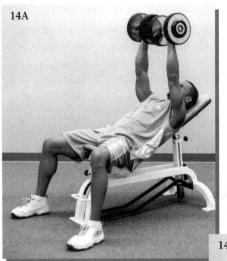

Starting Position:
Place your bench at a 45-degree incline. Slowly lay back on the bench and hold a dumbbell in each hand (close to your shoulders). With your elbows in tight to your body and palms facing in, push the dumbbells up above your sternum—in the center of your chest with your arms slightly bent. Rotate your palms so they are facing your knees.

Active Phase:
Slowly lower the weight until your elbows are at right angels or level with your body. Keep your wrists straight and in line with your elbows. Exhale as you push the weight up to the starting position. Keep your elbows slightly bent at the top.

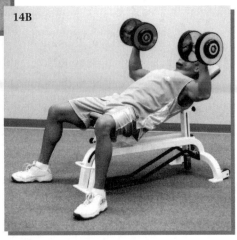

Performance Tip: Set your bench at a 30- to 45-degree incline. If it is set too high you will feel it more in your shoulders. Keep the weights in line with your chest rather than your chin. Be sure to stop when your elbows are level with your trunk.

Shoulders:

OVERHEAD SHOULDER PRESS

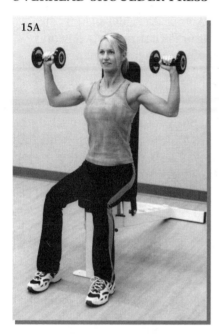

Starting Position:
Sit on the end of a bench and hold the dumbbells in each hand. Lift the weights up level with your eyes and position your arms at 90-degree angles with your palms facing out. Tighten your abs by pulling your bellybutton inward and keep your shoulders flat by sinking your shoulder blades into your spine.

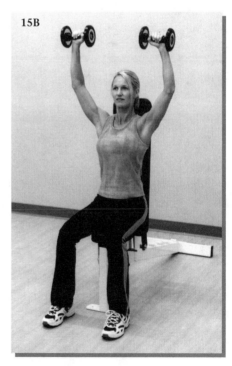

Active Phase:
Exhale as you press the dumbbells up toward the ceiling—until your arms are slightly bent. Keep space between the dumbbells above your head. Slowly lower the weight until the dumbbells are level with your eyes and your arms are at right angles.

Performance Tip:
Keep your wrists straight and in line with your elbows.
Be sure to stop before your elbows dip past your shoulder
to prevent unnecessary stress to the joint.

SIDE LATERAL RAISE

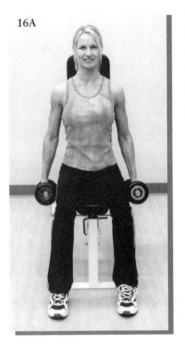

16A

Starting Position:
Sit on the end of a bench and hold a dumbbell in each hand. Tighten your abs and sink your shoulder blades into your spine to maintain proper posture. (This exercise can be per-formed seated or standing).

Active Phase:
Keeping your elbows slightly bent, exhale as you raise your arms until they are level with your shoulders. Slowly lower the weight to the starting position.

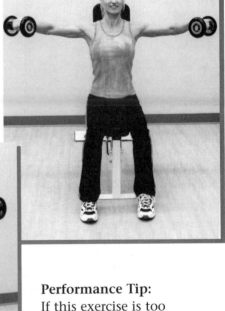

16B

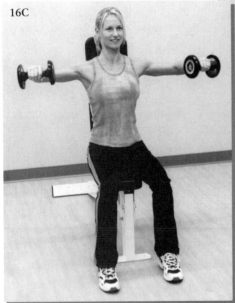

16C

Performance Tip:
If this exercise is too difficult or you feel any stress in your joints, bend your elbows to a 90-degree angle as in photo 16C.

Triceps:

LYING TRICEPS EXTENSION

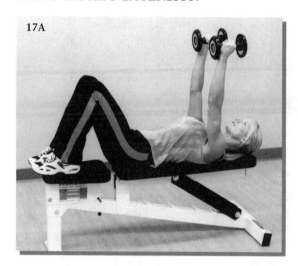

Starting Position:
Hold a dumbbell in each hand and lie on your back with your feet on the bench. Holding your elbows in tight to your body, and palms facing in, press the weight straight up above your chest. Position your wrists and elbows in line with your shoulders.

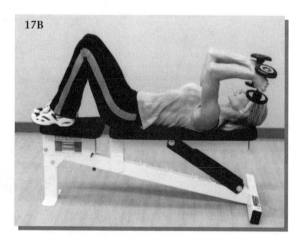

Active Phase:
Lower the weight while keeping your elbow and shoulders in place and descend to a 90-degree angle. Exhale as you lift the weight up to the starting position.

Performance Tip:
The nickname for this exercise is "skull crushers." Maintain space between the dumbbells to prevent accidental injury to your face.

KICKBACK

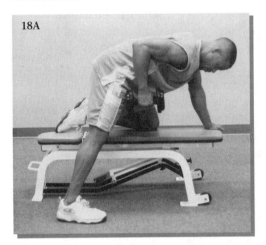

Starting Position:
Create a tripod for support by placing your left hand and knee on a bench and your right foot on the floor with your knee slightly bent. Holding a dumbbell in your right hand, lift your elbow up until it is level with your body and your arm is at a right angle.

Active Phase:
Keeping your shoulder stable, exhale as you extend your arm back until your elbow is just about straight. Slowly lower the dumbbell back to the starting position. When you have completed a full set, repeat on the left side.

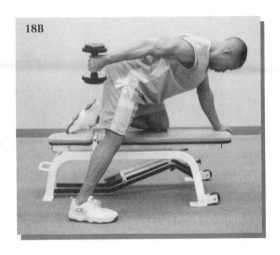

Performance Tip:
Stop before the dumbbell passes the 90-degree angle at the start and finish of the exercise. This will keep the load on the triceps and off the biceps.

Biceps:

BICEPS CURL

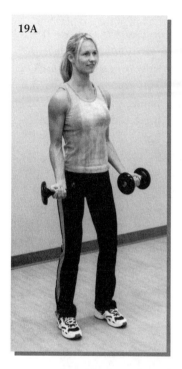

19A

Starting Position:
Holding a dumbbell in each hand, sit on the end of a bench with your palms facing out. Keep your elbows slightly bent and maintain proper posture by pulling your bellybutton in toward your back and sinking your shoulder blades into your spine.

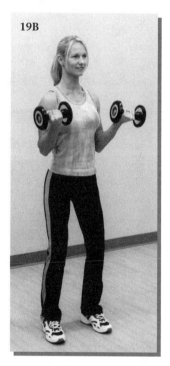

19B

Active Phase:
Keeping your elbows close to your sides, exhale as you lift the weight up toward your shoulders. Hold for one second at the top and slowly lower the dumbbells back to the starting position.

Performance Tip:
Keep space between the dumbbell and your shoulder at the top of the movement. This will keep the load on the muscle.

CONCENTRATION CURL

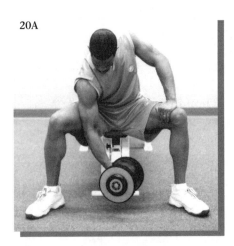

20A

Starting Position:
Sit on the end of a bench with your feet slightly wider than hip-width apart. Rest your left hand on your left thigh and lean forward, extending your right arm toward the floor. Grasp a dumbbell with your right hand and secure your elbow on the inside of your right thigh. Pull your bellybutton in toward your back and sink your shoulder blades into your spine.

20B

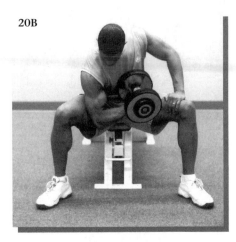

Active Phase:
Curl the weight in the direction of your left knee until the dumbbell is just in front of your chest. Slowly lower the weight back to the starting position. Exhale on the way up. When you have completed a full set, repeat on the opposite side.

Performance Tip:
Resist the temptation to rest your working arm on top of your thigh. This limits your range of motion and takes away from the intensity that gravity has to offer. Keep your spine straight and motionless during the entire range of motion.

Core-Abs:

OPPOSITE ARM/LEG LIFT

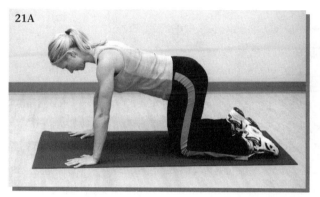

Starting Position: Begin on your hands and knees—quadruped position. Maintain a sturdy base of support by keeping your hands shoulder-width apart and your knees hip-width apart. Tighten your abs by pulling your bellybutton into your spine—again-gravity. Keep your hips and eyes facing the floor.

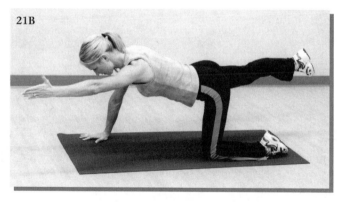

Active Phase: Lift your left arm and right leg simultaneously until they are both level with your trunk. Rotate your thumb up toward the ceiling and keep both hips facing the floor.Pause for one second at the top, then, slowly lower to the starting position. Repeat on the other side.

Performance Tip:
Maintain a flat back by keeping your abs contracted and hips facing the floor. Perform this exercise at a slow pace—take your time! This is an excellent exercise for anyone wishing to improve their balance, coordination and strengthen their back.

CRUNCH

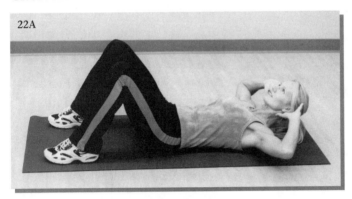

Starting Position: Lie on your back with your knees bent and your feet flat on the floor. Position your fingertips just behind your ears and lift your head off the floor. Press your lower back into the floor and pull your bellybutton in toward your spine.

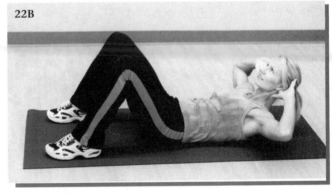

Active Phase: Exhale as you lift your shoulder blades completely off the floor by contracting your abdominal muscles. Hold for one second at the top and slowly descend to the starting position. For maximum results, keep your head off the floor throughout the set.

Performance Tip: Imagine an accordion coming together as you close the gap between your ribs and your hipbones. Keep your eyes on a spot on the ceiling to prevent excessive neck movement.

REVERSE CRUNCH

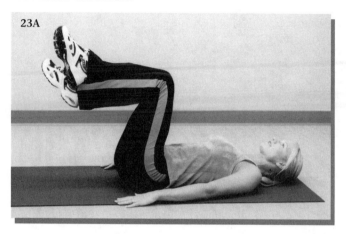

Starting Position: Lie on your back with your knees bent and lifted above your hips at a 90-degree angle. Relax the lower part of your legs so your feet drop toward your buttocks. Press your lower back into the floor and pull your bellybutton toward your spine. Place your hands by your sides (palms down) for balance and support.

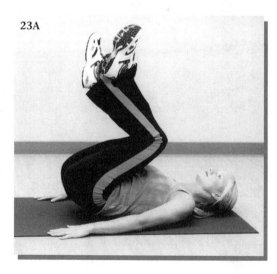

Active Phase: Exhale as you lift your knees toward your chest as high as you can without putting too much pressure on your hands. The goal is to get your buttocks completely off the floor. Slowly lower your body back to the starting position.

Performance Tip:
Keep your feet and lower legs relaxed to prevent momentum into the lift. Keep your lower back pressed into the floor at the start and finish of the exercise.

BICYCLE

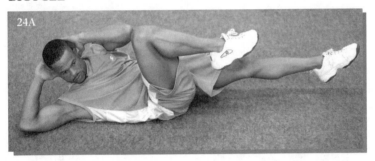

Starting Position:
Lie on your back with your knees bent and lifted above your hips at a 90-degree angle. Position your fingertips just behind your ears and lift your head off the floor. Extend your left leg out keeping your heels 6 to 12 inches off the floor.

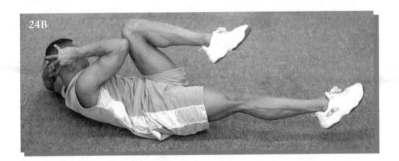

Active Phase:
Bring your left knee in toward your chest and raise your right shoulder off the floor toward your knee. Hold, and repeat opposite knee and shoulder.

Performance Tip:
Keep your elbows stable and focus on initiating the twist at your waist. Press your lower back into the floor and pull your bellybutton in toward your spine.

Strategic Stretching

It is no secret that flexibility is an important component of optimal fitness. Its benefits include an increase in synovial fluid in the joints, as well as improving coordination, balance, blood supply and nutrients to joints. Further, it helps to reduce the risk of injury, alleviate low back pain and possibly lower stress.

Few of us take the time to adequately improve our flexibility. To help you in your efforts, we have provided you with a variety of stretches that you can incorporate into your workout as well as make part of your daily routine. Be sure to warm up prior to stretching. You NEVER want to stretch a cold muscle or joint.

We encourage you to move into each position slowly and hold the stretch for at least 15 to 30 seconds. Unless you are an athlete training for a dynamic sport, it is also important that you remain still or static—that means no bouncing. If you feel pain beyond that of a slight discomfort, reduce the range of motion (ease up on the stretch). Also, it is not uncommon for you to experience some soreness the next day or so after stretching. Fortunately, you can expect the soreness to subside within a few weeks.

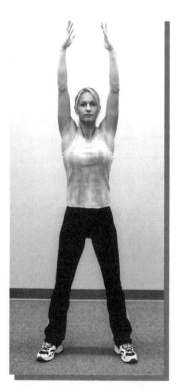

#1 OVERHEAD STRETCH (Lats)

Action:
Stand straight with your feet shoulder-width apart, hips facing forward, and abs tight. Raise both arms up toward the ceiling like you would first thing in the morning.

Tip:
Keep your weight evenly distributed on both feet and maintain the natural swayin your back without arching and leaning backward.

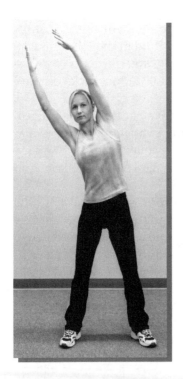

#2 OVERHEAD DIAGONAL STRETCH
(Lats and obliques)

Action:
Stand straight with your feet shoulder-width apart, hips facing forward, and abs tight. Raise both arms up toward the ceiling, elevate the shoulder girdle and gently lean to the right. Hold, then, repeat to the opposite side. You'll feel this stretch along the side of your trunk–lats and oblique.

Tip:
Rather than bending sideways at the waist, elongate your body and reach up and slightly to the side toward the area where the wall meets the ceiling.

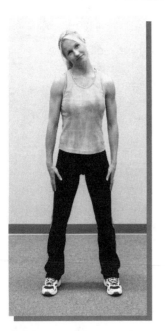

#3 NECK STRETCH
(Upper trapezius and levator scapula)

Action:
Keeping your shoulders square, slowly tilt your head to one side as though you want to touch your ear to your shoulder. Then, slowly tilt your head to the other side. This stretch is also great for stress relief because tension can be carried in this area.

Tip:
Keep your shoulders pressed down and gently tilt your head to the side. It is natural to want to lift both shoulders during this stretch. It may be helpful to hold on to the bottom of a table to help keep your shoulder pressed down.

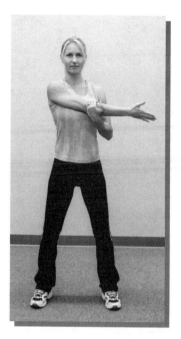

#4 SHOULDER STRETCH
(Rear deltoid and rotators)

Action:
With your shoulders pressed down, bring one arm across the chest parallel to the floor with the elbow slightly bent. With your opposite arm, trap the arm above the elbow, and apply gentle pressure. Perform this stretch on both sides.

Tip:
Keep your hips square and trunk stable—motionless.

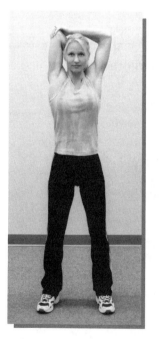

#5 TRICEPS STRETCH (Triceps)

Action:
Raise your right arm up over your head. Bend this arm at the elbow so that your hand drops behind your head. With your left hand, hold the bent elbow, and gently guide the elbow toward your head until you feel the stretch in the back of your arm. Perform this stretch on the left arm as well.

Tip:
It is important that you take your time and pull gently. If you aren't feeling the stretch, increase the bend in your elbow.

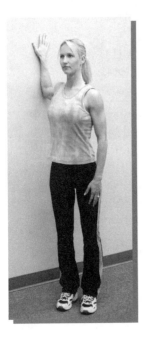

#6 CHEST STRETCH
(Pectoralis major, minor and the anterior deltoid)

Action:
Stand next to a wall (or stable surface) and hold your right arm at a 90-degree angle. Place your palm and forearm on the wall or solid surface. Lightly turn your body away from your arm—feel the stretch in your chest and shoulder muscles. Perform this stretch on both sides.

Tip:
Be careful not to over stretch by turning your body too much or holding your arm to high. Keep your elbow in line with your shoulder at a 90-degree angle.

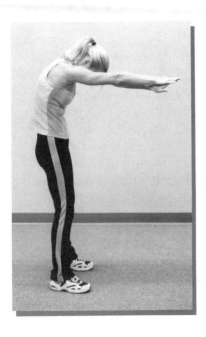

#7 UPPER BACK STRETCH
(Mid-trapezius, rhomboids and rear deltoids)

Action:
Standing upright with your feet hip-width apart, look down at the floor and reach both arms out in front of you. As you reach forward, round your chest so you feel the stretch between your shoulder blades.

Tip:
Press your shoulders down and keep your trunk upright by squeezing your glutes.

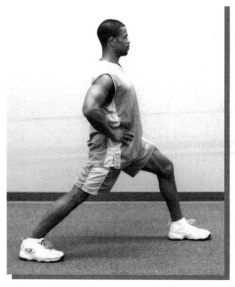

#8 RUNNER'S STRETCH (Hip flexor and calf - gastrocnemius)

Action:
Standing with your feet about shoulder-width apart, step forward with one leg while the rear leg remains straight with the heel firmly on the floor. Slowly push your hips forward, keeping your back straight. Perform this stretch on both sides.

Tip:
It is important to keep your back heel on the floor. If you slightly bend your back knee you can also stretch the deeper calf muscle—the soleus.

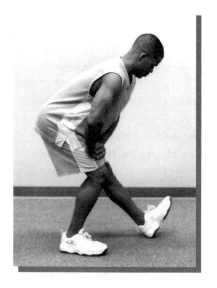

#9 STANDING HAMSTRING STRETCH

Action:
Standing with your feet about shoulder-width apart, step forward with one leg placing your heel on the floor while you transfer the weight to your bent back leg. Keeping your back straight, place both hands on the thigh of the bent leg and gently lean forward. Repeat on the opposite side.

Tip:
Stick your buttocks out and sit back on your hips. Keep your back flat and think about getting your belly button to the thigh of the extended leg.

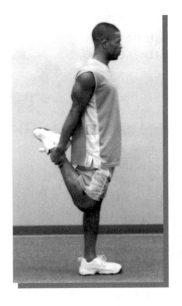

#10 QUADRICEPS STRETCH (Quadriceps)

Action:
Stand up straight, and slowly bend one leg and hold at the ankle. Position your bent knee next to the knee of your standing leg while you press your hips forward. For increased balance you can place one hand on a wall, chair, etc. Perform this stretch on both sides.

Tip:
Be sure to hold your leg at the ankle rather than the foot. Also keep space between your heel and glute and position your bent knee so it is pointing straight down to the floor to prevent over stretching the ligaments in your knee. Keep your hips pressed forward.

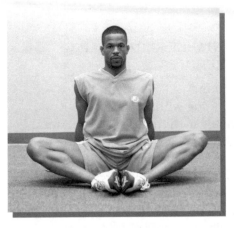

#11 BUTTERFLY STRETCH (Groin and thigh adductors)

Action:
While sitting on the floor with your back straight and hands placed behind you for support, bring the soles of your feet together in front of you—heels touching each other. Allow your knees to naturally drop toward the floor as you relax into the stretch. If you decide to use your hands to hold your ankles in place, it is important that you keep your back straight and your elbows inside your inner thighs.

Tip:
It is important that you keep your back straight and upright. Also, keep a gap between your heels and groin to prevent overstretching the ligaments in your knee.

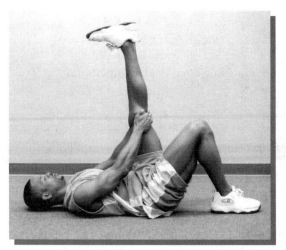

#12 LYING HAMSTRING STRETCH (Hamstring)

Action:

Lying on your back with both knees bent, keep one foot flat on the floor as you straighten out and extend the opposite leg up (vertical) over your hip. With both hands, hold on to the leg that is vertically extended and gently pull toward your chest. You will feel the stretch behind your leg in the hamstring. Perform this stretch on both sides.

Tip:
Keep your glutes on the floor and on the leg being stretched, keep your knee slightly bent.

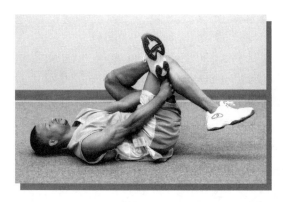

#13 GLUTE STRETCH— HALF-LOTUS (Glutes and hip)

Action:

Lying on your back with both knees bent, keep your right foot flat on the floor as you lift your left leg so that your ankle is able to rest on your right thigh. With both hands, reach your right leg behind your thigh and gently pull this leg off the floor toward your chest. You will feel the stretch in the hip and glute your left leg. Repeat this stretch on the rightside.

Tip:
This stretch is performed safety when your head is resting on the floor and both hands are wrapped around the thigh of the stationary leg. If your head lifts off the floor, place a pillow behind it for support.

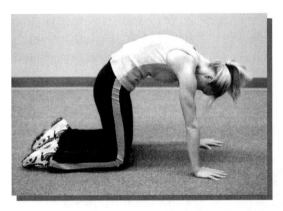

#14 CAT ARCH
(Erector spinae, mid-trapezius, and rhomboids)

Action:
Kneel on your hands and knees with your head, neck and back in alignment. Keeping your shoulders relaxed, lower your chin toward your chest, pull in your belly, and round your back, like a cat arching. You'll feel this stretch throughout your back and shoulders. Hold the arch in your back for a few seconds and then slowly return to the starting position.

Tip:
Press your back up toward the ceiling. Feel the stretch along the entire length of your spine.

Appendix D
Common Words and Terms

Abs: an abbreviation for the abdominal muscles. These include the rectus abdominus (the six-pack), and the external and internal oblique that run diagonally across the sides of the body.

Acute: a description of a condition that has a rapid onset and follows a short but severe course.

Aerobic: cardiovascular exercise where oxygen is metabolized for energy production and movement.

Amino acids: "building blocks" of the body. Besides building cells and repairing tissue, they form antibodies to combat invading bacteria and viruses; they are part of the enzyme and hormonal system; they build nucleoproteins (RNA and DNA); they carry oxygen throughout the body and participate in muscle activity. When protein is broken down by digestion, the result is 22 known amino acids. Nine are essential to include the amino acid, histidine; the rest are non-essential (can be manufactured by the body with proper nutrition).

Amenorrhea: abnormal suppression or absence of menstruation.

Anaerobic: the metabolic process that creates energy and movement without the presence of oxygen.

Anaerobic threshold: the point during high-intensity activity that the body no longer meets the demand for oxygen—anaerobic metabolism kicks in. Generally, the more fit the individual, the higher the anaerobic threshold.

Anorexia nervosa: an eating disorder characterized by a distorted body image, an intense fear of becoming obese, extreme weight loss and self-starvation.

Antioxidants: molecules that boost the body's defense system against free radicals. These include beta carotene, lycopene, vitamin C, E, sulfur and selenium.

Arteries: vessels that carry oxygenated blood from the heart to the tissues of the body.

Atherosclerosis: a specific form of arteriosclerosis characterized by the accumulation of fatty material on the inner walls of the arteries causing them to harden, thicken, and lose elasticity.

Atrophy: the condition in which muscle size is diminished due to lack of activity.

Barbell: the straight, long bar on which weight plates are loaded, used primarily for resistance training.

Beta-blockers: medications that "block" or limit the sympathetic nervous system. They act to slow the heart rate and maximum heart rate to prevent over-stressing the cardiovascular system.

Bioavailability: bio means life or living system, and available means ready for use. So bioavailability is the degree and rate at which a substance (such as protein) is absorbed into a living system or is made available to the body.

Blood pressure: the total pressure of blood that is exerted against the walls of blood vessels, arteries, capillaries, and veins, which is measured in mmhg (millimeters of mercury). It is recorded as the systolic and diastolic pressure.

Body composition analysis: a diagnostic check of the body's tissue proportions that divides your body into two parts: lean body mass and fat mass.

Body-fat percentage: determining how much of your total body weight is fat mass.

Body mass index: a mathematical formula that dates back to 1835, and is currently used to determine health risks such as cardiovascular disease, hypertension and high blood cholesterol to name a few. It is most commonly used as a relative measure of body height to body weight for determining the degree of obesity.

Bulimia nervosa: an eating disorder characterized by binge eating followed by self-induced vomiting or the use of diuretics or laxatives to prevent weight gain.

Calorie: the basic energy unit that the body needs in order to carry out physiological functions. Measured as the quantity of heat required to raise the temperature of one kilogram of water by 1°C from a standard initial temperature.

Cancer: a malignant cellular growth within tumors or cells in which cells continually divide and multiply at an uncontrollable rate. Caused by mutations within the cells DNA that translates to cancer. Mutations are caused by environmental, nutritional, and physiological stresses. Tumors can either be benign or malignant. Malignant cells are cancerous.

Carbohydrate: "carbo" refers to carbon, and "hydrate" to water, a combination of hydrogen and oxygen. This macronutrient commonly stated as "carbs" is derived from plants and is the body's primary energy source. Each gram of carbohydrate by weight provides four calories of energy.

Cardio: short for cardiovascular exercise, "cardio" is crucial for a healthy heart, lungs and vascular system.

Cardiovascular disease: general term for any disease of the heart and blood vessels. Includes: coronary artery disease, hypertension, stroke, congestive heart failure and peripheral vascular disease.

Cholesterol: a fat-like substance found in the blood and body tissues and in animal products. Although essential for the production of hormones and steroids, its accumulation within the bloodstream leads to atherosclerosis (narrowing of the arteries). There are two types of cholesterol: LDL and HDL.

Chronic disease: a condition that persists over a long period of time. It can be an injury, illness or a disease.

Circuit training: an exercise protocol where the participant moves through a series of exercise stations in a continuous non-stop fashion. Advantages include muscular endurance, aerobic conditioning and caloric expenditure.

Co-dependency: a relationship in which one person becomes dependent on someone or something other than himself or herself.

Complete proteins: foods that contain all of the essential amino acids.

Compound exercises: exercises where multiple muscles are stimulated and multiple joints are recruited to execute the movement. Example: squats.

Concentric phase: the part of the weight lifting movement phase where the muscle exerts force and shortens in length. Typically initiated when the movement moves against the force of gravity as in the upward movement of the bicep curl.

Cortisol: often referred to as the "stress hormone," it's an adrenal hormone which is secreted by the adrenal glands in response to any kind of physical or psychological stress.

Daily reference values: guidelines for dietary intake that are intended to serve as a yardstick for food comparisons, not as a strict dietary prescription. Measured in percentage values based on a 2,000-calorie diet.

Degenerative disease: a process of wear and tear that occurs with aging in virtually all individuals.

Diabetes Type 1: usually diagnosed in children and young adults and was previously known as juvenile diabetes and insulin dependence. In this type of diabetes, the body does not produce insulin. Insulin is necessary for the body to be able to use sugar. Sugar is the basic fuel for the cells in the body, and insulin takes the sugar from the blood into the cells. This is often a hereditary condition.

Diabetes Type 2: the most common form of diabetes. In this type of diabetes, either the body does not produce enough insulin or the receptor cites on the cells ignore the insulin. Characterized by high levels of blood sugar—often brought upon by a poor diet and obesity.

Diet: The usual food and drink of a person or animal.

Dumbbell: a weight that can be grasped within the grips of the hand intended for exercise purposes.

Eccentric phase: the part of the weight lifting movement phase where the muscle is elongated. Typically initiated when the movement is in the direction of gravity as in the downward movement of the bicep curl.

Empower: to equip or supply with ability; encourage action.

Endorphins: any of a group of peptide hormones that bind to opiate receptors and is found mainly in the brain. Endorphins reduce the sensation of pain and affect emotions. Endorphins are anti-stress hormones, help improve your memory, block the lesion of blood vessel and enhance our immune system.

Enzymes: proteins necessary to bring about biochemical reactions.

Essential fatty acids: the two main types of fatty acids that the body requires but can not manufacture on its own—linolenic (omega 3) and linoleic (omega 6) acids.

Exercise frequency: the number of specific exercise sessions within a specific time period. For example: perform resistance training two to three times per week.

Fat: an essential macronutrient that provides energy, protects organs, and provides cushioning and insulation. Each gram of fat by weight provides nine calories of energy.

Fiber: indigestible plant matter in carbohydrates. Primarily classified as soluble and insoluble.

Food: substance that comes from either plant or animal that provides the body with nutrients such as protein, carbohydrate, fat, vitamins and minerals for growth and the maintenance of life.

Food combining: the process of separating specific foods and eating a combination of certain ones at meals.

Food frequency: eating within a specific time period to regulate metabolism.

Fractionated oils: a manufacturing process that uses high temperatures or solvents to separate hydrogenated oil into liquid and solid parts. When listed on food labels, it indicates the presence of trans fat.

Free radical: aggressive chemicals that cause permanent damage when they react with cell components. They are atoms or molecules that have an unpaired electron that makes them highly reactive. Free radicals attack the nearest stable molecule and "steal" its electron. When a stable molecule is attached it becomes a free radical itself, creating a chain that can eventually cause cell damage. Free radicals are naturally and synthetically produced and are known to destroy tissues, cause cancer and advance aging.

Fructose: also known as fruit sugar, a simple sugar that is found within honey and fruits that is frequently used as a sweetener and preservative.

Functional exercise: any exercise that mimics real life movement patterns through the use of weights, or other exercise equipment. Stimulates development of muscles involved in common movement of the human body.

Gastrointestinal by-pass: a surgical process for obese people to drastically lose weight. Works by bypassing the stomach, duodenum, and portions of or most of the small intestine—where absorption of nutrients takes place. The general effect of this gastrointestinal bypass surgery is to generate mal-absorption of vital nutrients. Diarrhea, nutritional deficiencies and severe metabolic alkalosis are some complications. This bypass surgery is associated with significant morbidity and mortality.

Glucose: the simplest sugar that the body's cells will metabolize from all carbohydrate sources. It is the end product of carbohydrate metabolism and is the body's main energy source.

Glucose intolerance: also known as impaired glucose tolerance, it is a precondition to Type 2 diabetes where excess glucose circulates the bloodstream, but not at a high enough level to be defined as diabetes. Insulin is still released, but not enough to metabolize the circulating glucose.

Glycation: uncontrolled, non-enzymatic reactions of sugars with proteins. Notoriously known to advance the aging process because sugars attach to structural proteins forming undesirable by products known as advanced glycation end products, which are known to increase free radicals.

Glycemic index: a classification that measures the effect that 50 grams of specific carbohydrates have on blood glucose levels.

Glycemic load: a measure of a carbohydrate's glycemic index as well as the carbohydrate's serving. Glycemic load takes the glycemic index value and multiplies it by the actual number of carbohydrates per serving.

Glycogen: a substance made up of sugars. It is stored in the liver and muscles and releases glucose (sugar) into the blood when needed by cells. Glycogen is the chief source of stored fuel in the body.

HDL: high-density lipoproteins, also known as "healthy" cholesterol, which are known to carry cholesterol to and from the liver and remove excess cholesterol from the blood.

Heart attack: the damage that occurs to the heart when one of the coronary arteries becomes obstructed.

Heart disease: a structural or functional abnormality of the heart, or of the blood vessels supplying the heart, that impairs its normal functioning. Usually caused by excess accumulation of plaque along the artery walls. Heart disease is one of the leading causes of death in North America.

Homeostasis: the tendency toward stability and balance in normal body states.

Hormone: a naturally occurring substance secreted by specialized cells and organs for the regulation of bodily functions such as metabolic processes and growth.

Hydrogenated oils: the result of a manufacturing process where a hydrogen atom is mixed with unsaturated liquid oil from plants like corn or soy to make trans fat such as shortening and margarine that stay solid at room temperature. Their main function is to increase the shelf life of food products.

Hyperglycemia: the presence of abnormally high levels of glucose in the bloodstream.

Hyperinsulinemia: an endocrine disorder characterized by a failure of our blood sugar control system to work properly. It manifests when insulin progressively loses its effectiveness in sweeping the blood glucose from the blood stream into the 67 trillion or so cells that constitute our bodies. Insulin levels in the blood rapidly rise to damaging levels and, together with the resulting elevated glucose levels, account for much of the damage to our arteries and vascular system. When insulin loses its effectiveness this loss is not due to any change in the insulin produced by the pancreas. It is due to a change in the cellular metabolism of almost every cell in our body.

Hypertension: high blood pressure elevated above 140/90.

Hypertrophy: the enlargement of muscle cells in response to progressive resistance training.

Hypoglycemia: An abnormally low level of glucose in the blood.

Insulin: a hormone released by the pancreas that transports glucose in the bloodstream into cells for energy consumption. Known as the "key" for glucose to enter cells.

Intensity: the physiological stress on the body during exercise; an indication of how hard an individual is working.

Interval training: short, high-intensity exercise bursts followed by periods of rest.

LDL: low-density lipoprotein that contains more cholesterol than protein. Labeled "unhealthy" because it can deposit cholesterol in our arteries leading to a variety of cardiovascular diseases.

Lean body mass (LBM): the component of body composition that represents everything but fat; muscles, bones, organs, connective tissue, blood and water.

Lifestyle: an individual's whole way of living.

Lifestyle disease: the relationship between how you live your life, regardless of your genetic make-up or family history, and the development of preventable, yet chronic diseases such as Type 2 diabetes, heart disease and certain cancers to name a few.

Linoleic acid: also known as Omega-6 fatty acids. An unsaturated fatty acid considered essential to the human diet. Vegetables, fruits, nuts, grains and seeds are sources of these fatty acids.

Linolenic acid: omega-3 fatty acid. An unsaturated fatty acid considered essential to the human diet. Sources are cold-water fish such as salmon, mackerel, flaxseeds, pumpkin seeds and rapeseed oil.

Liposuction: surgical process where fat is removed from certain parts of the body using a suction process to eliminate the deposited fat.

Lycopene: a pigment or coloring that is found in tomatoes and some other foods. It gives tomatoes their red color. Lycopene is the most powerful of all carotenoid (or pigment) antioxidants. As an antioxidant, lycopene helps protect the cells of your body from the effects of harmful free radicals.

Macronutrients: the major nutrients that provide caloric value.

Meal: the food served and eaten in one sitting.

Metabolism: the entire network of physical and chemical processes involved in maintaining life. It encompasses all the sequences of chemical reactions that enable us to release and use energy from food, convert one substance to another, and prepare products for excretion and elimination.

Micronutrients: substances that are needed by the body (in very small amounts), because they cannot be synthesized in the body. This means that they must be provided by the diet. All vitamins and most minerals are micronutrients

Minerals: an inorganic substance that is required for the human body to carry out chemical reactions for stability, maintenance, and growth.

Muscle: the cumulative contractile components that create movement, support, and metabolic functioning of the human body.

Muscular endurance: the capacity of a muscle to exert a force repeatedly against resistance or to hold an isometric contraction over time.

Muscular strength: the maximum force that a muscle can exert against a resistance in one single maximal effort.

Neuromuscular adaptation: the ability of the muscle and nerves to generate a greater contractile force without risk of injury. This adaptation is primarily responsible for the initial strength gains in an untrained individual.

Nutrients: a source of nourishment, especially a nourishing ingredient in a food.

Obesity: an excessive accumulation of body fat. Usually defined as more than 25 percent body fat for men and over 30 percent for women.

Omega 3 and 6 fatty acids: known as linolenic and linoleic fatty acids respectively and are essential for optimal function of the human body and must be consumed through our diet.

Osteo-arthritis: a form of arthritis, occurring mainly in older persons, that is characterized by chronic degeneration of the cartilage of the joints. Also called degenerative joint disease.

Osteoporosis: a degenerative condition, in which the body slows down its absorption of calcium and characterized by the thinning of bones. Often leads to fractures because bones become brittle and weak.

Partially hydrogenated oils: also known as trans fats, partially hydrogenated oils are manufactured through a process where a hydrogen atom is mixed with unsaturated liquid oil from plants like corn or soy to make trans fats. These can be found in deep-fried foods, margarine, cookies, muffins, cakes, and pre-packaged foods like crackers, breads, cereals and most snack foods. Their main function is to increase the shelf life of food products.

Peripheral arterial disease: clogged or blocked arteries that affect the blood flow to the limbs.

Phytochemical: phyto is the Greek prefix for plant, which literally means to bring forth. Therefore, phytochemical have to do with the chemistry of plants, plant processes, and plant products. Carotenoids like lycopene are phytochemical. Some phytochemicals are chemopreventives—meaning they help prevent cancer.

Portion: an amount of food eaten as a meal or snack. A typical portion size of either a carbohydrate or protein is the palm of your hand (not to exceed the first knuckle) or a clinched fist.

Proactive: acting in advance to deal with an expected difficulty; anticipatory; a matter of taking action over becoming disabled.

Proprioception: the sense of body position in space; body awareness.

Protein: any of a group of complex organic macromolecules that contain carbon, hydrogen, oxygen, nitrogen, and usually sulfur and are composed of one or more chains of amino acids. Proteins are fundamental components of all living cells and include many substances, such as enzymes, hormones, and antibodies that are necessary for the proper functioning of an organism. Each gram of protein by weight provides four calories of energy.

Recommend dietary allowance (RDA): the RDA represents the establishment of a nutritional norm for planning and assessing dietary intake, and are the levels of intake of essential nutrients considered to be adequate to meet the known needs of practically all healthy people.

Repetition (reps): one complete action of an exercise.

Resistance training: often referred to as strength training or weight lifting, resistance training involves any physical training that uses weights—dumbbells, barbells and weight-lifting machines, to name a few—to perform isometric, isokinetic or isotonic exercises to strengthen and develop muscles.

Resting heart rate: the amount of heart beats in one minute at rest.

Resting metabolic rate (RMR): the minimum number of calories your body needs to support its basic physiological functions, including breathing, circulating blood and all of the numerous biochemical reactions required to keep the body alive.

Rheumatoid arthritis: an autoimmune disease that causes inflammation of connective tissue and joints leading to weakness, loss of mobility, and deformity.

Saturated fat: a fat that has all of its hydrogen bonds full. Known to raise LDL cholesterol and cause the formation of platelets in the arteries. They are solid at room temperature and usually of animal origin.

Self-esteem: how a person feels about himself or herself.

Self-concept: the mental image or perception that one has of oneself. Usually, our behavior is consistent with our self-concept.

Self-sabotage: auto-destruction.

Serotonin: the central nervous system neurotransmitter that modulates mood, emotions, sleep and appetite.

Set: the number of successive reps performed without rest.

Stroke: a sudden and often severe attack due to a blockage of an artery to the brain.

Superset: involves two exercises for different muscle groups performed back to back without rest.

Supplement: an erogenic aid; substances taken to enhance performance. The Dietary Supplement Health and Education Act of 1994 defined dietary supplements as a food category and a product intended to supplement the diet.

Target heart rate: the number of heart beats per minute that indicates appropriate intensity levels for an individual.

Toxins: a poisonous substance, especially a protein, that is produced by living cells or organisms and is capable of causing disease when introduced into the body tissues but is often also capable of inducing neutralizing antibodies or antitoxins.

Trans fatty acids: used as a preservative and as a binary agent, manufacturers take a healthy fat such as soybean oil and change its chemical composition in order to make it a solid. They are by-products of the hydrogenation process and known to cause diseases and cancers.

Unsaturated fats: fatty acids whose hydrogen bonds have not been saturated or occupied. A fat derived from plant and some animal sources, (especially fish), that is liquid at room temperature. Consuming foods that contain more unsaturated fats than saturated fats may contribute to reduced blood cholesterol levels.

Vegan: a pure vegetarian who excludes all animal-derived foods from the diet.

Vitamin: any of various fat-soluble or water-soluble organic substances essential in minute amounts for normal growth and activity of the body and obtained naturally from plant and animal foods.

Weight Lifting: see resistance training.

Wellness: the lifestyle of creating health and evolving physically, intellectually, emotionally, spiritually and socially.

Yo-Yo Dieting: a lifestyle of dieting in which the dieter will embark on several diets with the perpetual goal of losing weight. Often success is temporary and the dieter eventually gains the weight back.

Appendix E
Recommended Resources

We decided to provide this appendix because we wanted to share with you a few of our reliable sources. Keeping up-to-date with the science of nutrition, advancement of exercise, scientific studies and medical breakthroughs is no easy task. However, by subscribing to a couple of newsletters, reading a few of our recommended books and routinely visiting a few Web sites, including **wellnessweightloss.net**, you can remain in the know.

Also, we offer a free Internet newsletter, which we mail once per week. This newsletter includes healthy and delicious recipes, pertinent information on nutrition and exercise, motivational tips and more. To receive this free newsletter, visit our web site and follow the subscribe directions.

In addition to all that you will receive from our online newsletter, we have provided you with some of our favorite reference newsletters, books and Web sites. You can also refer to our links page on:

wellnessweightloss.net for updates on other resources.

NEWSLETTERS

We are constantly reading newspapers, magazines and books. However, two of the most consistent pieces of reliable literature we read, reference and recommend are the Wellness Letter and Nutrition Action Healthletter. Both newsletters are available to the general public and highly regarded and respected in the wellness, exercise and nutrition industry.

Wellness Letter
Attn: Subscription Department
P. O. Box 420148
Palm Coast, Florida 32142
Web site: http://www.WellnessLetter.com

Center for Science in the Public Interest
RE: Nutrition Action Healthletter
1875 Connecticut Ave., N.W., Suite 300
Washington, DC 20009
Web site: http://www.cspinet.org

WEB SITES

The following are some of our most frequently visited Internet sources. Each of these sites will help you in your journey. However, as with most things in life, we encourage you to use discernment.

Institute of Medicine of the National Academies:
    http://www.iom.edu
American Diabetes Association: http://www.diabetes.org
American Dietetic Association: http://www.eatright.org
American Heart Association: http://www.americanheart.org
The Journal of the American Medical Association:
    http://jama.ama-assn.org
National Institutes of Health: http://www.nih.gov
Vegsource Interactive, Inc.: http://www.vegsource.com
U.S. Food and Drug Administration: http://www.fda.gov
Centers for Disease Control and Prevention: http://www.cdc.gov
World Health Organization: http://www.who.int/en

SUGGESTED READING

There are hundreds of books that we could easily recommend, however, we have provided 12 of our favorites. We have both selected six books each that we hope you take time and read. Each of these books has influenced our work and make up a big part of our bibliography. We are recommending these books because they are enjoyable and informative. *Enjoy!*

Allen, James.
As a Man Thinketh.
Marina Del Rey: DeVorss & Company, 1983.

Bailey, Covert.
The Ultimate Fit or Fat.
Boston: Houghton Mifflin, 1999.

Chopra, Deepak.
The Seven Spiritual Laws of Success.
San Rafael: Amber-Allen Publishing and New World Library, 1994.

Cousins, Norman.
Anatomy of an Illness as Perceived by the Patient.
New York: Bantam Books, 1979.

Diamond, Harvey and Marilyn.
Fit For Life II: Living Health.
New York: Warner Books, 1988.

Huang, Chungliang Al and Lynch, Jerry.
Thinking Body, Dancing Mind: TaoSports for Extraordinary
   Performance in Athletics, Business, and Life.
New York: Bantam Books, 1992.

Margen, Sheldon and the editors of the
   UC Berkeley Wellness Letter.
Wellness foods A to Z: An indispensable guide for
   health-conscious food lovers.
New York: Health Letter Associates, 2002.

Miller, Jennie Brand, Wolever, Thomas M.S., Powell, Kaye Foster
   and Colaguiri, Stephen.
The New Glucose Revolution: The Authoritative Guide to the
   Glycemic Index--the Dietary Solution for Lifelong Health.
New York: Marlowe & Company, 2002.

Northrup, Christiane.
Women's Bodies, Women's Wisdom: Creating Physical and
   Emotional Health and Healing.
New York: Bantam Books, 2002.

Pert, Candace B.
Molecules of Emotion: The Science Behind Mind-Body Medicine.
New York: Simon & Schuster, 1999.

Robbins, John.
Diet for a New America: How Your Food Choices Affect Your
   Health, Happiness, and the Future of Life on Earth.
Tiburon: H J Kramer, 1987.

Robbins, John.
The Food Revolution: How Your Diet Can Help Save Your Life
   And The World.
Berkeley: Conari Press, 2001.

HEADQUARTERS

To learn more about the *"Fat That Doesn't Come Back"* seminar series, purchase audio and visual programs, and to contact Robert and Krista, the following is provided:

Wellness Weight-Loss
P. O. Box 187
Port Hueneme, California 93044
Office: (805) 642-8440
Web site: http://www.wellnessweightloss.net
E-mail: info@wellnessweightloss.net
Online Internet Newsletter:
http://www.wellnessweightloss.net/subscribe.htm

Appendix F
Acknowledgments

We have worked with many men and women over the years. Their experiences with diets and desire to thrive in life have significantly empowered us to write this book. As many of their personal stories are woven throughout this book and their names changed to protect their privacy—we express our sincere appreciation to each and every person who has shared their frustrations, emotional ups and downs, and successes with us.

We have chosen to publicly acknowledge key members of our team for their ongoing support and belief in our work. First, we would like to thank Anna Munson as she helped us kick-start this book by editing many of the initial chapters. We also would like to thank Kelly Dobbe who read, reviewed and helped us structure a big part of this book. Next, we have our editor, Gretchen Ditto, who has experienced the Wellness Weight-Loss process first hand. Without Gretchen on our team, this book would have remained in concept for many lingering years. Thank you, Gretchen.

After writing *Fat That Doesn't Come Back,* we asked a group of our clients and friends to read it and share with us their thoughts and constructive recommendations for the book. Taking the time out of their busy schedules to read our manuscript and offer suggestions has helped us communicate our message more clearly. Our sincere appreciation goes out to: Cara Cohen, Marrianne Merrill, Josue Cano and Hans Bloem.

We also thank the forerunners of this book: Christine Hall, who wrote the foreword; Brenda Watson, who wrote the preface; and Debi Mullens, who not only proofread the book, but added a special touch by writing, "How To Use This Book." In addition to the ongoing support we receive from clients, family and friends, we also thank our publicist, Kelley Donahue Johnson and Howard A. Fishman of the law offices of Armstrong Hirsch, Jackoway, Tyerman and Wertheimer for believing in us and our passion to help others create health daily and release fat that doesn't come back.

Last but not least, we are forever grateful to: Susan Pollard, whose friendship and encouragement helped to keep our vision alive; Michal Escobar, who captured the photograph for the book cover; Susan Stout, who designed our logo; and Christa Agostino, who not only proofread this book, but designed it from front to back.

The message in **Fat That Doesn't Come Back** is our gift to all who want to live a diet-free life and evolve with their lifestyle.

Appendix G
About the Authors

Robert Ferguson and Krista Clarke are the founders of Wellness Weight-Loss, a company dedicated to educating and coaching people of all ages in the areas of nutrition, exercise, and the psychology and strategies of creating a healthy lifestyle and releasing fat. Robert and Krista are both established fitness and health specialists with an emphasis on weight loss and coaching.

Recognized by many as the "Master Weight-Loss Coach," Robert is a former U.S. Marine, professional athlete and the host of *"The Robert Ferguson Show."* He has provided dynamic, entertaining and life-empowering seminars, lectures and workshops for thousands of people across North America since 1987.

Krista, a former fitness champion and long-time certified personal trainer is the star of *"Time To Tone"* where she inspires people of all ages to participate in resistance training. "Time To Tone" is an instructional series of videos, DVDs and technical manuals designed to entertain and educate the public on the benefits and proper techniques of resistance training. Krista, was born and raised in Canada, however, she currently resides in California with her husband and co-author Robert.

Robert and Krista are also the founders of the seminar series *"Fat That Doesn't Come Back,"* in which they motivate, inspire and coach participants on how to evolve with their lifestyle. In addition to coaching, lecturing and offering seminars worldwide, Robert and Krista are regular contributors to a host of periodicals on the subject of nutrition, exercise, health and weight loss.

Widely respected and sought after by celebrities, athletes and corporations for their ability to empower others toward a healthier lifestyle, Robert and Krista continue to coach and operate Wellness Weight-Loss in Ventura County, California.

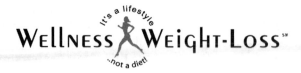